Pre- and Perinatal Massage Therapy

A Comprehensive Guide to Prenatal, Labor, and Postpartum Practice

Carole Osborne

second edition

Wolters Kluwer | Lippincott Williams & Wilkins
Health
Philadelphia · Baltimore · New York · London
Buenos Aires · Hong Kong · Sydney · Tokyo

Acquisitions Editor: Kelley Squazzo
Product Manager: Linda G. Francis
Development Editor: David Payne
Marketing Manager: Shauna Kelley
Primary Photographer: Al Gardner
Design Coordinator: Joan Wendt
Compositor: SPi Global

Copyright © 2012 Lippincott Williams & Wilkins

351 West Camden Street
Baltimore, MD 21201

Two Commerce Square
2001 Market Street
Philadelphia, PA 19103 USA
LWW.com

All rights reserved. This book is protected by copyright. No part of this book may be reproduced in any form or by any means, including photocopying, or utilized by any information storage and retrieval system without written permission from the copyright owner.

The publisher is not responsible (as a matter of product liability, negligence, or otherwise) for any injury resulting from any material contained herein. This publication contains information relating to general principles of health care that should not be construed as specific instructions for individual patients. Manufacturers' product information and package inserts should be reviewed for current information, including contraindications, dosages, and precautions.

Printed in China

Library of Congress Cataloging-in-Publication Data
Osborne, Carole.
Pre- and perinatal massage therapy / Carole Osborne. — 2nd ed.
    p. ; cm.
  Includes bibliographical references and index.
  ISBN 978-1-58255-851-6
 1. Massage. 2. Doulas. 3. Pregnancy. I. Title.
  [DNLM: 1. Massage—methods. 2. Pregnancy. WB 537]
  RG950.O78   2012
  618.2'4—dc22

2010043541

The publishers have made every effort to trace the copyright holders for borrowed material. If they have inadvertently overlooked any, they will be pleased to make the necessary arrangements at the first opportunity.

This book is dedicated to Josh and Elizabeth, whose gestations and births inspired my dedication to women and families.

And, in memory of Shirley Osborne (1921–2010), my sweet mama, whose unconditional love taught me the meaning of mothering and who forever stands securely behind me.

Foreword I

Michele Kolakowski, RMT, CD(DONA)

I purchased the first edition of *Pre- and Perinatal Massage Therapy* when it was published in 1998. For all the years of my private practice as well as teaching prenatal, labor, and postpartum massage therapy, Carole's book has been at my side like a trusted friend. Now years later, the book has lovingly been rubbed and sun kissed to a lighter shade. The pages are filled with tea stained rings from long days and late nights reviewing the perspectives and wisdom within. The book's spine is now shredding open from many travels, and pages 35 to 44 sometime tumble out. I have loved this book.

With my aging, well-loved first edition of *Pre- and Perinatal Massage Therapy* in hand, I called Carole a few years ago, and we shared our hopes and challenges for teaching pregnancy, labor, and postpartum massage into the future. With an increasing number of prenatal massage books and DVDs for students, practicing professionals, and educators to choose from, I told Carole how I still yearned for an expanded comprehensive textbook with specific topics and enhancements that would better prepare and sustain therapists in creative, passion-filled careers, and in turn, better serve a growing population of very diverse childbearing women. Carole's second edition of *Pre- and Perinatal Massage Therapy* has answered my hopes for the future.

Without a doubt, the second edition of *Pre- and Perinatal Massage* is the preeminent textbook and instructor resource package for massage therapy schools that want to launch, improve, or expand their maternity massage courses. Whether a basic 1-day course, a comprehensive 200-hour continuing education program, or something in between, *Pre- and Perinatal Massage,* the complementing Instructors' Resource Center and online ancillaries make for a flexible maternity massage curriculum of exceptional quality. Educators will appreciate the invaluable teaching tools created by Carole, an award-winning teacher with decades of experience in the classroom.

- Sample Syllabi for Various Length Courses and Class Planners
- Additional Online Topics Relevant to Pre- and Perinatal Massage Therapy
- Image Bank for PowerPoint and Other Visual Presentations
- Answers to Test Yourself and Test Bank Questions
- Discussion of "What Would You Do?" Features
- Over 90 Minutes of Video Clips of Techniques, Positioning and Draping, and Body Mechanics
- Sample Session Sequence Outlines for Pregnancy, Labor, and Postpartum

The second edition of *Pre- and Perinatal Massage Therapy* also features additional distinctive topics and enhancements that make it a "must have" reference for both the student and the practicing professional.

- This book has expanded, detailed explanations; photos and anatomical illustrations of safe client positioning; helpful therapist body mechanics tips; and dozens of effective prenatal, labor, and postpartum massage therapy techniques.
- "My Story" sidebars throughout the book are real-life experiences of women and professional therapists that punctuate and personalize key concepts of the book. "My Story" reminds the reader that each woman's pregnancy, birth, and journey in motherhood are unique.
- An extensive obstetrical glossary includes key terms related to the normal progression and complications of pregnancy, labor, and postpartum as well as relevant medications, procedures, and diagnostics and will assist therapists in utilizing correct medical terminology—an essential aspect of successful practice and coordinated, interdisciplinary care with other healthcare professionals.
- "What Would You Do?" sections throughout the book provide the reader with the opportunity for intuitive and critical thinking on key topics that are unique to the practice of pre- and perinatal massage therapy.

- "Points of View" sections highlight a variety of maternity massage educators' opinions on "hot topics" such as massage in the first trimester of pregnancy, appropriate abdominal and leg massage in pregnancy and the early postpartum weeks, safe client positioning during pregnancy, contraindications, and more. These sections are a superb way for therapists to educate themselves about these topics and to better inform their practices and education for new mothers. For massage therapists who work in spas, clinics, and hospitals, these discussions can also provide the basis for sound clinical practice decisions, procedures, and policies based on informed facts, not fiction and fear.
- Chapter 9 is a unique chapter filled with inspiring, thought-provoking, heartwarming, personal stories of practicing pre- and perinatal massage therapists from around the world. Carole also includes the survey results of 274 practicing massage therapists who specialize in pre- and perinatal massage therapy that gives voice to many perspectives and manifestations of careers being of service to childbearing women and their families.

In addition to celebrating the birth of *Pre- and Perinatal Massage Therapy*'s second edition, I want to express my heartfelt gratitude to Carole for her inspiration and compassionate support that has so positively influenced my career and that of thousands of other massage therapists and professionals. In turn, thousands of women and their children have also benefited from Carole's lifelong passion to humanizing the experience of pregnancy, labor, and postpartum with skilled, caring pre- and perinatal massage therapy. And like a pebble tossed into a calm pond, the ripple effects of her work will continue for generations to come. Carole, thank you for elevating our specialty once again with the second edition of *Pre- and Perinatal Massage Therapy* and perpetuating your amazing legacy and gifts as a teacher for the future. I look forward to many more cups of tea with this new second edition.

Longmont, Colorado

Foreword II

Penny Simkin, PT, CD(DONA)

It takes a village to have a baby*.

Pregnancy and childbirth represent a permanent transformation from woman to mother, fetus to infant, and man to father; other new roles are also created: co-parents, grandparents, siblings, and more. In fact, each birth causes a ripple effect that radiates outward from the family of origin to the community and beyond. In every culture, childbearing women are guided and advised through this transformation by a "village" of specialized experts. In North America, the "village" includes their medical caregivers or midwives, and some of the following: childbirth educators, nutritionists, yoga teachers, doulas, lactation counselors, mental health specialists, peer group facilitators, chiropractors, physical therapists, acupuncturists, and even numerous informative Web sites. Not the least of the special villagers are those special people addressed by Carole Osborne in this book—body workers and massage therapists.

The work of touch and massage uses the hands, the head, and the heart of the practitioner. The intimate nature of massage involves not only the intention but also the specific skills to nurture, heal, comfort, soothe, and relax the receiver, who places her trust in her massage practitioner and benefits emotionally and physically.

The childbearing year is a particularly vulnerable time for a woman. Her emotional and physical needs are uniquely altered; her whole body and mind are affected, with rapid changes of all kinds: weight gain, bodily discomforts, alterations in posture and balance, emotional lability, feelings of dependency, new perceptions of her self and her world, and reflections on her childhood and the way she was parented. The fetus within her and its safe passage become her major focus. She labors and gives birth, undergoing some of the deepest, most intense sensations and emotions she is likely ever to experience—excitement, anticipation, exertion, fatigue, fear, anxiety, vulnerability, pain, uncertainty, nakedness, exposure, unfamiliarity with her surroundings and her healthcare providers, and possible physical injury. The potential for everything from joy and triumph to disappointment and suffering exists. For a positive emotional outcome, she needs comfort, reassurance, and guidance, along with skilled maternity care, during childbirth.

Afterward, her body returns to a nonpregnant state, but now it feels very strange to her and may hold pain or a need to heal in some parts. Her "new" body produces breast milk and functions on much less sleep due to the constant need to care for her baby. Once again she is in a vulnerable emotional state, with no time for herself, possible psychological challenges, or lack of confidence in her mothering abilities.

What keeps women going during this time? How do they deal with these extraordinary challenges? The answer is that some people handle them better than others. The resilient, emotionally and physically healthy woman who has a healthy baby and an *adequate support system* weathers this time well with pleasing memories, a sense of accomplishment, and enhanced self-esteem. As one woman said, after giving birth, "After that, I knew I could do anything!" Those who lack some of these assets may look back on their childbearing experience with sorrow, guilt, shame, or anger. They may feel defeated, neglected, incompetent, and traumatized.

My own study, "Just another day in a woman's life?" (Birth 18(4):203–210), found that when women feel well-cared for by their healthcare professionals during childbirth, they feel a greater sense of accomplishment, higher self-esteem, and greater satisfaction with their birth experiences 20 years later (and probably longer) than those who did not feel well-cared for. All women had vivid, accurate, and poignant memories of their children's births and the professionals who cared for them. Those who reported low satisfaction with their children's births had negative memories of things that were said and done to them by their caregivers, and felt no sense of personal accomplishment.

The massage practitioner, by employing comforting and healing skills with a woman during the childbearing year, is in a perfect position to enhance not only the way the woman feels as she goes through it but also how she will look back on it in the future. The massage practitioner may not realize it at the time, but he or she will also be remembered by the woman for years to come. I think every massage therapist should ask himself or herself, while working with

---

*With acknowledgment of the African proverb, "It takes a village to raise a child," which inspired my rewording to focus on childbearing.

childbearing women, "How will she remember this?" The answer can be a guide to saying or doing things that will contribute to a good memory.

What a privilege it is for skilled, compassionate, and sensitive massage practitioners to offer their talents to women at this pivotal stage in their lives! How fortunate childbearing women are to have this service! Carole Osborne, a top authority in the field, models the expertise and compassionate understanding needed. Let her guide you to the joy and satisfaction of massage therapy for childbearing women.

Seattle, Washington

About the Author

Carole Osborne has been a somatic practitioner since 1974. Since she began developing infant and prenatal massage therapy in 1980, she has focused her bodywork career on maternity and somato-emotional applications of this work. In addition to private practice, she has worked in osteopathic, psychological, and women's medical settings primarily in San Diego, CA, and in her hometown of New Orleans, LA. She has trained thousands of therapists and other perinatal specialists in her advanced certification workshops held throughout North America and in the United Kingdom. She is also the author of *Deep Tissue Sculpting,* a contributing author to *Teaching Massage Therapy,* frequent contributor to professional publications, and cofounder of the International Professional School of Bodywork (IPSB) in San Diego, California. In 2008 the AMTA Council of Schools presented Carole with the Jerome Perlinski National Teacher of the Year Award, a high point of her 35 years as a somatic arts and sciences educator. In 2010 she was inducted into the World Massage Festival's Hall of Fame.

Acknowledgments

This is my fourth time "birthing" a textbook. I continue to be humbled and exhilarated by the process, and I am profoundly grateful to the "village" it takes. My deepest appreciation especially goes to:

My clients whose pregnancies, births, and postpartum experiences have given me the context to explore and confirm the possibilities of this work.

The 4500+ therapists who have studied this work with me, offering me innumerable lessons and refining my teaching and expressive skills. Special thanks to the several hundred who participated in our certified therapists' practice survey, and to Jane Serling, MSPH, who guided that survey's development and completion.

Those who helped create the foundations of this book, my career, and my fascination with nurturing the mother, especially my earliest collaborators and colleagues Sandy Karst, Ed Maupin, Bill Helm, Kate Jordan, Diana Panara, Ray Hruby DO, Barry Green, and Andy Sheets, the father of my children.

My current collaborators and fellow instructors of Pre- and Perinatal Massage Therapy workshops, Linda Hickey, Liz Ellis, and Jennifer Hicks, who help me keep the work vibrant and current.

Linda Hickey for co-writing Chapter 5, and for her invaluable contributions, feedback and encouragement throughout the book's conception and writing. She has stitched into it her passionate clinical and instructional excellence, and I am equally grateful for her abiding friendship.

Liz Ellis and Jennifer Hicks for their many contributions to the collective wisdom of this book and their dedication to the teaching of this work.

Ronnie Allan, Nanci Newton, and Anne Gilbert for generously persevering to convey the progression of our work through photographing their excellent sessions with their clients.

David Lobenstine for his enthusiasm and determination in mining the Internet and Columbia University for research gems.

Penny Simkin, for her wise and generous Foreword, our spirited discussions during brisk walks and leisurely meals, decades of support, and her example of a wise, humble, and consummate professional and mother.

Michele Kolakowski for her exuberant Foreword, thorough and brilliant reviewer's suggestions, and the ultimate gift to a teacher: taking her learning to places beyond her teacher's reach.

Sheila Kitzinger, Betty LaDuke, and Harriette Hartigan for kind usage of their inspiring art and photographs, and their championing of women's beauty and strength.

Marjeanne Estes, Body Therapy Associates Manager, for her steady presence and skilled steering of the business ship as I focused on writing, her stellar assistance in the classroom, and for a fierce and real friendship. "*Et toi!*"

Karen Lavelle, for many years reliable and capable management of the book division of BTA.

Cherie Sohnen-Moe, whose business consultations have helped ground and grow the bottom-line more than once.

The various perinatal healthcare professionals who ensured technical and factual accuracy and infused a positive perspective into my books, particularly, James Webber, MD; Diane Smith, midwife; Penny Simkin, PT and doula trainer; Liz Smith, prenatal anatomy and physiology instructor; Ana de Vedia, licensed acupuncturist and instructor; Pamela Ferguson, Shiatsu instructor; and the talented manuscript reviewers. This book would be a puny child without the enrichment of their knowledge and refinements.

Al Gardner, photographer and videographer, for capturing the facts and feelings of my work in appealing light and images, and for a friendship deeply rooted in our home soil. And Julius Evans, videographer, whose creativity and focus complemented Al so well.

The other photographic contributors, all of our vibrant models for photo and video, and the International Professional School of Bodywork (IPBS) in San Diego for space for the video shoot.

Ruth Werner and Tracy Walton for blazing the Lippincott trail, and encouraging me on that journey.

The Lippincott Williams and Wilkins team: Linda Francis, managing editor extraordinaire and gentle, yet iron-willed spirit, who transformed my words and vision into this reality with patience, flexibility, and kindness; David Payne, development editor, who made good information into better sentences and brilliantly tightened my rambling manuscript; Ed Schultz, Jr., video director; Julie Stegman, senior publisher;

and current and former acquisition editors Kelley Squazzo and John Goucher, respectively.

And finally, my deepest gratitude to those without whom this book's birth would be a hollow accomplishment:,my family and friends. Their love and reminders of Truth took me through turmoil and transition into the completion of this second edition. In addition to friends mentioned above, those who especially sustained me while tolerating more neglect than they deserved include: Josh, Elizabeth, Mama, Lynn, Sidney, Kate N., Beth, Diana, Maela, Leigh, Ed, and James. My Heart is Your Heart. We are One.

Photo credits:
Al Gardner
Ronnie Allan
Nanci Newton
Linda Hickey
Brandi Reichen
Jamie Dotan
Julie Howell
Andy Sheets
Jeff Tippit

Preface

Pre- and Perinatal Massage Therapy is a comprehensive guidebook to massage therapy for pregnant, laboring, and postpartum women. It provides a concise theoretical and practical foundation for massage therapists, and it equips them to safely weave appropriate therapeutic touch into modern maternity healthcare. It documents the benefits of massage and describes the relevant anatomical, physiological, emotional, and functional changes of the childbearing year. Featuring well-researched guidelines, it will prepare massage therapists to work cooperatively with others in the perinatal healthcare professions. Contributions to this book of many experienced massage therapists add a community perspective of this specialty area, unparalleled in other texts of its kind. Many maternity-specific massage and bodywork techniques are included in this book and are fully explained and illustrated. Marketing, ethical, and other business-related considerations, accompanied by a variety of profiles of successful pre- and perinatal massage therapists, bring it all into practice.

Course Applicability

I have written this book most specifically to inform and inspire advanced students in diversified curriculums that include both Western-originated and Asian-originated massage therapies. It is well suited for courses addressing special populations, from introductory modules to longer electives. Instructors and practitioners in continuing education seminars offering specialization and certification in maternity massage therapy will find concise, thorough, and practical depth and breadth. Individual practitioners can easily learn independently from its many features.

Spa managers, healthcare administrators, and mental health professionals seeking to create more well-rounded services for expectant women will find practical, reliable input. This book is also intended to provide doulas, midwives, nurse-midwives, obstetrical nurses, physicians, perinatal physical therapists, and childbirth educators the background to responsibly include skilled therapeutic touch as adjunctive patient care.

Practical and Humanistic Goals

The work in this book supports practitioners' educational and business goals. It also has the potential to positively change individual women and their families. It can begin to knit an ever-widening fabric of nurturing touch into communities and throughout our world, helping unite and transform our all-too-often violent, touch-aversive societies. It has the potential to provide comfort, growth, and pain relief and to support personal, interpersonal, and planetary development.

Gestation of the Second Edition

Over three decades as a massage and bodywork practitioner inform each reminder and instruction in this second edition. It carries my voice, that of a seasoned practitioner, teacher, and author; it also carries the voices of other therapists, their clients, and other perinatal authorities. Just as the first edition culminated a swelling creative urge, my passion for this work and dedication to developing a body of maternity massage therapy knowledge infuse this second edition. Over a decade later, massage therapy, this specialty field, and I are more mature, more demanding and discerning, yet more energized. This "offspring" inherits these traits.

● EXPANDED CONTENTS

As a second edition, *Pre- and Perinatal Massage Therapy* presents expanded content, both practical and theoretical. The four new chapters significantly expand content, elaborating on several topics skimmed or omitted in the first edition. These include the following:

- Positioning, draping, and therapist body mechanics
- Practical guidance for working with pregnancies when special needs arise, including gestational complications and high-risk factors and special populations of pregnant women

- Sensitive, appropriate inclusion of the oft-ignored interface between the body and emotions during the childbearing year
- A glossary of therapeutic massage and bodywork, anatomical, physiological, and other perinatal terminology, and common medications and procedures (an online obstetrical glossary will supplement this print glossary).
- The business considerations of marketing, recordkeeping, and interacting with other perinatal professionals, and the implications of ethical concerns for a successful practice
- Extended profiles and vignettes of practitioners' practices in a range of professional settings

Moreover, using examples, principles, and insight, common ethical issues have been interlaced throughout the book and its online resources, including the following:

- Scope of practice
- Professional boundaries
- Dual relationships
- Power imbalances
- Transference/countertransference
- Sexual issues
- Development of supervision groups and other forms of self-care

● WIDENED, UPDATED PERSPECTIVES AND RESEARCH

Obviously, a second edition offers the opportunity for improved accuracy and updating, and I have made many such improvements throughout the original five chapters. Since the first edition, the field of maternity massage therapy has seen notable growth. Results of an extensive survey of certified pre- and perinatal massage therapists reflect these developments. I have intertwined these insights into the technical and business sections, informing both with a contemporary practicality and relevancy.

Also, I have sought to create a current research view into the womb. I have culled facts and data relevant to a maternity massage therapy practice from newer, pertinent publications and from medical, psychological, midwifery, and somatic therapy research. Presented in a straightforward, accessible manner, these evidence-based data add currency and reliability to all recommendations, precautions, and contraindications.

Finally, where there are considerable differing opinions, I have included varied perspectives of other massage therapy and perinatal experts, sometimes those with considerably different viewpoints. These "Points of View" feature boxes and online discussions are intended to provoke thought and to reflect the evolving nature of the maternity massage therapy body of knowledge; "Points of View" topics include the following:

- Recommendations and precautions for safe leg and abdominal massage
- Massage therapy in the first trimester
- Effects of stress on prematurity and low birth weight
- Positioning requirements, particularly the prone position
- The benefits of perineal client self-massage
- Deep work on the lower back and sacrum
- Working with edema in pregnancy and postpartum
- Breast massage therapy

● INCREASED QUALITY AND QUANTITY OF HANDS-ON TECHNIQUES

What an improvement in the hands-on work in this edition! In three easily identified technique manuals, you will find new photographs, many embedded with relevant anatomical structures bringing greater precision and clarity to each. Most are included within the online video clips, organized into sample sessions. Additionally, verbal instructions have been revised to follow a thoroughly classroom-tested and logical format that deepens understanding and command of the techniques. This format includes the following:

- Techniques' intention, imagery, and source material
- Procedural steps
- Relevant precautions
- Hints for ease, effectiveness, or variation for body size and conditions

As in the first edition, this instruction carries the accessible, friendly tone of a caring, seasoned teacher. They are clear and easy for other instructors to teach from, and they offer multi-intelligence instruction. I have interlaced facts and data with personal expression to represent both the science and the art that are the essence of effective massage therapy. Moreover, I offer each technique as a possible procedure, with sequences as suggestions rather than rigidly proscribed protocols. Therapists can choose from sample sessions, but those sessions only come alive when infused with their own spirit, creativity, and individual response to their particular clients' needs.

In addition to these qualitative improvements, the quantity of techniques has also been increased in the second edition. I have added another 38 techniques for a total of 62. This increased number of techniques allows the following:

- A greater variety to choose from: complex to simple, superficial to deep, and physiological to energetic procedures
- A broader coverage of discomfort-specific techniques: every common discomfort associated with pregnancy, labor, and postpartum has at least one technique specifically designed for its relief.

● UPDATED ART AND DESIGN

The second edition features a completely new art program, including photos or illustrations for all techniques. Beautifully and simply rendered line drawings complement and clarify the textual content. Most technique illustrations even include embedded, relevant anatomical structures, increasing the effectiveness of this feature. In addition to the art, a completely fresh and updated design enhances the appearance of this book.

This edition retains the birth symbols, one of the most unique first edition art elements. These computer-generated versions of traditional textile designs adorn several features in the second edition. Women's hands have woven similar patterns, sometimes simple, often elegant, into textiles and other art for over 400 generations. The diamond shape at their center depicts feminine sexuality enclosing a smaller representation of the child within, with arm- and leg-like lines projecting from the sides. It is still the most frequently occurring iconic motif rendered in Eurasian and Indonesian art. (Concept developed from Allen M. *The Birth Symbol in Traditional Women's Art from Eurasia and the Western Pacific.* Toronto: The Museum for Textiles, 1981.)

An Overview of the Chapters

The first three chapters focus on why, when to, and when not to perform maternity massage therapy. The underlying rationales are presented first, followed by general and specific guidelines, precautions, and contraindications. Explanations accompany many photos to convey how to safely and comfortably establish the environment, set up and manage the equipment, and use proper therapist body mechanics and client positioning. Several decision-making tools and strategies will summarize these recommendations and give practitioners a thought process to follow as they apply the information to their work with individual clients.

The middle three chapters are the heart of the practical work, each ending with a technique manual. Readers can quickly access these hands-on sections using the colored bars edging these pages. Chapter 4 elaborates each trimester's maternal and fetal changes, women's physical and emotional experiences, and the accompanying pleasures, concerns, and discomforts that may follow. Practical considerations and guidelines for the therapist working in each trimester follow. A summary of recommended massage therapy for each trimester provides therapists with nondogmatic, nonprescriptive, but relevant hands-on guidance. The prenatal technique manual that completes this chapter complements this overview well. Here's where the practitioner will find detailed, step-by-step hands-on prenatal procedures, concisely and clearly explained and illustrated.

Chapter 5 is a journey through labor and birth, highlighting the significant and specific role of a massage therapist who is part of a birth team. Each stage and phase of labor brings challenges and excitement for the laboring mom. General guidelines direct therapists in safely and effectively meeting women in the intensity of their labor experiences. The Chapter 5 technique manual elaborates specific, labor-tested procedures that practitioners might need during labor's stages and for cesarean support. Special topics covered include self-care for therapists during the rigors of labor massage therapy, techniques to teach partners, collaborating with the medical or midwifery professionals, emotional issues, and ethics and maintaining professional boundaries while responding to the intimacy of labor and birth.

Chapter 6 explains the adjustments and healing of the immediate postpartum period, and the remaining time most women need for full recovery. This understanding of anatomy, physiology, structural adaptations, body use during infant care, and emotional concerns underlies the hands-on technique manual in this chapter. Moving past the first 4 weeks postpartum, you will find other suggestions and techniques for long-term recovery of function, gait pattern, postural integrity, abdominal and pelvic floor strength and function, and cesarean scar normalcy.

Most of *Pre- and Perinatal Massage Therapy* focuses on the roughly three quarters of pregnancies that follow normal, healthy development. My perspective is that of many perinatal experts: in most cases, pregnancy is neither an illness nor a medical emergency. I seek to empower women and their families by offering opportunities to develop trust in their bodies' inherent wisdom and to attune them internally. I encourage their thorough education in the wide range of healthcare and self-care options available, carefully considering their advisability in their unique pregnancies.

That said, practitioners need to be able to recognize the signs of deviations from the normal prenatal and postpartum adaptations women experience. When physicians diagnose or midwives determine that unhealthy conditions are occurring, they need to know how to adapt their therapeutic sessions. Chapter 7 is devoted to these topics, zeroing in on prenatal and postpartum complications and high-risk pregnancies. It also discusses other vulnerable groups and those requiring special considerations, including those with assisted conceptions, diversity of partners, and survivors of childhood sexual abuse. Emphasis is on relevant adaptations and implications for session work, communication and collaboration with perinatal healthcare providers and facilities, and scope of practice and other ethical guidelines. A special section on working with women on bedrest rounds out this chapter for women whose pregnancies have special needs.

Chapter 8 and its accompanying online business resource center move theory and technique out into the world of therapeutic bodywork and massage practices. The nuts and bolts, forms and records, promotional materials, and considerations for bringing this knowledge to clients are at its core. Whether working with the occasional client who is pregnant or growing a pre- and perinatal massage therapy specialization, the therapist will learn the business realities. Certified therapists around the United States, Canada, and the United Kingdom provided the multitude of materials in this chapter and the accompanying online business resource center that show promotions and client intake and interaction. A special section focuses on specific ethical issues that inevitably confront maternity massage therapists. Suggestions for educational materials, classes, and demonstrations show how to appropriately teach safe touch for pregnancy and labor to women and their partners.

Finally, Chapter 9 and the online business center profile in detail and with a comprehensive overview what a maternity massage therapy specialty practice really entails. Chosen from over 5,000 former students, several very successful practitioners share, in their own words, their development, successes, difficulties, inspirations, and wisdom. Among these contributors are an owner of a pregnancy massage therapy center and practitioners on staff at a hospital, an obstetrical office, and an interdisciplinary healthcare center. Therapists at maternity specialty spas and in their own private pre- and perinatal practices share tips, practical experiences, and stories. Synthesizing prior chapters' theory and technique with client interaction, this practical chapter would not be complete without hearing from expectant women themselves. Personal, moving stories in these moms' own words provide a fitting closure to the text.

Pedagogical Features

To make learning even easier, the following features are included in the book:

- **Chapter objectives** provide measurable learning goals for each chapter.
- **Key terms** stand out in boldface when first used, with definitions collected into an end-of-book glossary.
- **Reminder!** icons punctuate important safety considerations and key concepts.
- **My Story** paragraphs describe personal experiences of clients or therapists.
- **Points of View** sections present topics of controversy among perinatal authorities, replicating a discussion group, with opinions of others supplementing and/or contrasting my own.
- **Technique Manuals** provide illustrated, step-by-step instructions for performing specific massage procedures (primarily in Chapters 4 through 7).
- **What Would You Do?** features present a brief, realistic scenario that a massage therapist would likely face in practice, with critical thinking questions to consider. Sample responses to these questions are accessible online.
- **Chapter Summaries** provide a review of the content presented in each chapter.
- **Test Yourself** sections provide 8 to 10 short answer questions to facilitate review of each chapter's contents, with answers accessible online.
- **Icons** throughout the text point you to online video clips related to what you are reading.

Online Resources

An abundance of additional material is available by visiting our Web site at http://thePoint.lww.com/Osborne-Pregnancy2e (scratch-off code to access these materials is on the inside front cover).

The Professional Resource and Business Center on the Student section of the website includes the following:

- Video segments of techniques with several women at different stages of the childbearing year. Arranged in session sequences, these clips synthesize material from throughout the book. They include the following:
  - Review of procedural steps
  - Clarifications of the most important safety precautions and contraindications
  - Positioning and draping using the sidelying and semi-reclining positions
  - Massage therapist body mechanics
- Obstetrical glossary with additional medications and other medical interventions, tests, and terminology
- Postural and session photographs from 3 therapists' work in each trimester, and postpartum
- Suggested session sequences
- Articles and excerpts from contributing authors' and therapists' writings
- Marketing templates and examples
- An expanded list of contact information for resources, internet-based resources, and other information featuring United States, Canadian, and other worldwide companies, associations, and individuals, organized by those most relevant to therapists and to clients

Instructor's Resources include the following:

- Answers to review questions and possible responses to "What Do You Think?" features
- Syllabi for several courses of varying lengths
- Image bank for creating PowerPoint and other visual materials
- Test Questions

Summary Invitation

Britain's noted childbirth educator and author, Sheila Kitzinger, introduces her powerful anthropological survey, *Ourselves as Mothers*, with this statement:

> "To be a mother is to take on one of the most emotionally and intellectually demanding, exasperating, strenuous, anxiety-arousing, and deeply satisfying tasks that any human being can undertake."

To all reading this book, I would like to add the following:

To nurture the birth of a mother and of her baby with skilled touch is one of the most intellectually challenging, emotionally and physically demanding, humbling, and inspiring experiences that a somatic practitioner can engage in. Appropriate touch with childbearing women has the potential to positively change women, their families, and our world.

Throughout our history, human hands have woven the fabrics, shaped the vessels, nurtured the food, and cared for the individuals of our families and our communities. Nurturing, knowledgeable tactile communication has been vital to childbearing in most cultures for thousands of years. For millions of women, over thousands of years, touch has provided loving support and eased childbearing discomforts. During the last century, birthing has become increasingly medically managed, especially in many Western societies. While obstetrical innovations have reduced many perinatal risks, the texture of birthing, one of life's most touching female experiences, has become less tactile and less woman centered.

I invite you to join me in reversing this trend and in the rewarding, life-enhancing practice of pre- and perinatal massage therapy.

Carole Osborne
San Diego, California

Reviewers

Michele Kolakowski
Longmont, Colorado

Suzanne P. Reese
Ramona, California

Kala Spangler
Boulder, Colorado

Penny Bussell Stansfield
Hillsborough, New Jersey

Suzanne Yates
Well Mother
Bristol, United Kingdom

Contents

Forewords v
About the Author ix
Acknowledgments xi
Preface xiii
Reviewers xix

CHAPTER 1
Benefits of Prenatal and Perinatal Massage Therapy 1

CHAPTER 2
General Prenatal Guidelines, Precautions, and Contraindications 25

CHAPTER 3
Client Positioning, Draping, Body Mechanics, and Other Practical Considerations 46

CHAPTER 4
Trimester Recommendations 67

CHAPTER 5
Massage Therapy as Labor Support 105

CHAPTER 6
Postpartum Perspectives and Techniques 133

CHAPTER 7
Clients with Special Needs 152

CHAPTER 8
Business Considerations 171

CHAPTER 9
Profiles of Maternity Massage Therapists 187

Glossary 205
Index 211

Benefits of Prenatal and Perinatal Massage Therapy

Learning Objectives

After study of this chapter, you should be able to:

1. Describe the societal benefits of maternity massage therapy.
2. List six to eight potential beneficial outcomes for individual women of prenatal, labor, and postpartum bodywork.
3. Discuss research data that substantiate or point to possible positive effects of massage therapy during the childbearing year.
4. Explain to potential and current clients, their families, and healthcare providers the potential benefits of your work with them.

Let's announce it confidently and enthusiastically: Skilled, nurturing touch is good for moms and their babies! How do we know? We know it by feel, by testimony, and by objective data. Every day another massage therapist feels an expectant client's tension soften and her breath deepen. Her discerning eye sees a client's improving postural integrity, despite that swelling abdomen. You will find therapists' accounts of these and other positive effects in these pages. Clients regularly leave the therapy table proclaiming their increased comfort. They report in subsequent sessions their improved mood, sleep, and awareness. As complementary healthcare research expands, more data validate improved outcomes for moms, babies, and their families. Classic and contemporary research will be the other focus of this chapter.

Clients, other healthcare providers, and therapists need to know that maternity massage therapy does more than just pamper a women, although that, in and of itself, has value. When informed that it may improve both the mother and baby's well-being, women and their families more readily invest in massage therapy. Other maternity healthcare providers are seeking solutions to their patients' needs, but they want facts not just promotions about massage therapy's potential and safety. Your forthright presentation of well-founded theories and substantiated data, can improve trust, communication, and cooperation with these professionals. With a deeper understanding of the science behind your work, you reassure all involved that massage therapy is safe and helpful, and your work may become more effective too.

This chapter will highlight the wide range of benefits possible from massage during the **prenatal, perinatal**, and **postpartum** phases of women's normal reproductive lives. An extensive review of **obstetrical**, nursing, **midwifery**, physical therapy, **childbirth education**, animal studies, and touch therapy research forms its foundation. These data lead to working theories, formulated with the addition of the practical clinical experience of massage therapists, many of whom have worked in maternity massage therapy practices for 25 or more years. This body of knowledge is the embryo of an evidence-based specialization in prenatal and perinatal massage therapy. Hopefully, in decades to come, solid research will further validate these theoretical claims and heartfelt assertions, providing a comprehensive understanding of the value of this work.

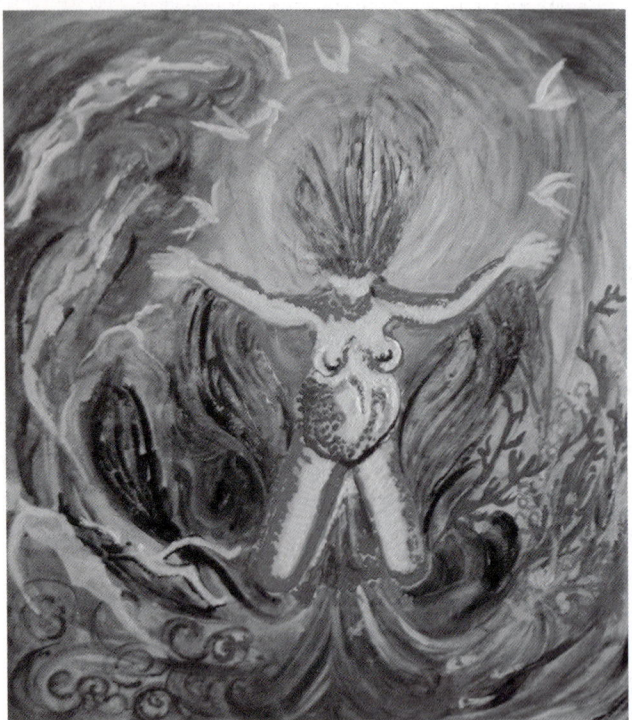

FIGURE 1.1 *Breaking Waters,* by Sheila Kitzinger. Used with permission of artist. All rights reserved.

Touching Humanity, One Mom and Baby at a Time

Nurturing touch during **pregnancy**, **labor**, and the postpartum period is not a new concept. Cultural and anthropological studies reveal that massage and movement during the childbearing experience was and continues to be a prominent part of many cultures' healthcare. India's ancient Ayurvedic medical manuals detail therapists' instructions for rubbing specially formulated oils into pregnant patients' stretched abdominal skin. Traditional sculptures depict Eskimo fathers supporting and lovingly stroking their wives' backs as attendants assist in the birth (Goldsmith 1984). In contemporary hospitals worldwide, birth **doulas** (labor assistants) or midwives hold and stroke laboring women through most of their labors (Klaus et al. 2002). Midwives, who for centuries have provided most of the world's maternity care, have highly developed hands-on skills. For billions of women, over thousands of years, touch has provided loving support and knowledgeable assistance and eased childbearing discomforts.

Anthropological studies indicate that most of the world's more peaceful cultures use touch prominently during pregnancy and early childhood (Prescott 2005). Studies correlating cultural anthropologists' data on infant physical affection and adult physical violence show an 80% correlation in 49 societies between high infant physical attention, including caressing and carrying the infant on the mother's body, and low crime and violence, including theft, torture, mutilation, and slavery (Prescott 2005).

The same researchers studied offspring separated from their mothers (loss of **bonding**/mother love), primarily with the famous Harry Harlow research monkeys. These young monkeys spent their formative periods of brain growth apart from their mothers. They were less capable of affection and pleasure and more inclined toward violence to self and others, depression, and isolation. Lack of sensory input of normal touching and rocking by the mother appears to damage the development of the neuronal systems that control affection and mediate violent behaviors (Prescott 2005).

World news reveals this problem daily and calls for solutions. Fortunately, many personal stories and slowly growing data suggest that massage therapy has some potential to reverse this trend, contributing to healthier moms and infants. Massage therapists and other touch professionals can contribute to a more peaceful world by caring and nurturing mothers through massage, thus enabling the mothers to be more able to care for and nurture their babies. For example, in one study, pregnant women massaged twice weekly for 5 weeks experienced less anxiety and less leg and back pain. They reported better sleep and improved moods, and their labors had fewer **complications**, including fewer premature births (Field et al. 1999). Less **prematurity** translates directly into less separation of mom and newborn, and more time and inclination toward the type of bonding that seems so integral to a culture that naturally expresses peace, love, and happiness.

Given this connection between touch and reduction of violence, massage therapists and other touch professionals working with women in their childbearing year can take great solace and pride in their contributions to more loving families, communities, and the world.

Stress Reduction and Relaxation

Most women regard motherhood as one of life's most precious opportunities. They and their families celebrate most pregnancies and lovingly welcome a new little one into the world. Often, however, this intense emotional investment is the very thing that makes the 40 to 42 weeks of pregnancy so stressful. Committed to the best for her baby, the mother can pressure herself in so many ways to be perfect. It's hard to eat right, exercise just enough, and maintain your job, especially when pregnancy's common discomforts develop. For those women who are less pleased with being pregnant, additional stress is likely. Where does expectant women's stress originate? How does it affect pregnancy outcomes? How can relaxation, particularly from massage therapy, reduce the negative effects of stress? These questions are addressed below.

● PREGNANCY: A TIME OF TRANSITIONS AND EXPECTATIONS

Although pregnancy is a welcome blessing for most, it brings with it many changes for all involved. As her body transforms, a woman must adjust to her altered physiological functioning. The shape of her pregnant body shifts, and her gait and other movement patterns usually alter. As her hair and skin change, she may feel as though she is no longer her former physical self.

Pregnancy is often a time of emotional upheaval and anxiety, as well as a time of euphoria and joy. In a single day, a pregnant woman's emotions may fluctuate tremendously. Her relationships to her mate, parents, friends, and coworkers change. Life issues that may have been repressed sometimes surface during pregnancy, including the legacies of physical and emotional abuse. Renegotiations of her degree of dependence and interdependence and her sense of her societal roles often arise at this time. A new baby can destabilize a woman's financial outlook and can especially strain a low- and middle-income family's budget.

At a time when every woman needs support, many American women find themselves isolated, without the community and familial support of former times and of other cultures. An alarming number of pregnant women also suffer abuse from their spouses (Mayo Clinic 2010). Single moms, lesbian parents, and handicapped and surrogate mothers often have additional challenges unique to their nontraditional situations. (See Chapter 7 for when special needs arise.)

Pregnancy is also a time filled with heavy expectations. With more birth control and lifestyle options currently available, many women have more apparent control over whether and when they become pregnant. Since the 1980s, more women have delayed pregnancy until their later twenties, thirties, or even into their forties (Harker and Thorpe 1992; March of Dimes 2010). Many women choose to have only one or two children that are more deliberately timed. Others are pregnant after years of investing thousands of dollars into getting pregnant via fertility treatments. All of these factors can result in pregnancies with greater significance and investment of emotional energy (Fig. 1.2).

Popular images in media create parental expectations of childbearing as a romantic, blissful time, but some women are not happy to be pregnant. Childbirth education and other instructional media sometimes cause an increase in performance anxiety. Consequently, some parents expect an "ideal" birth and anguish over anything that falls short of their expectations. Others cling to real or imagined promises of painless, risk-free labor through technology and pharmaceuticals to assuage their fears about the upcoming birth. Health issues increase the maternal and fetal risks for some so that these women are more apprehensive about their pregnancy's outcome (Ricci 2009).

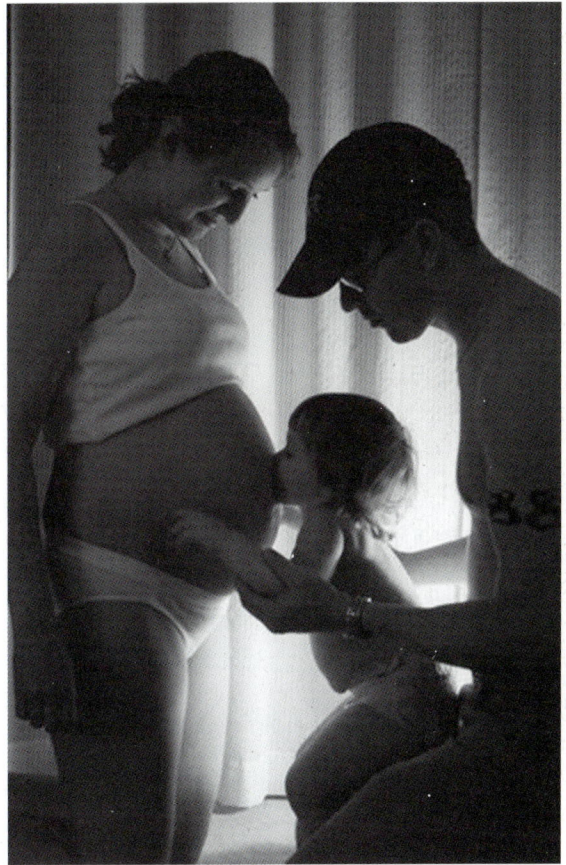

FIGURE 1.2 Joyful welcoming. Another pregnancy may be stressful, but it often brings families closer together as they prepare for and welcome the new baby.

REMINDER: Be prepared to support and care for women with a wide range of feelings about their pregnancies and from varying socioeconomic and familial support systems.

With all of these concerns, pregnant women usually experience increased stress. Stress activates the **sympathetic branch of the autonomic nervous system**. This increases adrenal production of stress hormones, creating a freeze, fight, or flight response. Such responses can be useful in responding to an emergency, such as applying the car brakes to avoid an accident or catching a falling child; however, such acute stressors and chronic sympathetic arousal provoked by ongoing worries and anxieties can have negative developmental impacts. Because these reactions prioritize blood supply to the extremities over the internal organs, stress can compromise circulation to the baby, perhaps as much as 65%, resulting in lower fetal heart rate and blood oxygenation (Gorsuch and Key 1974).

My Story

Massage therapy is so relaxing. I hadn't done much for myself since I became pregnant, and I can really see how it benefits me and my baby by loosening muscles and making me slow down.

—Melissa

Points of View: Stress, Prematurity, and Low–Birth-Weight

Some researchers believe that both neuroendocrine and immune system processes related to stress contribute to two of the most negative pregnancy outcomes, **prematurity** (Cooper et al. 1996) and **low–birth-weight** (Wadhwa et al. 2001). In addition, other studies point to stress as contributing to the following:

- Increased maternal heart rate, blood pressure, vomiting, nausea, **spontaneous abortion** (**miscarriage**), gestational **hypertension**, including **eclampsia**, and immune system dysfunction
- Interference with fetal brain and central nervous system development
- Higher incidence of miscarriage, prolonged labors with more complications, and **postpartum complications**
- Increased perinatal **fetal distress**, low–birth-weight, and infant irritability, restlessness, crying, and digestive disturbances (Cranden 1979)

Animal studies suggest that prenatal stress may have long-term effects in a child's life. Adolescent rhesus monkeys whose mothers were stressed during their pregnancies were not only more anxious, clumsier, sicker, and shier than control teen monkeys, but also slower to learn and unable to focus on tasks. Researchers speculated that their results might offer clues to one of the causes of attention deficit disorder (ADD) in children (Schneider 1999).

As compelling as these data are, not all authorities agree on such widespread connection between prematurity and prenatal stress and other related psychological factors. About half of the 20 studies in one review of research on prematurity and stress-related factors (social support, life events, anxiety, depression, and general stress) showed an association of the two (McCormick and Siegel 1999). Interestingly, it appears that both the physiological and affective effects of stress are lessened as a woman moves through her pregnancy, so that early prenatal stress may be more detrimental than that which occurs closer to **term** (Glynn et al. 2004). This also could explain some of the conflicting results in the review above. By adapting over time, this could be another physiological example of the body's wisdom in adapting to prenatal demands.

SUPPORT, RELAXATION, AND PRENATAL MASSAGE THERAPY

Learning how to relax and to focus internally are integral parts of childbirth education programs. Relaxation and self-awareness tend to create increased well-being for both the mother and the baby and increased chances for positive birth experiences. Women and their partners who learn relaxation techniques are better able to adapt to stress during pregnancy and labor, and in the days and years of parenting (Nichols and Humenick 2000; Hetherington 2007).

Individualized hands-on time with a somatic practitioner presents a unique and potent experience of support and relaxation for pregnant women. Massage therapy supports expectant women because it generally makes them feel good, function more effectively, or feel more optimistic. Certain types of massage therapy are intrinsically relaxing, encouraging a woman to turn inward, concentrating on her own body and mind rather than on external events, a particular sense of letting go (Samuels and Samuels 1996). That is soothing to most women and perfect preparation for coping with the demands of labor and birth.

In fact, in preparation for labor, perinatal specialists recommend women practice deep sustained levels of relaxation for 45 to 60 minutes without falling asleep, especially in the last 6 to 8 weeks of pregnancy (Samuels and Samuels 1996). This is the exact length of most massage therapy sessions. Massage therapy environments are very conducive to relaxation, providing a quiet, undisturbed place that encourages and sustains a deep, regular rate of breathing. Appropriate positioning for massage allows the muscles to relax, and a receptive, nurturing attitude on the part of the massage therapist provides an atmosphere that invites relaxation to take place.

In contrast to the effects of stress, support and relaxation activate the **parasympathetic branch of the autonomic nervous system**. This helps create physiological balance and encourages a healthy, smoothly functioning state. When relaxed, an expectant woman will have steadier blood pressure, pulse, and respiratory rates; regular blood flow to uterus, **placenta**, and fetus; and healthier immune system functioning, emotional states, and responses to stressful stimuli, and she will feel less fearful and anxious (Nichols and Humenick 2000) (Fig. 1.3).

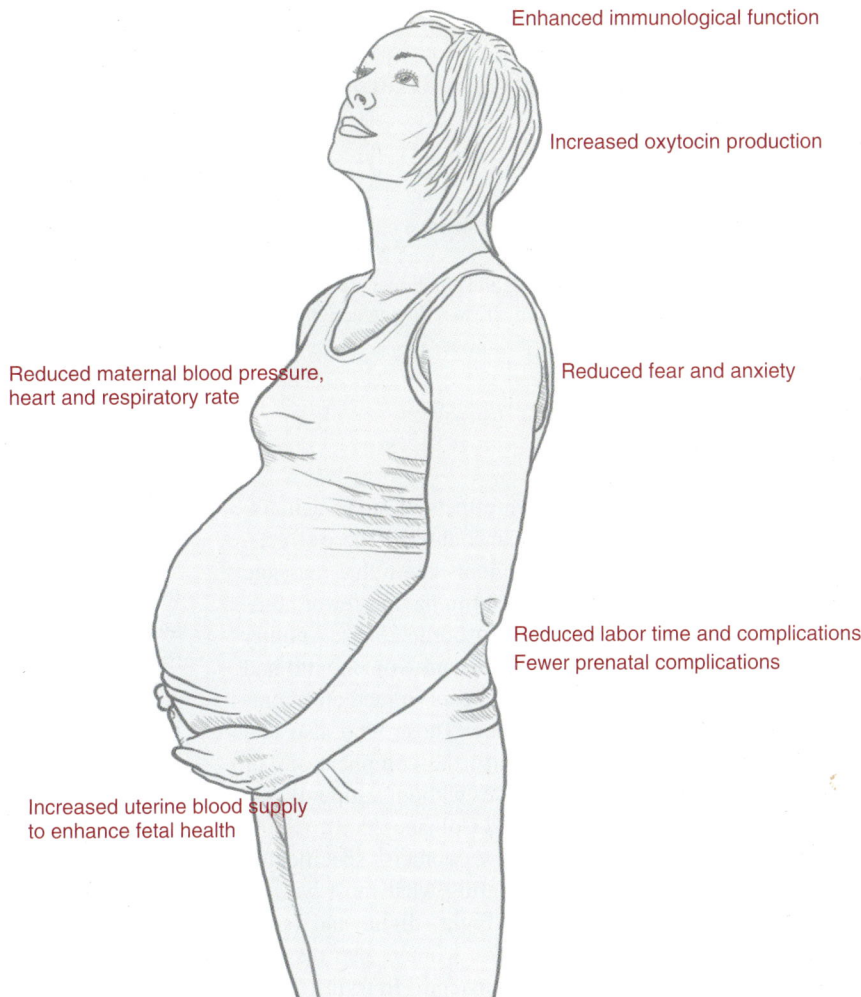

FIGURE 1.3 Possible maternal and fetal benefits of prenatal relaxation.

> **REMINDER:** *Increased relaxation facilitates healthy circulation to the uterus that improves fetal development.*

Even a single massage therapy session can create these results, as well as reduce the immediate pain level the mother might experience. Multiple sessions are potentially even more powerful in pain reduction and in diminishing anxiety and depression (Moyer et al. 2004). Research suggests that massage therapy sessions as brief as 6 to 20 minutes produce muscle relaxation (Longworth 1982; Field et al. 1992). In one small study, immediately after sexually abused women received 30-minute massages, twice weekly for 1 month, subjects reported feeling less depressed and anxious. Their decreased salivary levels of the primary stress hormone, **cortisol**, confirmed their perceptions. Over the study period, these women experienced a decrease in depression and in life-event stress. Although a control group practicing relaxation therapy also reported less anxiety and depression, their stress hormone levels did not change, and they reported an increasingly negative attitude toward touch (Field et al. 1997).

Massage can create the same positive physiological states and increased alpha brain wave activity as meditation. Massage movements provide variations in pressure, rhythm, and positioning that flood the sensory nerve pathways with input that increases body awareness and overrides signals of pain and stress (Juhan 1998).

A massage therapist provides not just soothing, nurturing touch; she also brings focused, individualized attention to her client's concerns. This regular, caring contact can be a vital component of a pregnant woman's support system, especially when family and friends are not providing such support. All therapists can offer attentive, nonjudgmental listening; those with complementary skills and training in counseling and emotional processing can offer additional sensitivity as women look to understand and assimilate the strong emotional states common during pregnancy. Massage therapists provide needed referrals to other professionals dealing with prenatal and perinatal health and emotional well-being. They also can educate women in body use that assists in managing and reducing stress.

> **Box 1.1**
>
> **Ways Prenatal Massage Therapy Provides Stress Reduction**
>
> 1. Nurturing, skilled touch
> 2. Individualized attention to needs
> 3. Emotional support, especially in the absence of supportive family and friends
> 4. Attentive, nonjudgmental listening and emotional processing
> 5. Education and encouragement in stress-reducing activities
> 6. Appropriate referrals to other specialists

However extensive the negative effects of stress actually are, it appears that proper support can counteract these effects. Many expectant massage therapy clients claim that massage therapy helped them in carrying to term, having fewer complications, and feeling more peace (Osborne 2009). Another study considered several hundred pregnant women who had many difficult life changes in the 2 years immediately preceding and/or during their pregnancy. Those who also had strong support systems had one-third the complications of those who experienced similar stresses without a support system (Nuckolls et al. 1972; Hobel and Colhane 2003).

As researchers zero in on how women, specifically, respond to stress, they are documenting what most women experience throughout their lives. Fight, flight, and fright aren't women's only stress reactions; women also respond with a pattern known as "tend and befriend." In trying times, women instinctively surround themselves with supportive people and care for others. Interestingly enough, the neuroendocrine core of this response may be **oxytocin** and other female reproductive hormones, the very substances responsible for gestational developments and mothering responses (Taylor et al. 2000; Moberg 2003). How appropriate, then, that they would seek out the nurturing care of a skilled and comforting massage therapist during this time of stressful and joyous transitions.

> **What Would You Do?**
>
> A new prenatal client spends her entire massage animatedly sharing the details of being pregnant. She also asks you many questions. You enjoy and share in her excitement, yet you realize after several sessions that she has talked throughout each session. Why is it important for her to turn inward and "focus" in her treatments? What can you do to encourage that—with your words, your hands, and the environment?

Improved Physiological Functioning

An expectant woman's endocrine system orchestrates a confluence of changes in every system of her body. Heightened levels of **progesterone**, **estrogen**, and other pregnancy-specific hormones prompt physiological adaptations that create and maintain the optimal gestational environment for a healthy newborn in the vast majority of pregnancies. The circulatory, respiratory, gastrointestinal, and urinary systems undergo the most notable of these physiological changes (see Fig. 4.2 for further details).

Massage therapy may supplement and reinforce these changes through generalized responses to stimulating the skin. While promoting normal prenatal physiology, it may help to minimize many of the secondary uncomfortable consequences of pregnancy. Some women may seek pharmacological and nonpharmacological relief for these secondary symptoms. Although massage therapy may help to reduce the intensity of, shorten the duration of, or alleviate these symptoms, it is not within the therapist's scope of practice to instruct clients to discontinue any medications.

● CIRCULATORY SYSTEM BENEFITS

Some pregnant women schedule massage therapy specifically to ease the discomforts of the normal effects of pregnancy on blood and interstitial fluid volume. Often they find relief from achy, swollen feet and legs; hand numbness and reduced function; and other normal circulatory discomforts (Osborne 2009). This section overviews prenatal circulatory physiology and reviews data and possible theories to explain this well-appreciated effect of prenatal massage therapy.

Normal Physiological and Mechanical Changes in the Circulatory System

To provide for fetal needs, the circulatory system makes brilliant adaptations. From as early as weeks 10 to 12, elevated estrogen and progesterone production increases total blood volume. It peaks by weeks 32 to 34 at 50% higher than nonpregnant levels. Levels of all blood components—white blood cells, plasma, serum protein, and serum enzymes—are elevated. Because red blood cells increase at a lower rate than these other elements, many women develop a physiological anemia. The positive result of all of these changes is more oxygen/carbon dioxide exchange, a higher supply of nutrients and hydration, and better waste product removal for both the mother and the fetus (Ricci 2009).

The heart actually enlarges slightly to accommodate this increased load, and by week 32, its output (stroke volume) is 30% to 50% higher than before pregnancy; it then declines to about a 20% increase at 40 weeks. Heart rate increases by 10 to 15 beats per minute, beginning in the second trimester and persisting to term. To help the vessels accommodate the load, progesterone causes peripheral **vasodilation** so that blood pressure actually declines slightly in pregnancy. Blood pressure is at its lowest during midpregnancy but maintains prepregnancy levels in the first and third trimesters in normal pregnancies. A significant rise in prenatal blood pressure can be indicative of gestational hypertension (Ricci 2009), a complication that needs close monitoring and care to prevent serious risk for both the mother and the baby (see Chapter 7).

Although most of these normal circulatory system changes go relatively unnoticed by the expectant mother, she is usually aware of the 40% increase in interstitial fluid volume over nonpregnant levels. By the third trimester, this increase often results in swollen legs and ankles (**edema**). Pelvic myofascial restriction and the mechanical effects of the weighty uterus contribute to this swelling, working much like a cork in a bottle of effervescent liquid, restricting femoral fluid return (Fig. 1.4). As a result, about 75% of women suffer normal, pregnancy-induced (nonpitting) edema in the lower extremities. This usually first occurs in the late second or third trimester. Some women can develop numbness, tingling, and burning sensations in the feet and lower legs as the extra fluid compresses on the tarsal nerve (**tarsal tunnel syndrome**). When this fluid increase pervades the pectoral girdle, **carpal tunnel syndrome** can develop with moderate to severe pain in the arms and hands, particularly in the middle and index fingers (Scheumann 2007).

Many women are self-conscious about the vascular effects of these changes when **varicose** and **spider veins** appear. Unfortunately, progesterone's wise relaxation of the smooth muscle walls of all vessels also challenges the integrity of the valves of the femoral, saphenous, and other leg veins. With uterine compression of the iliac veins and inferior vena cava restricting blood flow from the legs, increased **femoral venous blood pressure** distends the vessels, and **varicose veins** appear in many women's legs. A woman's heredity and diet, prolonged sitting or standing, and the position and size of her baby are important factors contributing to edema and varicose veins. Some women also develop vulvar varicose veins. Those higher levels of progesterone also dilate the peripheral blood vessels that can burst to form vascular spiders, areas of reddish broken capillaries on the legs, face, and upper body (Ricci 2009).

During pregnancy, the blood's clotting capacity increases to four or five times higher than nonpregnant levels. Because the clot-dissolving capacity (**fibrinolysis**) also decreases dramatically, women are less likely to hemorrhage during childbirth; however, they also are more likely to develop blood clots (**thrombi**), particularly in the legs and groin. Thrombi are also the result of the growing **gravid** uterus restricting iliac and femoral circulation and contributing to sluggish blood flow; higher progesterone levels relaxing vascular smooth muscles; and increased metabolic demands elevating blood and interstitial fluid volumes (Jefferies and Bochner 1991). Although these changes are mostly unnoticed by pregnant women, their therapists need to be ultraaware of this increased risk for clots, taking specific precautions during sessions (see Chapter 2).

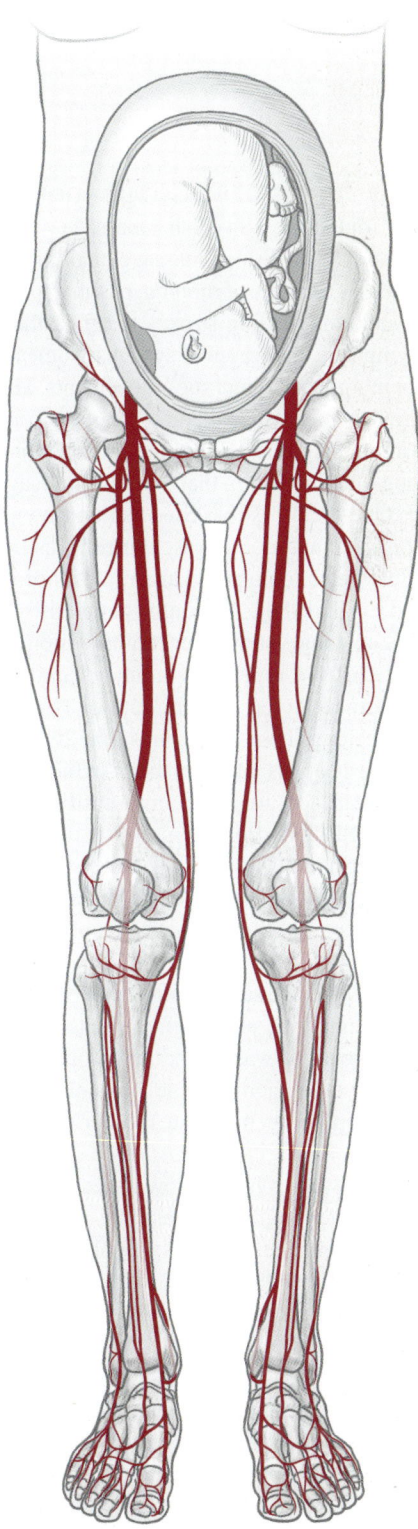

FIGURE 1.4 Leg edema. The enlarged uterus compresses iliac vessels, a major cause of normal edema in the feet and legs.

> ### My Story
>
> Before the massage, I had been holding water in my legs and feet. Afterwards, the swelling lessened, and my whole body felt very relaxed and ready for a peaceful nap.
>
> —Aletha

Circulatory Effects of Massage Therapy

Circulatory massage (Swedish massage or traditional European massage and Esalen massage, and lymphatic drainage massage) uses a variety of rubbing, pushing, pulling, lifting, percussive, and compressing strokes to affect the underlying muscular, lymphatic, and vascular systems. Some also use passive range of motion or "gymnastic" movements. The speed and depth of circulatory massage therapy can vary from very slow and soft to a more vigorous speed and/or deeper pressure.

It is a long-standing claim that Swedish massage increases circulation. One theory is that Swedish and lymphatic massage may produce autonomic vascular reflexes that promote delivery of oxygen and nutrients and removal of waste materials (Arkko et al. 1983). Manually pumped by effleurage, petrissage, kneading, and other compression techniques, lymph capillaries are repeatedly emptied and refilled, producing a sustained increase in the rate of lymph formation and removal. Along these same lines, one hypothesis about massage is that it opens capillary beds, which increases the total capillary surface area and temporarily increases both venous and capillary hydrostatic pressure to increase lymph filtration and formation (Foldi 1978); however, these are currently unvalidated theories (Weerapong et al. 2005).

If contemporary, well-designed research eventually validates these mechanism theories, this could provide further explanation of why massaged pregnant women report feeling better. An enhanced supply of nutrients and oxygen and accelerated removal of waste products promote cellular respiration. This would facilitate the physiological processes of gestation, improving both the mother's and the baby's tissue health.

Several older studies hint at how Swedish and lymphatic drainage techniques might decrease the negative effects of increased blood and interstitial fluid volumes that result in edema. Performed rhythmically, lymphatic strokes might work like a hydraulic pump shifting excess fluid from the tissues to the blood (Zanolla et al. 1984). The mechanical effects of compression strokes theoretically increase capillary blood flow and produce local vasodilation through increased histamine release. It is theorized that these effects also may be induced through the autonomic vascular reflexes described above (Linde 1989) (see online roundtable discussion regarding lymph and fluid movement at http://thePoint.lww.com/Osborne-Pregnancy2e).

Two particular small studies of specific applications of slow, rhythmic stroking to stimulate parasympathetic activity (Longworth 1982; Fakouri and Jones 1987) form the foundation of a protocol that many therapists are exploring for normalizing heart rate and blood pressure. This autonomic sedation series, detailed in the Chapter 4 technique manual, deserves further research, as it potentially could increase relaxation while contributing to the management or prevention of gestational hypertensive disorders.

Significant myofascial binding and soft tissue restrictions may reduce local circulation in both upper and lower extremities. **Deep tissue** work to the pectoralis major and minor and other pectoral girdle structures may help reduce carpal tunnel syndrome symptoms, especially when combined with circulatory techniques that might flush excess fluid from the arms. If myofascial restriction in the lower pelvic region is contributing to edema and varicose veins, careful, specific **myofascial** and/or **passive movement techniques** may help to relieve edema. Guiding women to more erect posture with less compression of the inguinal structures appears to help, too. Women derive most benefit from gentle leg and pelvic work while taking extreme caution to work safely there, as described in Chapter 2.

● RESPIRATORY SYSTEM BENEFITS

Although elevated progesterone production prompts a 30% to 40% increase in exchange of gases with each breath (**tidal volume**), most expectant women still tend to feel short of breath and often hyperventilate. This rapid, shallow, upper-chest breathing pattern is the result of the growing uterus restricting diaphragm excursion and chest expansion (Ricci 2009). Compensating for the enlarged abdomen and breasts, many women also lean back as though to prevent falling forward. This posteriorly shifts the upper thoracic area while the lower ribcage presses more anteriorly. A tendency toward anterior rotation of the pectoral girdle restricts ribcage expansion, further negatively impacting respiration.

With individual guidance in diaphragmatic or abdominal breathing, a pregnant woman can correct shallow, rapid, or **paradoxical** breathing patterns (abdomen contracts with inhalation, expands with exhalation). Diaphragmatic breathing promotes relaxation, reduces stress, and relieves the musculoskeletal strain of inefficient breathing on the neck, chest, and upper back. Although the inferior ribcage circumference expands during pregnancy, women often benefit from instruction in more lateral and posterior ribcage expansion to foster more costal, deeper diaphragmatic breathing patterns (Noble 1995).

Deep tissue massage, structural realignment guidance, passive and active movement, and **myofascial trigger point** therapy may improve breathing by correcting restrictive postural deviations and improving neck, abdomen, and chest mobility (Witt and MacKinnon 1986). Myofascial

> ### My Story
>
> *I had felt a stitch in my side for weeks. After last session's deeper breathing and those strokes on my ribs, that's gone. Relaxing and breathing to my baby seems to make this all more real to me, too.*
>
> —Kim

restriction, tender points, and habitual holding patterns in the scalenes, sternocleidomastoid, intercostals, pectoralis major and minor, levator scapula, rhomboids, trapezius, and serratus anterior require particular attention (Scheumann 2007; Osborne-Sheets 2002).

Many women have uncomfortable congestion in the nose and sinuses due to estrogen-induced increased vascularity in the respiratory tract. This worsens if a woman has respiratory allergies that she cannot medicate to control and when she has a cold. In this case, she will especially appreciate facial massage, emphasizing sinus relief with pressure points. You also can teach her self-massage that may help ease sinus discomforts. (Ferguson 1995).

● GASTROINTESTINAL SYSTEM BENEFITS

Progesterone seems to have one purpose for the digestive system: eek out every morsel of nutrition to grow a healthy baby. To do so, it relaxes the smooth muscle lining of most of the digestive system, and this decreases peristalsis. The resulting slower transition time of food through the gastrointestinal tract allows for maximal absorption. Unfortunately, secondary effects of elevated progesterone levels are not so welcome: constipation, **heartburn** or acid indigestion (pyrosis), and sometimes gall bladder disease.

Twenty-five percent of all expectant mothers are frequently constipated (Ricci 2009). Lethargic peristaltic activity, aided by compressed intestines that are dislocated by the growing uterus, means more slowly processed foods. The resulting higher water absorption, especially in combination with iron supplements, low-fiber foods, and any decreased activity level, creates bloating and strained bowel movements. Often hemorrhoids develop, too.

The enlarged uterus also presses on both the stomach and the gallbladder. In combination with a more relaxed esophageal sphincter, this allows stomach acid to regurgitate into the upper esophagus, bringing burning pain into the midchest and throat. More than 75% of all women have heartburn (**gastric reflux**), especially in later pregnancy and when lying down (Ricci 2009).

Estrogen, progesterone, and **human chorionic gonadotrophin (hCG)** are partially responsible for another common gastrointestinal complaint, nausea and vomiting (**morning sickness**). hCG maintains a woman's estrogen levels in early pregnancy, inhibits maternal rejection of the embryo as foreign tissue, and increases basal temperature. Its high level is suspected to be linked to "morning sickness," particularly common in weeks 2 to 14. Some women continue to feel sick throughout their pregnancies; some unfortunate women are nauseated all day and night (Ricci 2009).

Many massage techniques that therapists use to relieve constipation are not safe during pregnancy (see Chapter 2). As an alternative, **reflexive** techniques, including foot **zone therapy** (**foot reflexology**) and **acupressure** or other Asian body therapies, may positively influence gastrointestinal functioning. Although there currently is little research to validate its effectiveness, many therapists and clients report good results from work on specific zones in the feet and hands (see Fig. 4.50) and along certain meridians from Asian medical traditions (Flocco 1993; Ezner 2000; Wang et al. 2008). One study suggests that nausea can often be reduced with daily acupressure to the PC-6 point on the forearms, two fingerwidths superior of the wrist (Belluomini et al. 1994).

Although some of these gastrointestinal discomforts are difficult to avoid or alleviate, it seems reasonable to theorize that massage therapy may counteract their negative nutritional impacts. Several studies of premature infants and cocaine-exposed premature infants documented significant weight gain for massaged infants when compared with unmassaged control infants. Researchers have proposed that massage increases vagal nerve activity, which stimulates production of food absorption hormones (Wheeden et al. 1993). Extrapolating from these infant studies, similar Swedish massage strokes might improve pregnant women's nutrient use.

● SKIN STIMULATION

Perhaps one of the most significant benefits of prenatal massage therapy is the simple and profound effect of skin stimulation. Ashley Montagu, anthropologist and "skin scholar," describes the brain as "the inside layer of the skin, and the skin the outside layer of the brain". Embryological development shows the relevance of this analogy, as the skin tissue is the first to differentiate, and it evolves out of the same tissue as the brain (Montagu 1978).

As "professional skin stimulators," massage therapists can look to a variety of classic animal studies that document the widespread importance of skin stimulation through touch, including the animals' own licking behaviors. Laboratory animals require a minimum level of routine care, but some enjoyed the equivalent of regular massage as their handlers petted and held them. In one study, post-thyroidectomy rats that were stroked and handled by caretakers suffered 13% mortality, as compared with a 79% mortality among those receiving routine food and cleaning only (Ruegamer 1954). Certainly birth is only partially comparable to such surgery, but, especially for traumatic or surgical births, the comparison may hold some validity.

Gentled or stroked rats and mice in many other experiments demonstrated significant differences from nongentled control groups. Pups of gentled rats and mice opened their eyes sooner after birth, were more active, developed motor coordination earlier, and weighed more at weaning. Stroked animals had stronger immune systems and showed 50% more synaptic junctions. They were more sexually active. Socially more dominant, they were curious, calmer, and better problem solvers, with superior mothering skills.

These rats' superior motor, mental, and social development lasted their entire lives. The positive results of tactile stimulation increased when the handlers stroked these animals throughout their maturation. The nongentled control animals in these studies were more excitable, timid, and fearful. They tended toward rage reactions in response to frustration, and they often bit each other and their caretakers (Weininger et al. 1954; Rosen 1957; Denenberg and Karas 1960; Tapp and Markowitz 1963; Juraska et al. 1980; Meaney et al. 1985; Pauk et al. 1986; Meaney et al. 1989). Add these studies to the results discussed earlier, and the argument for the peacemaking potential of prenatal massage therapy grows even stronger.

More directly relevant to maternity massage therapy, consider the many negative effects observed when pregnant rats couldn't self-stimulate by licking. An experimental group of expectant rats wore large collars that restricted their characteristic licking of their swelling abdomens and teats. The collared rats' mammary development was 50% less than that of the control rats. These mothers randomly and ineffectively attempted to build their nests, where they delivered fewer live offspring than control mothers. Avoiding contact with their litters, they neglected cleaning the afterbirth and licking their young. Fewer pups survived the neglect, and their mothers had difficulties in nursing them. Because their placentas were very poorly developed, researchers postulated that the skin stimulation of licking promoted the secretion of the vital hormones for healthy pregnancies (see Fig. 4.2 and online resources for more information on endocrine production and placental functions at http://thePoint.lww.com/Osborne-Pregnancy2e) (Roth and Rosenblatt 1996).

From these studies, it would be reasonable to suggest that:

- Skin stimulation stimulates the brain, creating positive effects in all body systems of both the mother and the baby.
- Touch during pregnancy promotes production of hormones, especially progesterone, estrogen, **human placental lactogen**, and **prolactin**, and that improves pregnancy outcomes and produces appropriate mothering behaviors. (See online resources for more information on prenatal and perinatal psychological benefits of touch at http://thePoint.lww.com/Osborne-Pregnancy2e.)
- Massage and other touch therapists inherently provide pregnant, laboring, and postpartum women with these general physiological benefits.

> **REMINDER:** *Skin stimulation = brain stimulation = improved placental functioning = improved hormonal production.*

Pregnancy brings skin changes in texture, oiliness, and pigmentation (Fig. 1.5). As the abdominal skin stretches over the expanding uterus, it can become dry, itchy, and taut. She may develop stretch marks (**striae gravidarum**) on her abdomen, breasts, and other areas where weight and size increases are most dramatic. Darker patches may develop across her cheeks and nose (**chloasma**), and a dark line known as the **linea nigra** runs from her pubic bone to her umbilicus. Many women appreciate the soothing effect of oils and other specifically formulated lubricants used during massage therapy.

● URINARY SYSTEM BENEFITS

Pregnancy's effects on the urinary system are the source of many jokes, but it's no joke to expectant women. Urinary frequency is highest in the first trimester and in the final weeks of pregnancy, particularly after the baby's **engagement** or **lightening**, when its head (depending on the baby's **position**) drops firmly against the mother's cervix, further compressing the bladder. **Sidelying** sleeping in later pregnancy allows greater blood circulation from the legs, increasing renal perfusion and filtration; most women complain of getting up four or more times a night to use the toilet. Decreased bladder tone and longer emptying time are other bothersome complaints. The swelling uterus compresses both the bladder and its ureters, slowing urination and reducing bladder space. Progesterone enlarges the kidneys and ureters, accommodating their increased workload. Urinary output is 40% to 60% greater, initially because of hormonal fluctuations and later in pregnancy due to increased fluid and waste product removal. All of these factors increase the likelihood of bladder and kidney infections during pregnancy (Ricci 2009).

As pregnancy progresses, weight gain also strains the pelvic floor muscles (Fig. 1.6), reducing their sphincter and supportive capacities. Many women leak small amounts of urine when laughing, sneezing, or coughing (**urinary stress incontinence**). If a woman does not maintain and regain muscle tone, this condition may worsen from the inherent stretching and possible damage to the pelvic floor musculature while giving birth.

Though outside the scope of practice of massage therapists, partner or self-massage of a woman's pelvic floor muscles may ready the area for birthing, as can numerous, daily repetitions of **pelvic floor (Kegel) exercises**. Tightening these muscles as though stopping urine flow and doing a variety of other strengthening exercises improve their tone and vascularization. (See Chapter 5 for further discussion.) Pelvic floor exercise also expands a woman's awareness and control of her pelvic floor, skills especially helpful during

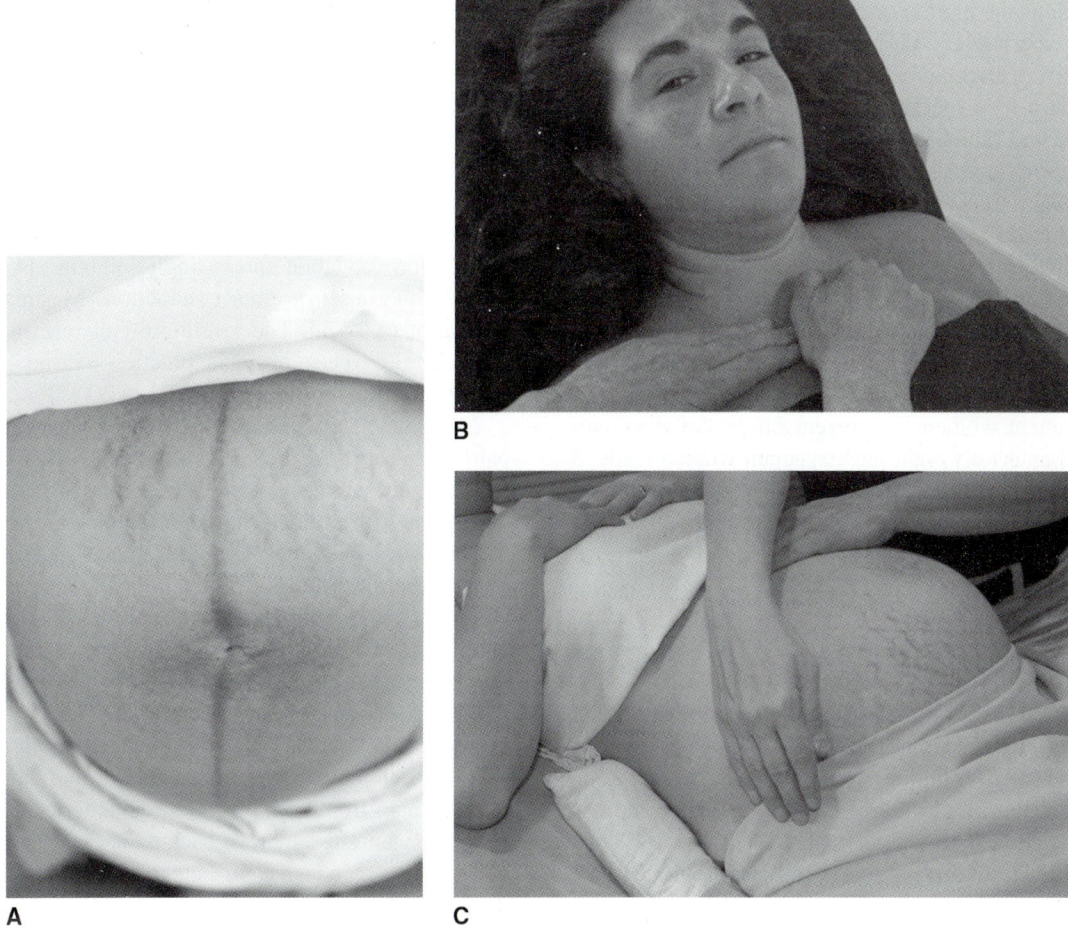

FIGURE 1.5 Common effects of pregnancy on skin. **A.** Linea nigra (Reprinted with permission from Ricci SS. Essentials of Maternity, Newborn, and Women's Health Nursing. 2nd Ed. Philadelphia: Lippincott Williams & Wilkins, 2009). **B.** Facial melasma (chloasma or the "mask of pregnancy"). **C.** Striae gravidarum (stretch marks).

labor and birth (Noble 1995; Franklin 2003). Some therapists report that reflexive techniques on the feet, hands, and energy meridians may enhance bladder and kidney function (Ezner 2000).

Reduction of Musculoskeletal Strain and Pain

In a recent survey of prenatal and perinatal massage therapists, they cited relief from musculoskeletal aches and pains as the primary motivator for their clients seeking therapy. Therapists reported the following areas, in descending order of frequency, as the most problematic: lower back, upper back/neck and shoulder pain, sacral and pelvic pain, sciatica and similar sensations, and abdominal pain (Osborne 2009). Fewer than half of pregnant women escape the inevitable strain of their growing bellies on their structural balance. The progressive growth, hormonal influences, and weight gain prompt back and pelvic pain, as well as other localized musculoskeletal discomforts (Fig. 1.6). A good massage is often just what an expectant woman's muscles and joints need.

● PRENATAL STRUCTURAL BALANCE

More anterior weight generally challenges a pregnant woman's structural integrity. As pregnancy progresses, her pelvis will tend to anteriorly rotate, spilling the uterus forward against the abdominal walls. This increases the lumbar curvature and stretches the abdominal muscles, usually separating the rectus abdominis at the **linea alba** (**diastasis recti**) by the third trimester. To compensate, she leans her upper ribcage more posteriorly, and her head and neck jut forward anterior of the optimal vertical line.

These compensations strain all of the posterior musculature, creating fatigue, tightness, excessive fibrous buildup (**fibrosis**), and hyperirritable, tender points that refer pain to distant sites (myofascial trigger points). Excessive lumbar lordosis shortens the hip flexors, iliopsoas, and tensor fascia latae; it also shortens the thoracolumbar fascia, decreasing spine flexibility. Enlarging breasts pull her pectoral girdle so that it sags into forward rotation, with tight pectoral muscles and stretched rhomboids. Increased uterine weight also strains the pelvic floor.

Many women broaden their standing foundation, and chronic tension builds in the piriformis and other external hip rotators. With the knee and foot no longer aligned with the hip joint, the iliopsoas cannot efficiently stabilize or flex the pelvis when walking. In compensation, the gluteus medius must first abduct the thigh for the quadriceps to complete a step. This creates the characteristic waddling gait of many pregnant women. To prevent falling forward with the increased anterior weight, the expectant woman tends to hyperextend her knees, and her weight will collapse into the medial arches of her weary feet (Fig. 4.9) (Noble 1995).

● BACK AND PELVIC PAIN IN PREGNANCY

These postural adjustments and the recommended weight gain of 25 to 30 lb can destabilize and painfully strain and compress the weight-bearing joints and associated myofascial structures identified in Figure 1.6. Pain in the pelvic region that started during pregnancy or within the first 3 months after delivery, and for which no clear diagnosis is available, is known as **peripartum pelvic pain syndrome (PPPPS)**. Women feel the greatest discomfort around the sacroiliac (SI) joint, lumbosacral joint, and pubic symphysis, but other pelvic and leg regions are sometimes achy, too (Figs. 1.6 and 1.7) (Howard 2000).

At the SI joints, the relationship of the ilea and sacrum shifts dramatically when the enlarged abdomen protrudes anteriorly. As the pelvis anteriorly rotates, the ligaments of these deep pelvic joints are compressed, strained, and can become hypermobile or hypomobile and painful in response. The long dorsal SI ligament seems to be particularly sensitive, and it is the site of pelvic pain in as many as 76% of women with pelvic pain (Vleeming et al. 2002). SI joint strain may refer pain into the buttocks and lower lumbar regions and as far as the lower extremities (Slipman et al. 2000).

Some women have severe lumbosacral joint compression, causing pain from lumbar nerve root impingement. Often this pain is constant, unilateral, and movement sensitive, and it can be felt on any part of the pelvis (Howard 2000). Besides the femoral external rotation previously described, the hip joints often feel compressed, with little space for free movement. Exceeding the recommended weight gain multiplies all of these strains.

As early as the 10th week of pregnancy, the hormones progesterone and **relaxin** begin softening the body's connective tissue. This allows more pelvic flexibility and space to accommodate the developing fetus and especially its passage through the pelvis during birth; however, the pelvis is not the single target for these hormones' softening effects. Laxity in ligaments, tendons, and fascia contributes to joint instability and strain on all joints, particularly weight-bearing structures, especially in the lumbar spine and pelvis. Many women report feeling as though they have become "a loose goose," walking like Dorothy's scarecrow friend in the classic 1950s movie, *The Wizard of Oz*.

Progesterone and relaxin also work synergistically to help maintain the pregnancy, and they soften the cervix in preparation for labor. Interestingly, relaxin also is thought to delay the onset of labor contractions by suppressing the release of oxytocin. The leveling off of relaxin production at about 30 weeks prompts practice uterine contractions (**Braxton-Hicks contractions**) (Ricci 2009).

Many women report their first incidence of chronic back pain during a pregnancy. Forty-eight to fifty-six percent of all expectant women experience some back pain, especially during the fifth through the ninth months. Of these women, 50% suffer pain in the SI area, 25% in the upper back, and 25% in the lower back. Though buttock and posterior thigh pain may occur, only about 1% have true sciatica (Ostgaard et al. 1992). Onset of pelvic pain is most common prenatally in the second trimester, but women are nearly as vulnerable in the first 3 months postpartum.

As detailed above, posturally induced strain to localized segments of the posterior musculature and ligaments and referred pain from both posterior and anterior trigger points create concentrated areas of back pain. Poor abdominal tone and diastasis recti also contribute to back pain. A fetus with a preferred uterine position often overburdens the favored side of the back, making it tired and sore from the unbalanced weight load. Some women develop temporary scoliosis from fetal positioning preferences.

Clients often describe the generalized back pain of pregnancy as fatigue, tightness, and achiness. A woman frequently feels SI pain as chronic soreness in the upper, medial quadrant of the buttocks, across the iliac crest, or at the posterior iliac spine of the pelvis, which radiates for several inches. Prolonged periods of standing or sitting, wearing high heels, and insufficient back support while seated can all create strain to these joints softened by relaxin and stressed by any pelvic rotation. Occasionally one SI joint's hypomobility will result in excessive mobility in the other. That hypermobility creates a sharp, stabbing posterior pelvic pain when the client rolls from a supine position, including your massage table (Noble 1995).

Pain from other pelvic joints varies with the source. (Fig. 1.7) Achiness in the center of the sacral and lumbar areas may indicate strain and compression of the lumbosacral joint. Sharp, stabbing anterior pain in the center of the pelvis indicates instability of the pubic symphysis known as **symphysis pubis dysfunction or pelvic girdle instability**. Softened by progesterone and relaxin, this joint is vulnerable to horizontal sheering strains that can be excruciating when movements elevate or depress one side of the pelvis. Trigger

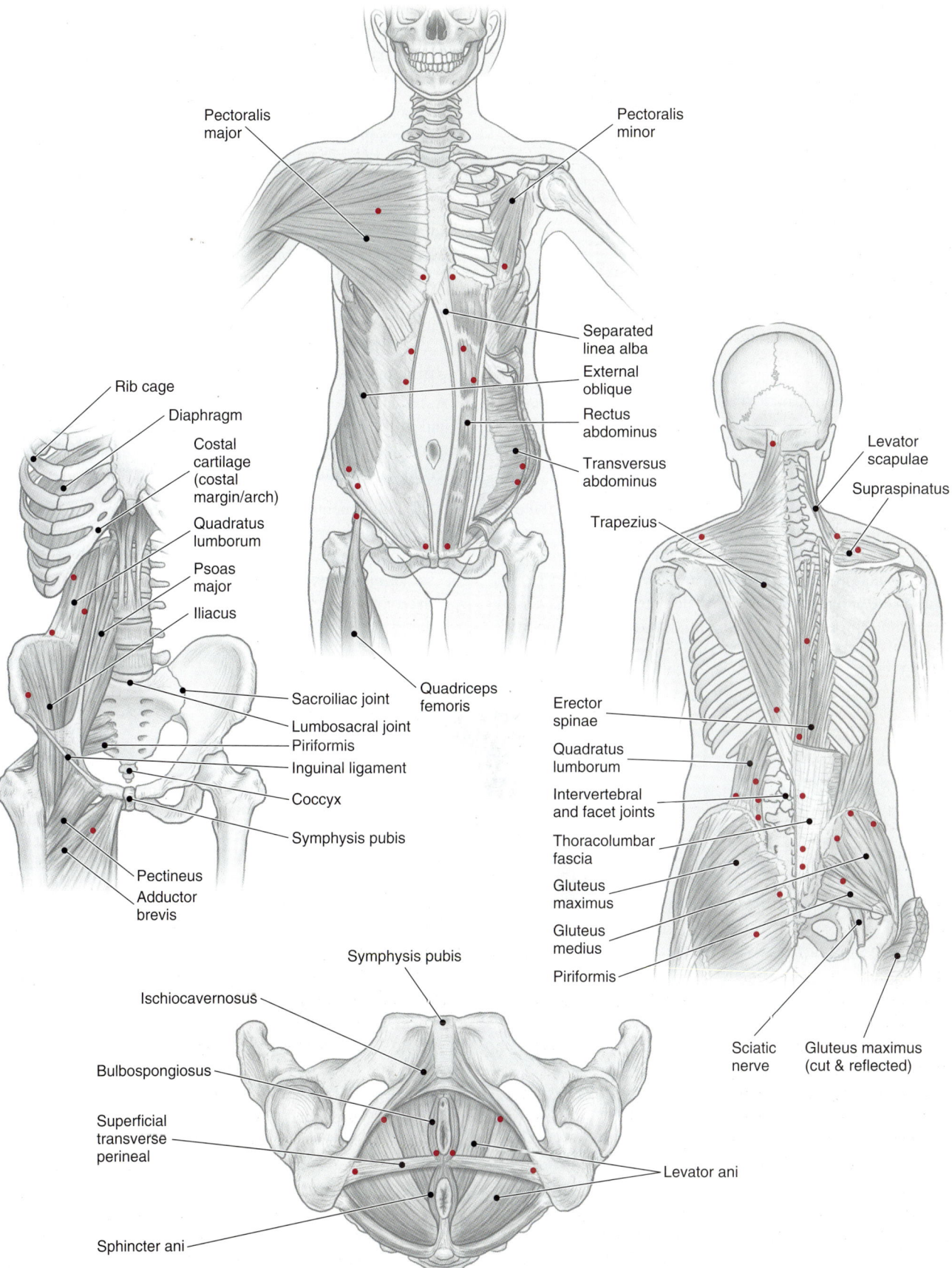

FIGURE 1.6 Joints and muscles most directly affected by pregnancy. Some common trigger points are marked with a red dot. Many trigger points are found bilaterally though they may only be indicated unilaterally in this illustration.

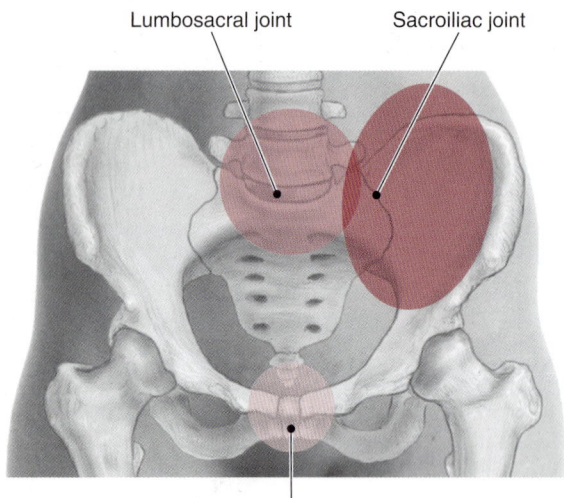

FIGURE 1.7 Areas of joint pain in the pregnant pelvis. *Shaded areas* indicate possible pain range radiating from strained pelvic joints. Density of shading correlates to the likelihood of pain, with the least likely being the lightest shaded area.

points and fatigue of the gluteus medius also contribute to back and pelvic pain (Fig. 1.7) (Noble 1995).

The growing uterus itself is part of the pelvic pain picture. During pregnancy, the pregnant uterus blossoms from a plum-sized pelvic organ to watermelon proportions. Reaching the xiphoid process level by the ninth month, the supportive structure of its eight **uterine ligaments** suspends the uterus in the pelvic cavity (Fig. 1.8). Formed of thickened layers of external uterine connective tissue, these ligaments include the following:

- Two broad ligaments proceeding laterally and attaching in the anterior, internal lower iliac region that also support the ovaries and fallopian tubes
- Two round ligaments extending from the anterior, superior uterine surface near the broad ligament, continuing through the inguinal ligament and attaching in the connective tissue of the labia majora
- Two sacrouterine ligaments continuing from the posterior uterus attaching to the posterior pelvic cavity wall and anterior surface of the sacrum at S2 and S3
- A small anterior ligament attached to the bladder and one from the posterior uterus to the rectum

As uterine growth inevitably stretches these ligaments, distortion and pull of their fascial continuations seem likely. These changes can result in pain referring from their attachment sites in characteristic fascial pain patterns as follows (Fig. 1.8):

- Broad ligaments: low back, buttock, and sciaticlike pain
- Round ligaments: diagonal pain from top of the uterus to groin; usually one-sided, depending on fetal position; sometimes as extensive as the vulvar and upper thigh fascia
- Sacrouterine ligaments: achiness just lateral to or beneath the sacrum and in the lower back

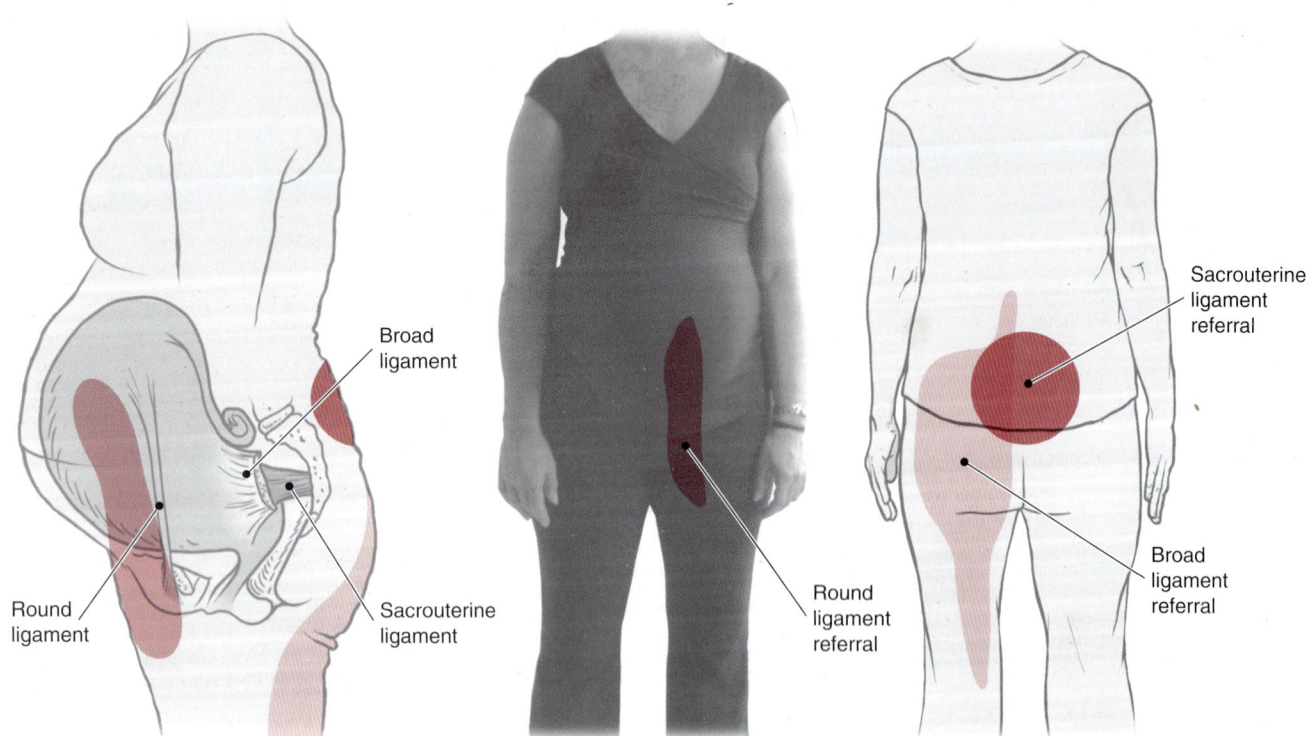

FIGURE 1.8 Uterine ligaments and their typical zones of referred pain. The sacrouterine ligament (*darkest area*) is more problematic in the third trimester, whereas round ligament pain (*medium area*) is more common in the second trimester. Broad ligament pain (*lightest area*) occurs more in the sixth month and can continue onto the lateral thigh, as well.

Occasionally, women feel pain in one or both buttocks that is not exclusively from the broad ligament. Pain radiating down the posterior leg can result from severe postural imbalance in the lumbar spine. More commonly, chronic piriformis tension may entrap and compress the sciatic nerve (**piriformis syndrome**). From either source, this pain burns, sometimes worsened by tingling, numbness, and weakness in the legs. Some women have coccygeal and other pelvic floor pain, too (Fig. 1.6).

● OTHER PRENATAL MUSCULOSKELETAL COMPLAINTS

Although not as common as back and pelvic pain, many expectant women complain of pain in the feet, calves, knees, thighs, and hips. Edema produces some of this achy, sore, tense feeling, as does strain to the muscles and joints of the feet and legs. Numbness around the medial malleolus and medial plantar aspect of the foot can occur if edema compresses the tibial nerve (**tarsal tunnel syndrome**). Cramping in both the gastrocnemius/soleus group and the peroneals torments some women's sleep, as do the vibrations and irritated feeling of "**restless legs**." Compression of knee and ankle joints results in soreness and fatigue. Hip joint discomfort and stiffness caused by compression and chronic external femoral rotation often become more severe in later pregnancy when sleeping positions are restricted to sidelying or **semireclining**. Some women have pain and numbness on the anterolateral side of the thigh thought to be caused by compression of the lateral cutaneous femoral nerve by the inguinal ligament and nearby fascial sheaths (Herman 2004).

Pregnancy often worsens prior postural imbalances and injuries such as lumbar and cervical lordosis, scoliosis, disc dysfunctions, and **thoracic outlet syndrome**. When poor posture compresses the brachial plexus, women feel a characteristic pain, numbness, or tingling in the entire hand and along the arm; however, edema-dependent carpal tunnel syndrome pain happens more frequently. Ribcage pain may occur as organ space diminishes in later pregnancy. As the lower circumference widens and the ribs spread, they can painfully strain abdominal attachments and intercostal muscles. Myofascial trigger points develop, referring pain into the mid and lower back and sometimes throughout the ribcage. The baby may intensify this discomfort with frequent kicks and strenuous stretching movements (Noble 1995). (Fig. 1.6).

Headaches are common and often musculoskeletal in origin, referring from tension, strain, and trigger points,

> **REMINDER:** To successfully address peripartum pelvic pain syndrome you must use a multifaceted approach to the many possible pain sources: joint structures and movement, uterine ligaments, muscular trigger points, tension and fibrosis, fascial binding and disorganization, and hormonal effects.

My Story

I came in with a splitting headache, but during the massage I could really feel my neck and shoulders relaxing in places that I didn't even know were tense. The visualization exercises helped too. I loved when the therapist held the baby up for me and took the weight off my spine!

—Tiffany

especially in the neck and upper back. They often increase in intensity and frequency if the woman tends to hyperventilate because the scalenes lift the upper ribcage and tug on their cervical origins. Other hormonal effects on blood vessel dilation and increased mucous production in the sinuses make sinus headaches more common, too (Gibbs et al. 2003).

● MASSAGE THERAPY AND PAIN CONTROL

Given the far-ranging scope of these many structural changes, expectant clients' interest in massage therapy is understandable. Eighty-one percent of prenatal sessions are given in the second and third trimesters, when these types of musculoskeletal discomforts tend to increase. A knowledgeable maternity massage therapist may help her clients to prevent, reduce, and manage pain by supporting and encouraging the body's adaptation to the many myofascial and proprioceptive transitions (Osborne 2009).

Recent research is accumulating a small and growing body of data regarding the effectiveness of massage therapy for reducing pain. In one of the few well-structured studies of massage and pregnancy, massaged women reported less back pain and a similar reduction in leg pain, among other benefits, compared with those who had an equal amount of relaxation therapy (Field et al. 1999). Depressed second trimester women had similar reductions in pain when they received massage therapy rather than relaxation sessions or normal prenatal care (Field et al. 2004). Another study looked at subacute low back pain, unrelated to pregnancy, and found improved function, less intense pain, and a decrease in the quality of pain when compared with several control groups (Pryde 2000). All of these studies were small, consisting of 26, 84, and 91 subjects, respectively, but the results mirror the practical experiences of massage therapists in a variety of settings. These therapists reported that approximately 95% of their clients felt less pregnancy-related pain and discomfort following a massage session (Osborne 2009).

One of the most comprehensive metaanalyses of massage therapy research confirmed these therapist-reported impressions. Looking at over 37 studies, reviewers found that a course of massage therapy treatments brought less

> **My Story**
>
> *I was unable to relate to my pregnant friend's severe back pain because, fortunately, I learned ways to prevent backaches from my massage therapist. What pain I had was extremely mild and handled weekly in my sessions.*
>
> —Jennifer

pain perception (Moyer et al. 2004). Not included in this study was another small sample-size study, this time looking at massage effects on lumbar muscle fatigue. Although not confirmed with electronic measuring instruments, subjects' feelings of fatigue were significantly lessened after only 5 minutes of massage rather than just resting after exertion (Tanaka et al. 2002).

Several theories attempt to explain the mechanism that creates this welcomed relief, but none have substantial scientific validation. Some suggest that massage reduces pain by alleviating painful stimulation and altering the processing of painful input (see Chapter 5 for discussion of the gate theory of pain control processing). Others speculate that it may affect the conduction of pain impulses in the peripheral nerves (Quebec Task Force on Spinal Disorders 1987). Perhaps the kneading and stretching of contracted muscle create inhibitory reflex responses from tendon proprioceptors that relieve muscle spasm. Another explanation is that pain-mediating endocrine responses reduce the perception of pain.

Until sufficient data confirm why it works, massage therapists can use several methods to prevent and reduce pain in their prenatal clients. **Resisted movements**, rhythmic **passive movements** (including small-amplitude **Trager** movements), and osteopathic **strain and counterstrain** and **muscle energy** techniques are all effective in pain management (Quebec Task Force on Spinal Disorders 1987). Deep tissue work and other forms of **myofascial release** may reduce pain by elongating shortened, bunched connective tissue (Osborne-Sheets 2002), and deep **cross-fiber friction** may reduce pain and the restricted range of movement of fibrosis (Cyriax 1984).

Myofascial pain syndromes (trigger points) are especially common for the woman coping with pregnancy's structural stresses. These hyperirritable spots are quite painful when pressed, and they generally create a characteristic referred pain in some other location, sometimes very distant from the trigger point.

Trigger points, caused by trauma, poor posture, or by muscle chilling, fatigue, strain, or tension, develop or worsen during pregnancy. Most pregnancy-induced trigger points appear in the musculature of the abdomen, ribcage, upper and lower back, neck, and legs (Fig. 1.6). Focused pressure and massage over the trigger point, combined with appropriate stretching and other treatment options (myofascial trigger point therapy), can reduce the pain associated with these points by relieving tissue ischemia and allowing restoration of normal tissue blood supply (Howard 2000). (See Chapters 2 and 5 for abdominal precautions.) Pregnant women welcome the lessening pain these techniques can bring.

In addition to hands-on techniques, educational activities also help reduce pain and decrease stress on structures. Correct and safe abdominal strengthening activities and body-use guidelines for walking, sitting, sleeping, carrying, and other daily activities will further reduce strain in the neck, back, and pelvis. Introducing more efficient movement patterns enhances and reinforces the effectiveness of hands-on therapy (Noble 1995).

Labor Preparation

Physical flexibility and kinesthetic awareness may equip a woman to more actively participate in the birth process. Muscle and joint pliability helps ensure the advantages of more movement and positioning choices to actively birth her baby (Ricci 2009). Open hip joints, supple adductors, hamstrings, and calf muscles, and resilient postural muscles can respond more positively to the urge of many laboring women to walk, squat, rock, lunge, kneel, or stand during all or part of labor. Any structure connecting to her pelvis needs length and pliability. At the very least, women birthing vaginally must be able to open their thighs to allow the baby's passage.

The same massage therapy methods useful for pain control may be effective in increasing flexibility, especially passive and assisted resisted stretching, deep tissue work, and osteopathic soft tissue treatments (Scheumann 2007). Many women enjoy exercise and stretching, and they find these activities to be safe, successful labor preparation. They can participate in fitness or yoga programs led by instructors with specialized prenatal training. Including some strengthening and aerobic exercise helps ready them for the athletic challenges of labor and birth (Noble 1995). Of course, they should consult with their prenatal healthcare provider concerning the advisability for them of prenatal exercise. (See online resources for more on prenatal exercise at http://thePoint.lww.com/Osborne-Pregnancy2e.)

Creating an awareness bond with her body is one of the many potential benefits of prenatal exercise and bodywork. As a result of the "feedback loop" of the sensory-motor

> **My Story**
>
> *I believe that massage therapy helped me so much while I was pregnant. My body would relax, and I'd be so centered within myself and able to focus and go inside, which made a big difference during labor.*
>
> —Andrea

system, increased bodily awareness creates increased sensory awareness and control of muscles (Juhan 1998). Heightened familiarity with her internal landscape means a woman may be more likely to make the labor journey with more ease, less pain, and with an adventuresome spirit.

The variety of stimuli introduced by bodywork techniques is one way that this feedback loop becomes activated. There are modulations in depth, direction, and duration of touch, especially in Swedish, deep tissue, and reflexive modalities. Kinesthetic input varies with changes in speed, rhythm, and intensity of passive and active movements. All of these experiences create a rich influx of information and corresponding responses and awareness in the client's body and mind. The result may be heightened perception, new body understandings, and specifically localized awareness.

As she participates in prenatal massage therapy sessions, there are numerous opportunities to help her connect with and express her physical awareness and her emotional flows. As she learns to more fully express her sensations and her needs as a client, she can improve her ability to more effectively communicate with her family and the labor professionals she employs. She is then more likely to be able to access her feelings and assert her needs during labor. Women with previous traumatic births or other physical and/or emotionally traumatic histories often need particularly sensitive attention to effective expression (see Chapter 7).

To birth with less effort, the musculature of the back, abdomen, and pelvic floor must remain relaxed to allow the uterus to labor without resistance. Relaxation here allows the baby to press more firmly against the cervix. The laboring woman should scan for and recognize tension throughout her body. Her labor may be easier if she knows how, through imagery, hypnosis, or conscious control, to release tension. Sometimes she must use specific muscles, such as the diaphragm, abdominals, or pelvic floor, in a precise, controlled manner. She can develop all of these abilities during prenatal bodywork. Education in diaphragmatic breathing, pelvic floor strengthening, perineal self-massage, and abdominal strengthening is particularly useful in developing awareness and control in these vital birthing muscles (see Chapter 5) (Noble 1995).

Most clients gain self-awareness, relaxation, and emotional support from receiving therapeutic bodywork during pregnancy. This contributes to the development of a woman who is more able to access those inborn skills and intuitions that have evolved over the millennia of humanity's existence and women's experiences of giving birth (Samuels and Samuels 1996) (Fig. 1.9).

Teaching massage to partners and others who will attend a woman's birth furthers their preparedness of labor. These family or friends can accompany her to a session to watch and practice simple, yet effective massage movements. Some therapists teach a segment in a childbirth education class or organize separate classes for small groups of women and their loved ones to learn labor massage possibilities. (See Chapter 5 and online resources on Childbirth Education Class Presentation Plans at http://thePoint.lww.com/Osborne-Pregnancy2e.)

Labor Facilitation

Massage therapists who attend births bear witness to the potential benefits of their skilled touch: it can contribute to shorter, less painful labors with fewer complications, less use of medications, and fewer interventions to normal birthing. Of course there are no guarantees for these benefits, but at the least, it usually can help improve both the mother's and her infant's physical and emotional well-being. Regardless of the labor difficulty, grateful new mothers send gift baskets with notes attesting to some version of, "I couldn't have done it without you." What these women inherently and personally know, contemporary research has yet to scientifically and conclusively verify; however, the hints of efficacy and the popularity with laboring women are compelling. Providing the option for such powerful, nonpharmacological pain management is a critical step toward the goal of a more mother-friendly model of maternity care (Budin 2007).

● TIMELESS TOUCH FOR LABORING MOMS

Historically and culturally, family members and maternity professionals have traditionally massaged mothers and their babies through the birth passage. Skim any history of childbirth (Cassidy 2006) or anthropologists' studies (Goldsmith 1984) and those pages overflow with images of laboring women soothed and reinforced by skilled and loving hands. When pain or stress intensifies, the impulse to reach out to reassure and assist a birthing woman comes naturally. Of course, not all laboring women want to be touched, but most appreciate reassuring touch at some point in their labors.

Those same publications also document Western cultures' last two centuries of movement away from "high touch" and toward "high tech" birthing. Modern monitoring, pharmacology, and surgical procedures have benefited many women and their families. They have also contributed to a birthing milieu that, for many, feels impersonal, disempowering, and statistically not as safe as many believe (Budin 2007).

● RESEARCH ON TOUCH IN LABOR

Several studies show preliminary validation of women's perceptions that rubbing and massage therapy specifically improved their ability to cope with labor, reduced labor pain and time, met their emotional and physical needs, and provided relaxation (Simkin and O'Hara 2002). The Touch Research Institute at the University of Miami had a massage therapist teach partners massage for during labor. Those mothers whose partners massaged them during labor experienced decreased

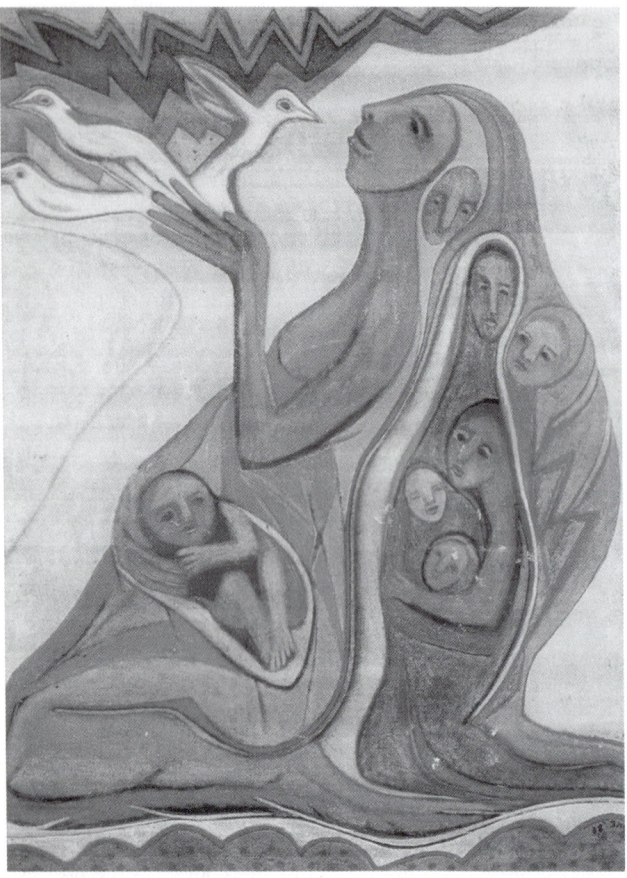

FIGURE 1.9 Activating the ancient mother archetype. Massage therapy can help women connect with "women's wisdom" by encouraging a turning inward. "Jamaica: Tomorrow, Homage to Edna Manley." Acrylic painting by Betty LaDuke. Used by permission of artist.

levels of anxiety and pain. Massaged women in this small study needed less medication, and their labors were shorter than those of the control group receiving routine obstetrical care only (Field et al. 1997).

In another study, birthing partners learned a 30-minute massage routine from a nurse who massaged the women in their early first-stage labor. The partners repeated the massage in active and transition stages. Naturally, pain levels and anxiety increased as labor progressed for the massaged group and for the control group, who had no massage, but less so for the massaged group. Those who were massaged had fewer pain reactions; fully 87% of the massaged women were more satisfied with their partners' support, and they found the massage to be helpful (Chang et al. 2002). This study only included 60 women, a familiar shortcoming of massage research.

Another study of 75 laboring women zeroed in on the effectiveness of massage to **acupressure** point SP-6. Compared with those who were simply touched at this point, those women who actually received acupressure sensed less labor pain, and their labors were shorter (Lee et al. 2004).

A third small study compared acupressure to points LI-4 and BL-67, (see Figs. 2.7 and 2.8 for specific locations of these points) light skin stroke on the area, or conversation for the same amount of time. The acupressure group reported less pain, but there were no verified effects on uterine contractions (Chung et al. 2003).

A nursing study of touch during active labor had nurses provide laboring women a high degree of nurturing and reassuring contact, such as stroking the brow and hand holding, in addition to the clinical necessities of pulse taking and cervical exams. After three contractions, they then offered only clinical touch for three contractions. During the three contractions of high contact, both pulse rate and systolic blood pressure dropped, and women appeared to be more comfortably coping with their labors than at other times (Birch 1986).

Perhaps the most compelling, reliable data are those collected in studies involving professional labor support. Also known as birth doulas, labor support professionals are women whose role is to provide physical and emotional support throughout labor. A doula typically spends most of her time stroking, kneading, holding, and physically and/or verbally comforting her charge. In a metaanalysis of six studies conducted worldwide, this consistent physical presence, nurturing touch, and emotional support created the following benefits for the experimental group compared with the control groups:

- 25% shorter labors
- 40% less use of **pitocin** (labor stimulant)
- 30% decrease in all pain medication use, including 60% decrease in requests for **epidurals**
- 40% less need for **forceps**
- 50% fewer **cesarean section births**
- Improved infant **Apgar scores**
- Enhanced family social adjustment postpartum (Klaus et al. 2002)

Though none of these studies has focused on the effects of a highly trained massage therapist on labor outcomes, results comparable to the birth doula studies seem likely. Meanwhile, practice files of prenatal massage therapists are full of detailed anecdotal evidence of easier, more satisfying, and healthier births when they are part of a birthing team (Fig. 1.10).

The long-term value of appropriate labor massage therapy is undeniable. More women express satisfaction with their childbirth experience and its impact on their lives when they are emotionally supported during labor. In addition, the quality of the woman's relationship with her maternity healthcare provider and the degree of participation she has in decision making have more long-term impact than the management of labor pain. In fact, nurturing care correlates more significantly with this satisfaction than the ease of the physical process of labor, even in long, complicated births (Green et al. 1990; The Nature and Management of Labor Pain 2003).

Practicing therapists have found many massage therapy techniques as effective during labor as they are prenatally.

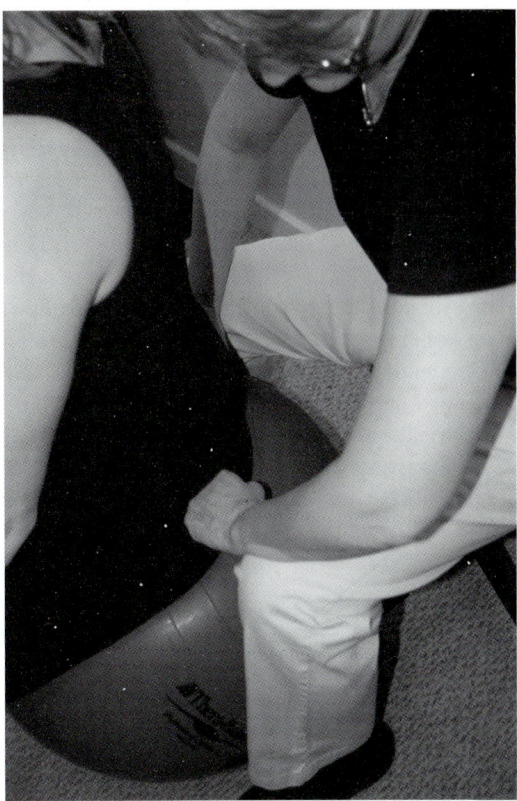

FIGURE 1.10 Labor massage. Skilled, comforting touch of doulas and massage therapists may help to ease labor pain.

Some general massage techniques reduce stress and promote relaxation. Deep tissue work and stretching may relieve muscle tension, cramping, and other soft tissue discomforts. The focused, calm presence that a therapist surrounds her client with often supports the physiological and emotional needs that naturally arise during labor and birth. Stress can significantly reduce blood flow to the uterus, and it may contribute to long, slow, highly painful, unproductive labors. A massage therapist may promote a level of relaxation that facilitates labor and allows a woman to explore the many aspects of the labor process. (See Chapter 5 for specific techniques.)

Encouraging Nurturing Maternal Touch

How important is cuddling, stroking, and carrying of a baby? Despite providing food and shelter, American orphanages of the early 1900s had infant mortality rates of 95% to 100%; the little ones there died of tactile and vestibular starvation (Montagu 1978). More recently, widespread media coverage publicized the developmental tragedies of children neglected in communist-regime Romanian orphanages (Settle 1991).

Here's what research on our mammalian cousins showed: the need for cutaneous stimulation compelled monkeys separated from their natural mothers to choose a softer, cuddly mother substitute with poor milk supply over a wire surrogate with outstanding and reliable nutrition. When mice that were handled during their infancy became moms, they nursed, cleaned, and cared for their young better than those in unstroked control groups (Montagu 1978).

So why wouldn't a mother who loves her infant not hold and care for her child? First, nurturing, respectful touch is an experience often lacking in the technological, touch-aversive cultures. Some women, like the research animals described above, have instead experienced neglect; impersonal physical contact; physical, sexual, and emotional abuse; and other negative developmental impacts. This deprivation may leave women without a fully embodied sense of appropriate, loving touch (Montagu 1978; Simkin and Klaus 2004).

Massage practitioners have the opportunity to positively impact their clients' nurturing skills. They can become role models from whom their pregnant clients learn loving, appropriate touch. Nursing studies show that both first-time and experienced mothers progressed similarly in touching their newborns. Initial touch was with tentative fingertips, then fuller hand contact, and finally complete arm embraces, leading to "molding" of the two to each other. This sequence was completed more slowly or was interrupted or aborted by those women whose prenatal and perinatal care consisted only of routine, impersonal touch. Researchers concluded that "appropriate, meaningful touch of pregnant and laboring women leads to touching babies in meaningful, effective, and caring ways," thus facilitating the transformation of a daughter into a mother (Rubin 1963, 1975, 1984).

In addition, massage therapists may teach women and their partners simple prenatal and labor massage techniques. Therapeutic procedures requiring refined palpatory skills and advanced anatomical knowledge are best in the hands of touch professionals; however, nonprofessionals can safely rub and knead family members, as long as important safety precautions are included in instruction (see Chapter 5 and online resources at http://thePoint.lww.com/Osborne-Pregnancy2e). Prenatal and labor massage instruction may prepare and empower partners and other loved ones to offer meaningful physical nurturing to the mother. If she feels satisfied with her partner's support, this usually helps to create a positive start for the new family's life together.

My Story

We wanted a gentle, unmedicated birth, but 16 hours of intense labor almost ended in a cesarean. My therapist used every massage technique to keep my hips relaxed, pressed on them, and cradled me on my side to help the baby come out.

—Pat

To further nurturing touch in the family, many maternity massage therapists enjoy teaching parents infant massage. Even simple sequences of effleurage, kneading, and raking can have significant health benefits to all babies, but particularly to those with health challenges. Premature infants who received 15-minute massage and movement sequences three times daily gained 47% more weight, secreted higher levels of cortisol and human growth hormones and were more active, alert, and relaxed than unmassaged control premature infants. They went home from the hospital an average of 6 days earlier. These babies' superior development continued through the 6 months of follow-up study, regardless of whether the massage was continued at home (Field et al. 1986). This study and numerous others (Solkoff et al. 1969; Rice 1979; Rausch 1981; Scafidi et al. 1986, 1990; Gunzenhauser 1990; Holst et al. 2002; Feldman 2002) support the benefits of skin-to-skin contact and massage for infants and for their caretakers, making a convincing case for the advisability of including infant massage instruction in prenatal and perinatal massage therapy practices. (See online resource: Infant Massage Instructional Programs at http://thePoint.lww.com/Osborne-Pregnancy2e.)

> **REMINDER:** Humans need nurturing touch to survive and to thrive.

Postpartum Recovery

Even new moms who have experienced massage's many benefits often neglect their self-care during the postpartum period; less than 25% of the prenatal clients of most of the surveyed perinatal massage therapists returned for massage therapy (Osborne 2009). That means that they miss the many emotional, physiological, and functional benefits of knowledgeable postpartum bodywork described below.

● FACILITATING EMOTIONAL ADJUSTMENTS

After childbirth, many women have an intrinsic need to tell their birth story. Some women retell the details repeatedly, oftentimes unsolicited by family and friends. This storytelling can seem most urgent when the outcome of labor and birth was not as anticipated, or when there was a significant feeling of loss of control. The psychological repercussions of childbearing profoundly influence the mother and each individual family member, her friends, and other associates. The psychological integration of her childbearing experience is a critical aspect of postpartum recovery. This is particularly important for women who have been depressed or who are slipping into postpartum mental illnesses (Simkin 1996).

Massage therapists can provide a professional yet caring opportunity for postpartum women to talk freely. Within a therapeutic session, many women will celebrate their accomplishments and unburden themselves of the fear, sadness, and anger often generated during labor. This may help them to begin to let go of muscular tension, frozen expressions and gestures, and unresolved issues. This is also an opportunity to relate any frustrations and concerns about infant care and their transition into mothering. Listening compassionately and attentively, a therapist can identify those who may need the assistance of mental health professionals and refer them appropriately.

● PHYSIOLOGICAL POSTPARTUM RECOVERY

In addition to providing emotional support, postpartum massage therapy facilitates physiological recovery of the exhausted postpartum woman. Labor is usually an athletic test of a woman's strength and endurance that can result in various muscular aches and pains. Circulatory, deep tissue, trigger point, and other reflexive massage methods may help to cleanse metabolic wastes and medication residues from tissues. This type of physiological assistance is especially helpful for postcesarean mothers who are recuperating from major abdominal surgery, as well as the strain of pregnancy. Sequential and appropriate therapy to the incision site may speed healing and reduce fibrous buildup in and around the scar (Andrade and Clifford 2008).

Constipation, difficulty urinating, uterine cramping, and perineal soreness are common in the days and weeks postpartum. Skin rolling, trigger point therapy, and Swedish abdominal techniques reduce these pains and aid in rehabilitation of the abdominal skin, muscles, and organs. Reflexive techniques to feet, hands, connective tissue, and energy meridians may enhance metabolic functioning, systematically and in individual organs (Ezner 2000).

● REESTABLISHING POSTURAL INTEGRITY AND REDUCING LABOR AND INFANT CARE PAIN

Labor sometimes worsens pain originating in prenatal postural imbalances. Women need particular attention to their back, abdominal, and pelvic floor areas. Additional structural stresses occur to the upper body during the many hours of nursing, lifting, and other childcare tasks (Pirie and Herman 2003). By reducing tension in postural muscles, reeducating

> *My Story*
>
> *I learned so much in my massages about appropriate levels of touch and so many techniques I can use to get in touch with my baby in the womb and for after she's born.*
>
> —Sara

My Story

I had two miscarriages prior to receiving bodywork. Through the course of my sessions, I discovered a lot of stored-up feelings regarding a child I'd carried and delivered many years prior to these losses. I was able to process my feelings regarding that baby and the feelings around the miscarriages. My next pregnancy produced my precious Brittany.

—Debbie

My Story

After my cesarean section, I came in a week later to get a massage. My recovery was quicker this time than it was for my previous two cesarean sections. Scar tissue was minimized by the massage work that was done to the incision in later sessions. It was also a great support to me to have someone to confide in as far as the nursing.

—Maria

the mother about the use of the iliopsoas muscles for both pelvic alignment and efficient gait, and encouraging proper body mechanics, a perinatal massage therapist offers relief from postural and mechanically induced postpartum pain (Fig. 1.11). For the fullest postpartum recovery, most new mothers should receive regular massage therapy for a full year after their baby's birth.

What Would You Do?

You are invited to attend a conference for public health nurses in your community as part of their continuing education program. How would you describe the benefits of massage therapy during pregnancy to this group?

CHAPTER SUMMARY

Parents, maternity healthcare providers, and massage therapists can feel confident and enthused about the likely positive effects of prenatal and perinatal massage therapy. For most, skilled, empathetic touch therapy offers far-reaching, multidimensional beneficial influences to individual women, their families, and the human family.

Below, note what research, observation, or clients' testimonies suggest that touch may accomplish on various levels:

In Society:

- Develops individuals more capable of love and pleasure.
- Builds less violent, more respectful cultures.

During Pregnancy:

- Reduces stress, promotes relaxation, and facilitates transitions through emotional support and physical nurturing.
- Reduces negative effects of changes to the circulatory system, including edema, varicose veins, and if blood pressure increases.
- Facilitates hormonal, respiratory, gastrointestinal, urinary, and other physiological processes during pregnancy.
- Reduces musculoskeletal strain and pain.
- Contributes to developing flexibility and the kinesthetic awareness necessary to actively participate in the birth process.
- Fosters nurturing maternal touch and healthy bonding.

In Labor:

- Contributes to shorter, less painful labor.
- Reduces labor complications, medications, and interventions.
- Improves infant well-being, mother's satisfaction with birthing, and family formation.

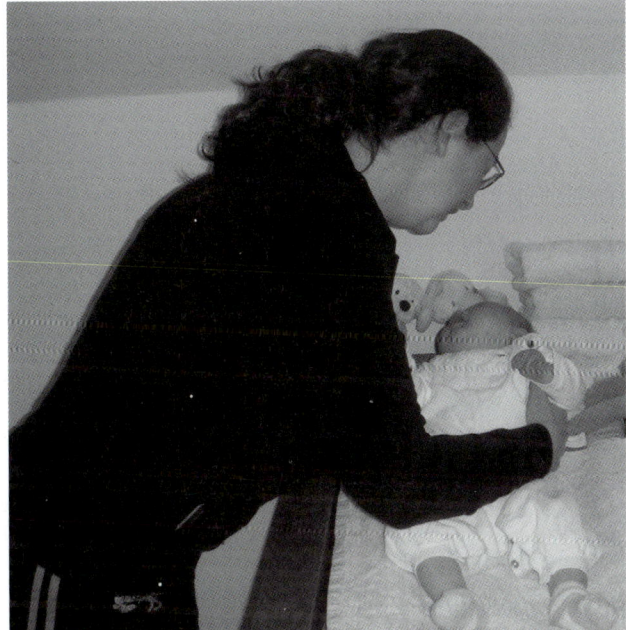

FIGURE 1.11 Postpartum structural stresses. Newborn care often stresses the lower back, pectoral girdle, and neck due to prolonged static neck flexion and repeated lifting and carrying of the infant.

In the Postpartum Period:

- Facilitates postpartum emotional, physiological, and family adjustments.
- Reduces musculoskeletal and organic pain.
- Promotes structural realignment of the spine and pelvis and reorganization of movement.
- Contributes to rehabilitation of abdominal skin, muscles, and organs.
- Promotes recovery from cesarean birth, including healing of the incision.
- Relieves muscle strain caused by childcare activities.

Test Yourself

For answers, visit the website at http://thePoint.LWW.com/Osborne-Pregnancy2e!

1. List five benefits of relaxation practice in pregnancy.

2. What are some of the possible negative effects of stress during pregnancy?

3. What effect do the following hormones have on the mothers' body?
   A. Estrogen
   B. Progesterone
   C. Relaxin

4. How might she experience the increased levels of relaxin and progesterone in her body?

5. Explain the causes of normal edema in pregnant women's legs.

6. How might massage during pregnancy affect the baby, during the pregnancy and after?

7. List the uterine ligaments that are believed responsible for some of the pelvic and back pain experienced by most pregnant women.

8. What joints are most likely to produce peripartum pelvic pain?

9. What are some of the possible positive benefits of having a massage therapist at a woman's labor?

10. Describe some of the conclusions about benefits of skin and vestibular stimulation that come from animal studies.

REFERENCES

Andrade C-K and Clifford P. Outcome-Based Massage: From Evidence to Practice. Second Edition. Baltimore: Lippincott, Williams and Wilkins, 2008.

Arkko PJ, Pakarinen AJ, Kari-Koskinen O. Effects of whole-body massage on serum protein, electrolyte and hormone concentrations, enzyme activities, and hematological parameters. Int J Sports Med 1983;4:265–267.

Belluomini J, Litt R, Lee K, et al. Acupressure for nausea and vomiting of pregnancy: a randomized, blinded study. Obstet Gynecol 1994;84:245.

Birch E. The experience of touch received during labor. J Nurse-Midwifery 1986;31:270–275.

Budin W, ed. Advancing normal birth. J Perinat Educ 2007;16:1.

Cassidy T. Birth: The Surprising History of How We Are Born. New York: Atlantic Monthly Press, 2006.

Chang MY, Wang SY, Chen CH. Effects of massage on pain and anxiety during labour: a randomized controlled trial in Taiwan. J Adv Nurs. 2002 Apr;38(1): 68–73.

Chung UL, Hung LC, Kuo SC, Huang CL. Effects of LI4 and BL 67 acupressure on labor pain and uterine contractions in the first stage of labor. J Nurs Res 2003 Dec;11(4):251–260.

Cooper R, Goldenberg R, Das A, et al. The pre-term prediction study: Maternal stress is associated with spontaneous preterm birth at less than thirty-five weeks gestation. Am J Obstet Gynecol 1996;175:1286–1292.

Cranden A. Maternal anxiety and obstetric complications. J Psychos Res 1979;23:109.

Cyriax J, Coldham M. Indications for and against deep friction. Textbook of Orthopaedic Medicine. Volume 2 Treatment by Manipulation, Massage, and Injection. 11th Ed. Toronto: Bailliere-Tindal, 1984.

Denenberg VH, Karas GG. Interactive effect of age and duration of infantile experience on adult learning. Psychol Rep 1960;7:313–322.

Ezner S. Reflexology: A Tool for Midwives. Pymble, Australia: Suzanne Ezner, 2000.

Fakouri C, Jones P. Relaxation RX: slow stroke back rub. J Gerontol Nurs 1987;13:32–35.

Ferguson P. The Self-Shiatsu Handbook. New York: Berkely Publishing, 1995.

Feldman R, Eidelman A, Sirota L, and Weller A. Comparison of Skin-to-Skin (Kangaroo) and Traditional Care: Parenting Outcomes and Preterm Infant Development. Pediatrics July 2002;110:1, 16–26.

Field T, Schanberg S, Scafidi F, et al. Tactile/kinesthetic stimulation effects on preterm neonates. Pediatrics 1986;77:654–658.

Field T, Morrow C, Valdon C, et al. Massage reduces anxiety in child and adolescent psychiatric patients. J Am Acad Child Adolesc Psychiatr 1992;31:125–131.

Field T, Hernandez-Reif M, Hart S, et al. University of Miami School of Medicine, Touch Research Abstracts, 1997.

Field T, Hernandez-Reif M, Taylor S, et al. J Psychos Obstet Gynecol 1997;18(4):286–291.

Field T, Hernandez-Reif M, Hart S, et al. Pregnant women benefit from massage therapy. J Psychos Obstet Gynecol 1999;20:31–38.

Field T, Diego MA, Hernandez-Reif M, et al. Massage therapy effects on depressed pregnant women. J Psychos Obstet Gynecol 2004;25:115–122.

Flocco O. Randomized controlled study of premenstrual symptoms treated with reflexology. Obstet Gynecol 1993;82:906–911.

Foldi M. Anatomical and physiological basis for physical therapy of lymphedema. Experientia 1978;33(Suppl):15–18.

Franklin E. Pelvic Power: Mind/Body Exercises for Strength, Flexibility, Posture and Balance. Hightstown NJ: Princeton Book Company, 2003.

Gibbs RS, Karian BY, Haney AF, et al. Danforth's Obstetrics and Gynecology. Baltimore: Lippincott Williams & Wilkins, 2003.

Glynn L, Schetter C, Wadhwa P, et al. Pregnancy affects appraisal of negative life events. J Psychos Res 2004;56:47–52.

Goldsmith J. Childbirth Wisdom. New York: Congdon and Weed, 1984.

Gorsuch R, Key M. Abnormalities of pregnancy as a function of anxiety and life stress. Psychos Med 1974;36;353.

Green JM, Coupland VA, Kitzinger JV. Expectations, experiences and psychological outcomes of childbirth. Birth 1990;17:15–24.

Gunzenhauser N, ed. Advances in touch: New implications in human development. Pediatric Roundtable #14, 1990.

Harker L, Thorpe K. The last egg in the basket? Elderly primiparity: a review of findings. Birth 1992;19:1.

Herman H. Pregnancy and Postpartum: Clinical Highlights Seminar. San Diego, 2004.

Hetherington S. A controlled study of the effect of prepared childbirth classes on obstetric outcomes. Birth 2007;17(2):86–90.

Hobel C and Colhane J. Role of Psychosocial and Nutritional Stress on Poor Pregnancy Outcome. J. Nutr. 133:1709S–1717S, May 2003.

Holst S, Uvna's-Moberg K, Petersson M. Postnatal oxytocin treatment and postnatal stroking of rats reduce blood pressure in adulthood. Autonomic Neuroscience: Basic & Clinical 2002;99(2):85–90.

Howard F. Pelvic Pain: Diagnosis and Management. Baltimore: Lippincott Williams & Wilkins, 2000.

Jefferies W, Bochner F. Thromboembolism and its management in pregnancy. Med J Aus 1991;155:253.

Juhan D. Job's Body: Handbook for Bodyworkers. Expanded Edition. Barrytown: Station Hill Openings, 1998.

Juraska, J, Greenough W, Elliott C, et al. Plasticity in adult rat visual cortex: An examination of several cell populations after differential rearing. Behav Neural Biol 1980;29:157–167.

Klaus M, Kennell J, Klaus P. The Doula Book: How a Trained Labor Companion Can Help You Have a Shorter, Easier, and Healthier Birth. New York: DeCapo Press, 2002.

Lee MK, Chang SB, Kang DH. Effects of SP6 acupressure on labor pain and length of delivery time in women during labor. J Alt And Comp Med 2004;10(6): 959–965.

Linde B. Dissociation of insulin absorption and blood flow during massage of a subcutaneous injection site. Diabetes Care 1989;6:570–574.

Longworth J. Psychophysical effects of slow stroke back massage in normotensive females. Adv Nurs Sci 1982;4:44–61.

March of Dimes. Birth Rates by Maternal Age. Available at http://www.marchofdimes.com/peristats/level1.aspx?dv=ms&reg=99&top=2&stop=2&lev=1&slev=1&obj=1. Accessed February 14, 2010.

Mayo Clinic. Domestic Violence Against Women: Recognize patterns, seek help. Available at: http://www.mayoclinic.com/health/domestic-violence/WO00044. Accessed February 14, 2010.

McCormick MC, Siegel J. Prenatal Care: Effectiveness and Implementation. Cambridge: Cambridge University Press, 1999.

Meaney, M, Aitken D, Bodnoff S, et al. The effects of postnatal handling on the development of the glucocorticoid receptor systems and stress recovery on the rat. Prog Neuropsychopharmacol Biol Psychiatr 1985;7:731–734.

Meaney MJ, Aitken DH, Sharma S, et al. Neonatal handling alters adrenocortical negative feedback sensitivity and hippocampal type II glucocorticoid receptor binding in the rat. Neuroendocrinology 1989;50:597–604.

Moberg KU. The Oxytocin Factor. Tapping the Hormone of Calm, Love, and Healing. Cambridge: DeCapo Press, 2003.

Montagu AM. Touching: The Human Significance of the Skin. New York: Harper & Row, 1978.

Moyer C, Rounds J, Hannum J. A meta-analysis of massage therapy research. Psychol Bull 2004;130:3–18.

Nichols F, Humenick S. Childbirth Education: Practice, Research and Theory. 2nd Ed. Philadelphia: W.B. Saunders Co., 2000.

Noble E. Essential Exercises for the Childbearing Year. 4th Ed. Harwich: New Life Images, 1995.

Nuckolls K, Kaplan BH, Cassel J. Psychosocial assets, life crises and the prognosis of pregnancy. Am J Epidemiol 1972;95:431.

Osborne C. Pre-and perinatal massage therapy: survey of massage therapists, 2009. www.bodytherapyassociates.com. Accessed June, 2010.

Osborne-Sheets C. Deep Tissue Sculpting. 2nd Ed. San Diego: Body Therapy Associates, 2002.

Ostgaard HC, Andersson GBS, Karlsson K. Prevalence of back pain in pregnancy. Spine 1992;17:53–55.

Pauk J, Kuhn C, Field T, et al. The positive effects of tactile versus kinesthetic or vestibular stimulation on neuroendocrine and ODC activity in maternally deprived rat pups. Life Sci 1986;39:2081–2087.

Pirie A and Herman H. How to Raise Children Without Breaking Your Back. Second edition. W. Somerville, MA: Ibis Publications, 2003.

Prescott JW. Prevention or Therapy and the Politics of Trust: Inspiring a New Human Agenda. Psychotherapy and Politics International 2005;3:194–221. DOI:10.1002/ppi.6. http://www.violence.de/prescott/politics-trust.pdf. Accessed 2/6/2009.

Pryde M. Effectiveness of massage therapy for subacute low-back pain. A randomized controlled trial. Can Med Assoc J 2000;162(13): 1815–1820.

Quebec Task Force on Spinal Disorders. Scientific approach to the assessment and management of activity-related spinal disorders. Spine 1987;12(Suppl 1):524.

Rausch PB. Effects of tactile and kinesthetic stimulation on premature infants. J Obstet Gynecol Neonat Nurs 1981;10:34–37.

Ricci S. Essentials of Maternity, Newborn, and Women's Health Nursing. 2nd Ed. Baltimore: Lippincott Williams & Wilkins, 2009.

Rice R. The effects of the Rice sensorimotor stimulation treatment on the development of high-risk infants. Birth Defects Orig Artic Ser 1979;15:7–26.

Rosen J. Dominance behavior as a function of early gentling experience in the albino rats. Toronto: MA thesis, University of Toronto, 1957.

Roth LL, Rosenblatt JS. Mammary glands of pregnant rats: development stimulated by licking. Science 1996;264:1403–1404.

Rubin R. Maternal Identity and the Maternal Experience. New York: Springer Publishing, 1984.

Rubin R. Maternal tasks in pregnancy. Matern Child Nurs J 1975;4:143–153.

Rubin R. Maternal touch. Nurs Outlook 1963:11:828–831.

Ruegamer B, Benjamin. Growth, food, utilization, and thyroid activity in the albino rat as a function of extra handling. Science 1954;120:184–185.

Samuels M, Samuels N. The New Well Pregnancy Book. New York: Fireside, 1996.

Scafidi FA, Field TM, Schanberg SM, et al. Effects of tactile/kinesthetic stimulation on the clinical course and sleep/wake behavior of preterm neonates. Infant Behav Develop 1986;9:91–105.

Scafidi FA, Field TM, Schanberg SM, et al. Massage stimulates growth in preterm infants: A replication. Infant Behav Develop 1990;13:167–188.

Scheumann D. The Balanced Body. Baltimore: Lippincott Williams & Wilkins, 2007.

Schneider ML, Moore CF. Prenatal stress and offspring development in nonhuman primates. In: Tremblay RE, Barr RG, Peters RDeV, eds. Encyclopedia on Early Childhood Development [online]. Montreal, Quebec: Centre of Excellence for Early Childhood Development; 2003:1–5. Available at: http://www.child-encyclopedia.com/documents/Schneider-MooreANGxp.pdf. Accessed Oct. 27, 2010.

Settle F. Musica, Da? My experience in a romanian orphanage. Massage Ther J 1991:64–72.

Simkin P, O'Hara M. Nonpharmacologic relief of pain during labor: systematic reviews of five methods. Am J Obstet Gynecol 2002;5(Supp 1186):S131–S159.

Simkin P. The experience of maternity in a woman's life. J Obstet Gynecol Nurs 1996;25:247–252.

Simkin P and Klaus P. When Survivors Give Birth. Seattle: Classic Day Publishing, 2004.

Slipman C, Jackson H, Lipetz J, et al. Sacroiliac joint pain referral zones. Arch Phys Med Rehabil 2000;81(3):334–338.

Solkoff N, Yaffe S, Weintraub D, et al. Effects of handling on the subsequent development of premature infants. Develop Psychol 1969;1:765–768.

Tanaka T, Leisman G, Hidetoshi M, et al. The effect of massage on localized lumbar muscle fatigue. BMC Complem Altern Med 2002;2:9.

Tapp J, Markowitz H. Infant handling: effects on avoidance learning, brain weight, and cholinesterase. Science 1963;140:486–487.

Taylor S, Klein L, Lewis B, et al. Biobehavioral responses to stress in females: tend-and-befriend, not fight-or-flight. Psychol Rev 2000;107:411–429.

The Nature and Management of Labor Pain. Part 1. Nonpharmacologic Pain Relief. Am Fam Physician 2003;68(6):1109–1112.

Vleeming A, De Vries H, Mens J, et al. Possible role of the long dorsal sacroiliac ligament in women with peripartum pelvic pain. Acta Obstet Gynecol Scand 2002;81(5):430–436.

Wadhwa P, Culhane J, Rauh V. Stress, infection and preterm birth: a biobehavioral perspective. Paediatr Perinat Epidemiol 15;2:17–29.

Wang MY, Tsai PS, Lee PH, et al. The efficacy of reflexology: systematic review. J Adv Nurs 2008;62:512–520.

Weininger O, Mc Clelland W, Arima K. Gentling and weight gain in the albino rat. Can J Psychol 1954;8:147–151.

Wheeden A, Scafidi F, Field T, et al. Massage effects on cocaine-exposed preterm neonates. J Develop Behav Pediatr 1993;14:318–322.

Witt PL, MacKinnon J. Trager psychophysical integration: a method to improve chest mobility of patients with chronic lung disease. Phys Ther 1986;66:214–217.

Zanolla R, Monzeglio C, Balzarini A, et al. Evaluation of the results of three different methods of post-mastectomy lymphedema treatment. J Surg Oncol 1984;26:210–213.

For additional resources, please visit http://thePoint.LWW.com/Osborne-Pregnancy2e!

General Prenatal Guidelines, Precautions, and Contraindications

Learning Objectives

After study of this chapter, you should be able to:

1. List the safety concerns related to different positions during the weeks and trimesters of pregnancy.
2. Adapt your depth of pressure and speed to a beneficial level for prenatal clients.
3. Explain the safety concerns related to prenatal leg and abdominal massage.
4. Identify other body areas where you need to make specific prenatal adaptations of massage techniques.
5. List adaptations to Swedish, deep tissue, movement, reflexive, and other methods that help ensure safety and effectiveness prenatally.
6. Recognize physiological changes that are not part of normal pregnancy progression.
7. List conditions that are classified as high risk and therefore more likely to create maternity complications.
8. List lifestyle and health history factors that warrant some additional concern and adaptation for prenatal massage therapy.

With so much potential benefit in receiving prenatal and perinatal massage therapy, why would a woman hesitate to receive regular sessions? Other than financial considerations, most women's ultimate concern with any pregnancy-related decision is, will this be safe for my baby? Women, their partners, and their healthcare providers need assurance that massage therapy will create expected benefits safely. To deliver that assurance, you must assess appropriateness of massage therapy for the individual woman and her needs. You need to understand when various positions on a therapy table and chair are safe and comfortable. You will be more technically effective with an understanding and an honest assessment of your skill base in the types of therapeutic massage and bodywork that can most effectively address the joys and challenges of pregnancy. (See Chapters 5 and 6 for labor and postpartum precautions and guidelines.) You need to understand why and learn how to adapt your touch to prenatal physiology and functioning. These adaptations include depth of pressure, pain level, precautionary areas, and specific methodological variations needed.

Some form of massage therapy will be safe for virtually every expectant woman. The skill you will develop in this chapter is determining how to touch and when during a pregnancy. To be safe, you need to be able to recognize when a pregnancy is not proceeding normally or more likely to develop problems. Chapter 7 will guide your work when these special needs arise.

Prenatal and perinatal massage therapy does not replace medical or midwifery prenatal care; it is collaborative with a woman's healthcare provider. Whether in independent practice or under direct medical supervision, remember to seek consultation when you need it, especially if a woman's pregnancy is high risk or she develops or has had complications.

> **REMINDER:** *Some form of massage therapy will be safe for virtually every woman when you follow safety guidelines.*

Who Can Receive Prenatal and Perinatal Massage Therapy?

Most pregnant woman can safely benefit from some type of therapeutic massage and bodywork. After all, pregnancy is not an illness. Pregnant women are not fragile, vulnerable to any pressure beyond that which would break a porcelain doll. In fact, many women feel that they are most sturdy, energetic, and fierce when pregnant. Depending on the adaptability of the mother's body to pregnancy's demands, both the mom and the baby can safely receive some form of massage therapy in each trimester. Remember that she may have other non–pregnancy-related injuries or conditions that need your consideration in determining whether to work with her and, if so, what type of work to use. In some sessions, pregnant women will prefer to relax and zone out; other times they enjoy engaging actively, learning more about their bodies or exploring fears and concerns.

Points of View: Is Massage Safe in the First Trimester?

Many massage therapy schools teach their students to delay prenatal sessions until after the first trimester. Usually, the rationale is that such delay avoids the possible association of any pregnancy loss, more common in the first trimester, with massage procedures. This is a wise legal precaution, especially when many schools' prenatal curricula are brief and/or lacking in depth. The safety of prenatal massage is relative to the therapist's applied knowledge. In the unlikely event that it would become necessary, a therapist with only minimal perinatal knowledge might find it difficult to muster a viable defense.

However, there is no substantive evidence to support the claim that massage is unsafe for first trimester pregnant women, when appropriate guidelines are followed. Some erroneous reasons given for the first trimester contraindication are that it will cause miscarriages or detach the placenta. There is no evidence that either possibility is likely if a therapist works superficially on the abdomen and avoids specific types of work on contraindicated points (see sections in this chapter for specific guidelines). Related to comfort, some teachers claim that massage in the first trimester will worsen nausea. Others say to not massage at all if a woman is nauseated. Again, when performed within informed guidelines given later in this chapter and in Chapter 4, this should not be a concern; in fact, parasympathetic responses might calm a queasy stomach. Of course, if she is vomiting or extremely nauseated, she is not likely to want to receive a massage.

To be more confident in the safety of your work and more specific in your effectiveness, do a personalized assessment of each potential client. Whether a continuing or new client, determine her general health history and the progress of her pregnancy. (See Chapter 8 and online resources at http://thePoint.lww.com/Osborne-Pregnancy2e). When she has signs of possible complications, has conditions putting her at higher risk of complications, or has other health issues, communications with her maternity healthcare provider also would be prudent. Ask her to get consent or seek consultation yourself to learn of any recommendations or limitations for her specific situation. Once you determine the personalized specifics of her pregnancy, use the general guidelines and specific modifications recommended in this chapter and Chapter 4 to tailor your work to her. Remember to update that assessment at each session with her to be current with her needs.

My Story

When I first met Sharon at the upscale day spa in Maryland where I worked, she returned her health form to me with nothing written on it. In fact, she gave the receptionist a hard time feeling that we were prying into her business; after all, she only wanted a massage.

So I simply asked if she would tell me whether she was over 35. I went on to explain how massage could certainly address a whole host of issues, but that if she had a problem with her pregnancy, then I would be better able to serve her knowing her state of health. I could then ask more questions that might lead her to see her doctor before her next scheduled monthly visit. She was dumbstruck that so much information went into performing a prenatal massage, and I was grateful that I had the knowledge to care for this woman.

—Mia Harper, Annapolis, MD

> **REMINDER:** *You may prefer to delay massage until a woman is into her second trimester; however, first trimester massage therapy is usually safe if performed according to recommendations.*

Positioning Safety and Guidelines

The practical question most therapists consider first when contemplating massaging pregnant women is how to accommodate that ripe belly. When accustomed to the **supine** (face-up) and **prone** (face-down) positions, both you and your client may feel limited to these options.

Safety, comfort, and therapeutic effectiveness issues will determine your use of both prone and supine client positions during pregnancy (Fig. 2.1). These same considerations point favorably to working throughout much of pregnancy, while clients lie on their sides. Remember that the guidelines below are not hard and fast rules, particularly regarding their timing. Individual needs, as well as twins and other multiples, change the timing of the recommended positions.

● PRONE

Let's face it: many women are belly sleepers and prefer to not give up that comforting position even for their massage. And massage therapists are more accustomed to working on a client's back while she is prone. But are these reasons to use the prone position throughout pregnancy? Although stomach sleeping may be a safe, comfortable resting position (Ricci 2009), once you apply sufficient pressure for an effective massage, it is no longer a reliably comfortable and safe position; neither is a ¾ prone position. The two most important problems with prone positioning are strain to the posterior structures and increased pressure inside the uterus (**intrauterine pressure**) (Fig. 2.2). Let's first consider the strain to the posterior structures.

Prone positioning on a flat therapy table can exert strain on the lumbar, pelvic, and uterine structures. Prone positioning shortens posterior musculature, compresses and anteriorly displaces the lumbar vertebrae and lumbosacral junction, rotates and strains the sacroiliac joints, and increases strain on the sacrouterine ligaments. With all of these affected structures, prone position, particularly in later pregnancy, often aggravates the very causes of many women's back discomfort. Although some women feel comfortable, many find breast, sinus, and other discomforts distracting from the full positive effect of their massage session.

Pillows or specialized equipment that is marketed for pregnant clients may mitigate these problems to some extent. However, one-size cutout tables or prone cushions don't fit all bellies, especially with multiples and various breech fetal positions. Nothing—not pillow props; cushions; pregnancy pillows; tables with cutout ovals, with or without a sling or net designed to support the belly; or most massage chairs—can completely solve all of the problematic aspects of prone positioning for massage therapy sessions. If the client is cushioned sufficiently high enough to keep pressure off of the uterus, then further strain to posterior structures and the taxed sacrouterine ligaments is likely. To prevent that strain, the belly must rest against the table, and that increases intrauterine pressure, especially as you apply sufficient pressure to address the posterior structures therapeutically. It's the proverbial "catch-22."

Lumbar and pelvic pain is one of the top three reasons women come in for massage therapy sessions (Osborne 2009). No matter how well-intended, even the best prone propping

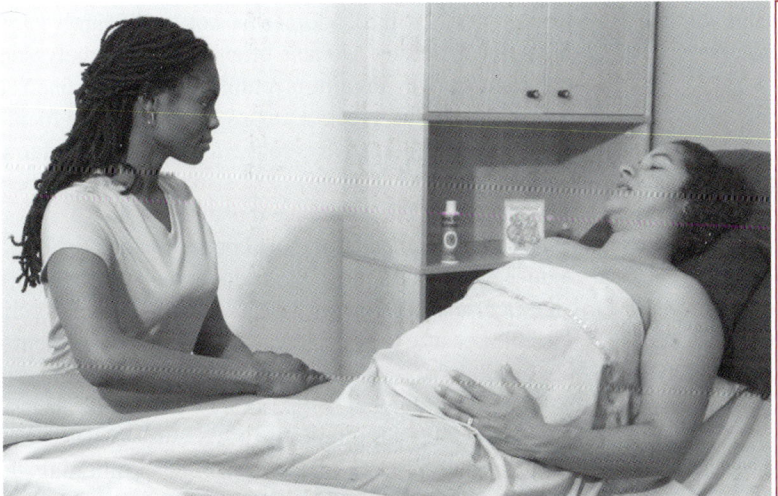

First trimester
- Supine, sidelying, semireclining, prone, or in a chair, depending on client comfort.
- Adapt for breast tenderness and other comfort and safety concerns, especially if using prone.

Second trimester
- Prone position is not recommended, even with specialized equipment.
- Supine - use pillow under right lower torso, up to week 22. After 22 weeks, only use semireclining and sidelying positions to prevent supine hypotensive syndrome; chair okay.
- Adapt for breast tenderness, SI joint, and other comfort and safety concerns.

Third trimester
- Sidelying and semireclining positions only; chair okay.
- Adjust for comfort and safety concerns.

FIGURE 2.1 Prenatal massage positioning overview. Comfort, safety, communication, and therapeutic effectiveness considerations underlie recommendations for positioning clients on massage therapy equipment.

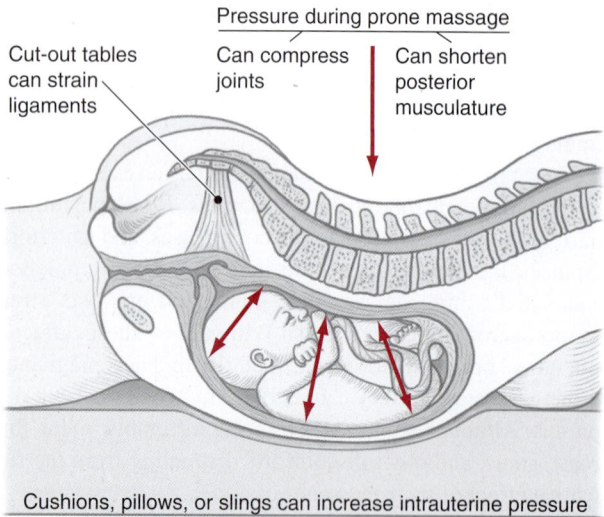

FIGURE 2.2 Effects of improper prone positioning. Both safety and comfort issues may arise when women lie on their swelling bellies to receive typical massage therapy sessions.

solution to maintain pelvic and lumbar alignment doesn't relieve strain from all achy structures. The **Contoured body-Cushion** (see online resources), when used appropriately as described in Chapter 3, can be a useful equipment for prenatal and postpartum work. When used under a prone client, it supports the pelvis at the anterior superior iliac spine (ASIS), normalizing the lumbar curve and helping to prevent lumbar and sacroiliac (SI) joint strain; however, it does not protect the vulnerable sacrouterine ligaments from strain. When this or any similar supports lift the prone pelvis sufficiently to prevent pressing the gravid uterus against the therapy table, they leave the uterine weight dangling from these ligaments. Any anterior pelvic misalignment in her daily activities is already straining anterior sacral attachments of these ligaments and the associated connective tissue matrix wrapped around the pelvis. They can become noticeably achier during a session, especially for the length of time and with the amount of pressure often needed to work effectively on the posterior body.

Now let's consider the increase in intrauterine pressure. The prone mom's torso weight presses her abdomen into the table or into any additional supportive device beneath it. This will increase the amount of pressure the uterine contents exert against the inner walls of the uterus. The amount of increase depends on the surface firmness and the mom's weight. As you press on her back with any but the lightest touch, your body weight further increases that pressure. If you use deeper pressures, especially in the problematic lumbar and pelvic areas, the pressure could be considerable.

So how safe is the prone position for massage therapy on pregnant women? That is a question with no direct data to supply a confident answer. Here are some considerations, though. Pregnancy enhances uterine muscle contractibility. Increase in intrauterine pressure, due to tight clothing, excessive amniotic fluid, and other causes, irritates the uterine muscles (Ricci 2009). These smooth muscles contract when irritated. Because the uterine muscles are already in a hypercontractile state, those contractions can potentially develop sufficient strength and regularity to threaten the pregnancy.

Keep in mind that avoiding increased intrauterine pressure is of particular relevance when there are placental abnormalities or a higher risk of such conditions (see Chapter 7 for details). Also, be extra cautious if there is heightened concern about fetal blood supply, **uterine competence**, and/or a history of miscarriages. Women diagnosed with these conditions are often uninformed about their impact on receiving massage therapy. Some of these problems go undetected until the woman is specifically screened for them or until bleeding, cramping, or other overt signs of problems have occurred to warrant further diagnosis.

On the other hand, in most uncomplicated, low-risk pregnancies, a mild, temporary increase in intrauterine pressure, such as occurs while resting briefly prone, is acceptable. During the first 13 weeks, the anterior iliac spines usually protect the uterus from increased pressure. Use the prone position in the first trimester if you or your client prefer, but remember that, even in the first trimester, this can be problematic when the embryo is larger than normal, with twins or other multiples, and when the mother is obese. Use **sidelying** and semi-reclined positions after the first trimester with all pregnant clients to avoid any risk of excessive intrauterine pressure.

> **REMINDER:** Prone positioning in second and third trimesters can increase intrauterine pressure and/or strain ligaments and muscles.

In addition to these safety concerns, there are some other equally compelling comfort reasons to use alternatives to prone positioning throughout pregnancy. Prone positioning exerts pressure on sensitive, enlarged breasts even in the first trimester, when the abdomen is not significantly larger. In fact, first trimester women often have extremely sensitive breasts. One way to minimize this pain when prone is to use a cushion that has breast recesses carved into the foam foundation. Other alternative is to use a pillow or rolled towels at the clavicles and at the lower ribs so the breasts lie between. This sometimes helps reduce this discomfort.

Pregnant women have more congestion due to hormonally induced increased mucous production. Women with colds, allergies, and other sinus conditions are particularly uncomfortable because their healthcare providers advise them to discontinue use of most medications that alleviate congestion.

On the emotional side, some women are uneasy and uncomfortable with "lying on my baby." Usually, the confines of face cradles and other prone positioning devices hamper verbal and emotional sharing, an important part of stress reduction and of a nurturing massage experience for many.

The prone position also is the least therapeutically effective position in which to receive a massage session. Stomach sleeping often creates or contributes to back pain, hip and neck dysfunctions, and other musculoskeletal misalignments (Pirie and Herman 2003). Why would you want to contribute to your clients' problems by using this position? Equally as relevant, you will probably have more access to more actively engage the tissue and movement of problematic posterior, hip, and shoulder trigger points, fascial shortening, and muscular tension working from the sidelying and semireclined positions rather than from prone.

In summary, to be sure of the safety and comfort of every pregnant woman and to improve session outcomes, eliminate the prone position after the first 13 weeks, regardless of your or the client's perception or preferences in this regard. Use caution and make reasonable adaptation for its use in the first trimester.

● SUPINE AND SEMIRECLINING

The decision over whether to use prenatal supine positioning should be based mostly on safety considerations related to maternal and fetal circulation. The inferior vena cava is the major vessel of blood return, receiving blood from the lower body through the iliac veins. It runs up the right sides of the vertebral bodies along the posterior abdominal wall. In the first trimester, the uterus hasn't grown beyond the pelvic cavity, and it is not very heavy. Once past 13 or so weeks, the weighty uterus and its contents rest against the common and interior iliac veins and the inferior vena cava when an expectant woman lies on her back. Extended vena cava compression will result in low maternal blood pressure and decreased maternal and fetal circulation (**supine hypotensive syndrome**) (Fig. 2.3). Some women report uneasiness, dizziness, weakness, nausea, shortness of breath, or other discomforts when lying flat on their backs, although others seem entirely content. However, with or without notable negative maternal effects, decreased fetal circulation can occur, particularly if the placenta is embedded posteriorly (Ricci 2009).

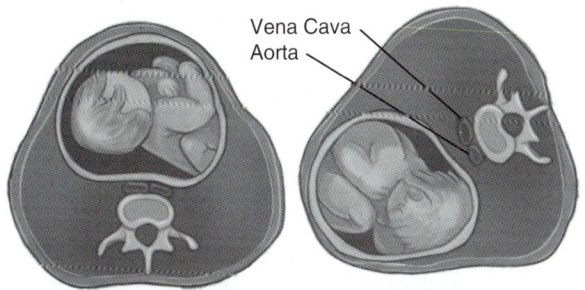

FIGURE 2.3 Supine hypotensive syndrome. The enlarged uterus compresses the inferior vena cava in an unadapted supine position (left). In sidelying position (right), torso vessels are free of the weight of the uterus and its contents (a total of as much as 4 to 5 lb even at week 22), improving blood flow to the mother and the fetus. (Used with permission from Ricci, p. 267.)

Some authorities advise pregnant women to never lie supine even when resting or sleeping (Callahan and Caughey 2007), primarily when there is increased concern about fetal oxygenation because of complications. Others only caution pregnant women to avoid supine exercising for a prolonged time during the second and third trimesters (Gibbs et al. 2008). From these parameters, it appears safe throughout pregnancy for most women receiving massage therapy to lie on their backs briefly, for 2 to 5 minutes. Of course, if she becomes uncomfortable, or if her healthcare provider places greater restrictions on supine positioning, change position.

In the second and third trimesters, be prudent in using the supine position, taking mitigating measures for more extended anterior work. An option in early second trimester of a single gestation pregnancy includes the use of pillow support under the right side of the lower torso to shift uterine weight toward the left, thus reducing compression of the vessels. After 22 weeks, the rapidly expanding uterus will compress a sizeable section of the vena cava, even with the pillow under the right pelvis. Also, decreasing levels of amniotic fluid toward term make a tilt toward the left less effective. Instead, you need to elevate her torso to a semireclined position, assuring an angle of 45 to 75 degrees from her hip to her head.

If a woman has multiples or is overweight, switch to a semireclined position after the first trimester. Other women who might prefer the **semireclining** position, regardless of the week of their pregnancy, are those with heartburn, who are short of breath, and those who are obese. Use the sidelying position as both a prone and supine alternative. (See Chapter 3 for detailed instructions to create all recommended positioning adaptations.)

There is also a comfort concern with the prolonged supine position. More than 3 to 5 minutes on her back can aggravate the expectant woman's SI joints and cause back pain. This more typically occurs if the back is poorly supported, if she is on an inadequately padded table, or during the last trimester. Supine positioning can create an immediate, painful, locking sensation in the upper buttock and iliac crest, usually on one side. This is caused by imbalance and strain to the SI joints, particularly if one SI joint is hypomobile and the other is hypermobile (Noble 1995). Because hard surfaces are more problematic than soft ones, 3 inches of triple-density foam padding is a minimum requirement on massage therapy tables used prenatally.

For client comfort and safety, support and reduce lumbar lordosis, when needed, in the supine position. You can best accomplish this with sufficiently high knee bolsters to help mechanically relax the lumbar area against the table. Don't forget to put another pillow under her calves and feet to level them with the knees and help relieve edema.

> **REMINDER:** *When supine, use a pillow under the right lower abdomen (weeks 13–22) or prop the client in a semi-reclined position to prevent supine hypotensive syndrome.*

● SIDELYING

The sidelying (lateral recumbent) position offers maximum safety and comfort throughout all pregnancies (Fig. 2.4). When sufficiently supported by pillows, bolsters, and/or positioning systems (see online resources list), most women can relax well in this position. (See Chapter 3 for detailed guidelines and illustrations.) The sidelying position minimizes uterine ligament and musculoskeletal strain. It prevents increased intrauterine pressure, increased sinus pressure, and pressure on the breasts, and it tends to encourage emotionally helpful conversation. Lying on one's side can offer the psychological comfort of a position that is reminiscent of the fetal position. Nestled comfortably on her side, she may feel more able to talk about her excitement, and her concerns, without the obstruction of a face cradle, as when prone, or the confrontational effect of talking face-to-face, as when supine or semireclining.

Physicians and midwives recommend the sidelying position for sleeping and resting to help ensure placental and fetal circulation. The uterine and other abdominal organs' weight falls to the supporting pillow in this position rather than compressing the abdominal organs and vessels (Fig. 2.3). When complications occur and in many high-risk pregnancies, women's healthcare providers often limit them to the left sidelying position. Left sidelying allows maximum maternal cardiac functioning and fetal oxygenation (American College of Obstetricians and Gynecologists 2009).

Unfortunately, many pregnant women make the overly cautious and ultimately uncomfortable conclusion that all women should lie exclusively on their left sides. It is not only perfectly safe for most to lie on either side, but sleep and digestion can improve when women sleep on both sides. Unless her physician or midwife requires otherwise, feel confident to prop your clients on whichever side she prefers or that will afford you best access to problematic areas. Divide your session time between left and right sidelying positions. Because they might sleep mostly on their left sides, often women need the left side worked more extensively.

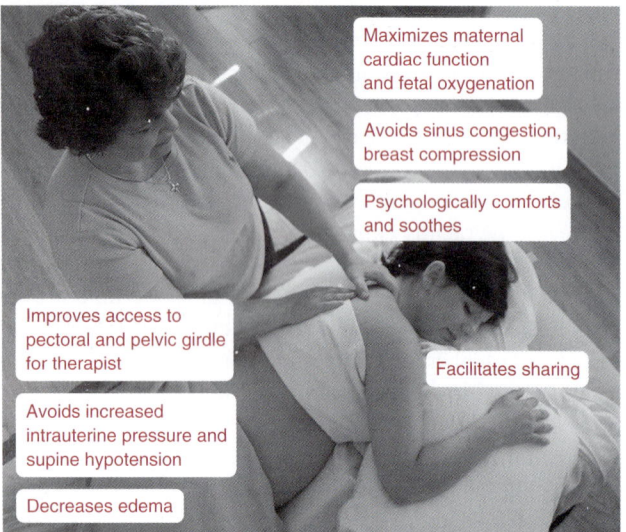

FIGURE 2.4 Advantages of sidelying positioning. With properly used supportive equipment, sidelying positioning for massage therapy offers benefits to the mother, the fetus, and the therapist.

Points of View: Positioning

All maternity massage instructors agree on one aspect of prone positioning: after the first trimester, a woman should not lie prone directly on a massage table without some type of accommodating equipment. Where differing opinions arise is regarding whether any types of supports sufficiently reduce the major problematic aspects of second and third trimester prone positioning: increased intrauterine pressure and strain to the posterior structures of the spine and pelvis. Some encourage prone positioning using specially contoured cushions, claiming that these supports will prevent these problems during a session. Unfortunately, there is no published evidence to confirm or negate this safety concern for the length of most massage therapy sessions. They may be comfortable for those massage therapists and other providers, such as chiropractors and physical therapists, who do very brief prone treatments (Stillerman 2008).

Recommendations for supine positioning have some variance among instructors. Some advise to never use supine without modifications to prevent supine hypotensive syndrome, even in the first trimester. Given the small weight of the fetus (1 oz) and the size of the gravid uterus (4 inches high and barely wider than the pubic bone) at the end of the first trimester, significant compression of the vena cava is highly unlikely before 14 to 20 weeks, except when there are multiples.

Among instructors who advise use of supports under the right side, as described above, there are small variances as to when to move the client from this modified supine to semireclining: at 14 weeks, 18 to 20 weeks, and as late as the last couple of months (Stager 2010; Stillerman 2008; Yates 2010). At 20 to 22 weeks, average fetal growth results in the uterus reaching maternal umbilicus level and wide enough to press weightily on the iliac veins and the inferior vena cava. This would be the point at which positioning her semireclined would get the desired effect of directing uterine weight more toward the pelvic floor. Requiring additional supports under the right side when the client is semireclined is an unnecessary redundancy that makes stability in this semisitting position more tenuous. Placement of this wedge or blanket varies for different instructors, with some suggesting that it be under the shoulder through iliac crest. Because the vena cava splits deep into the pelvic region as the common and then internal and external iliac veins, continuing the support down to the right hip seems more accurate.

> **REMINDER:** Sidelying is the recommended and safest position for prenatal massage therapy.

In summary, the recommended and safest position for prenatal massage therapy is the sidelying position, regardless of possible inconvenience to or preference of the practitioner (Figs. 2.1 and 2.4). Another safe option, although generally not as comfortable for the expectant client, is seated massage therapy on either a household chair or a stool. Massage chairs are a safe alternative only when the pregnant client rests her back against the pad normally used for chest support, for the same reasons as described in the prone positioning discussion above. (See Chapter 3 for details.)

Effective Methodologies for Prenatal and Perinatal Massage Therapy

Most basic massage therapy training programs teach at least one therapeutic method readily adaptable for maternity care. Even simple Swedish massage routines and introductory deep tissue or neuromuscular techniques will reduce stress, nurture, and help relieve backache and painful hips. What some schools lack are the time and, sometimes, expertise to adequately convey the prenatal physiological, functional, and emotional changes to make safe and effective adaptations to routine protocols. You'll find such information in these pages.

Choose from the wide-ranging variety of therapeutic massage and bodywork techniques (**somatic practices**) for your maternity work (Box 2.1 and online resources further define these practices). There's no single method or procedural sequence that is *the* ideal prenatal or postpartum session. To limit yourself in that way would deprive women of the extensive benefits of the many somatic practices available to the professional massage therapist or bodyworker. Identify which of the methods listed you are knowledgeable and skilled in. During the childbearing year, you will need to significantly modify some of the techniques and eliminate others. Use this text's guidelines and precautions to carefully evaluate the physiological, structural, and psychological impact of every technique from any method you contemplate using. See Box 2.3 for critical reminders about making technique choices and modifications.

In later chapters, you will learn many specific prenatal and perinatal techniques from a variety of methodologies. You can incorporate them into most standard routines you practice or use the suggested sequences outlined with Chapter 4 materials online. You also can see some of these techniques in the online videos. Let these images spark your creativity and personalize your approach to your clients.

As with all hands-on skills, your education will be more complete if you also participate in a comprehensive educational program that includes demonstrations, supervised

---

Box 2.1

An Alphabetical List of Applicable Somatic Therapies

(Subtypes are listed under generic categories as appropriate. This is a partial list, focusing on the methodologies with which the author is most familiar. See glossary and online box for definitions and further information.)

- **Circulatory Massage:** Lymphatic Drainage, Swedish Massage
- **Craniosacral Therapy:** Biodynamic Craniosacral Therapy
- **Cross-Fiber Friction (Deep Compression Massage)**
- **Deep Tissue Massage:** Deep Tissue Sculpting, Kinesis, Myofascial Release, Structural Integration, Skin Rolling
- **Joint Mobilizations:** Assisted-Resisted Stretches, Passive Movements, Positional Release, Range of Motion (Swedish Gymnastic Movements), Rhythmic Deep Tissue Blends, Sensory Repatterning, Stretching, Traction, Trager work
- **Reflex Massage:** Acupressure, Shiatsu, and other Asian Body Therapies, Connective Tissue Massage (*Bindegewebsmassage*), Reflexology (Zone Therapy), Trigger Point Massage (Myofascial Trigger Points, Neuromuscular Therapy)
- **Somato-emotional Processing:** Somato-emotional Integration, Somato-emotional Release.

---

hands-on practice, and feedback on specifically adapted, clinically tested techniques. See the online resources at http://thePoint.lww.com/Osborne-Pregnancy2e for some suggestions.

Pressure, Speed, and Moderating Pain Level During Sessions

If advisability and positioning are the earliest concerns for therapists, generally the next is appropriate pressure and pain levels. Some therapists feel that pregnant women seem so vulnerable, yet their training recommends working very deeply for certain methods to be effective. With maternity massage, you will need to find the pressure and speed that are "just right." Some types of techniques and areas, such as abdominal effleurage, need to be superficial, touching only into the skin and superficial fascia. Others, such as deep tissue and trigger point work, need therapeutic depth, but no deeper than what the client experiences as pleasure at the borderline of pain; therapeutic depth becomes a secondary issue in the medial leg and abdomen, as explained below. Usually, if you work more slowly, including when entering and exiting from the body, your touch will be more soothing and easier for the client to receive deeply.

Always learn the client's pressure preferences, perception of pain, tension level, and needs in a given body area. Her general health, injuries, or other safety considerations discussed later in this chapter often dictate lighter pressures than those used with nonpregnant clients.

Table 2.1 Number Scale Method of Labeling Pressure/Pain Level

Pressure/Pain Level	Description
0	Pressure only
1–5	Pressure perceived as pleasurable
5.5–7	Increasing pressure is beginning to change from purely pleasurable into mild discomfort; however, that discomfort still feels good
7.5–10	More pain than pleasure, becoming intolerable at 10

My Story

I loved my first experience with massage therapy. I definitely feared it would be too harsh; it was nothing like that. It was warm, attentive, and wonderful. I wished it would go on forever. I felt more balanced, and the specific tight areas I had just melted as my therapist worked gradually deeper.

—Roselle

Provide her with a reliable means to express her experience, such as a number or color-coded scale. This allows her to communicate beyond generalized responses such as "that feels okay." Some therapists are successful with a number scale method of labeling pressure/pain level usually graded as presented in Table 2.1.

A good alternative involves imagery rather than numbers. Pregnant women often relate better to right-brain metaphors than left-brain linear concepts, as pregnancy expands right-brain functioning (Jones 1987). Try using a color scheme for pleasure/pain feedback that follows the common correlation of a traffic light, shown in Table 2.2.

Remember that pain level is a function of both depth and speed of pressure into tissues. Gradually adding your body weight to your working tool often develops client receptivity, with tissues yielding and inviting greater depth. When tissues open before your hands, rather than you forcing your hands into tight areas, you can work with greater depth, more ease, less pain, and usually a more participatory client. When you develop aware clients, not only will their sessions become more pleasurable for them, but they will also learn more about themselves in the process. An actively participating client also means that your work will be less effortful for you, physically and emotionally.

Mechanical considerations, such as table height, positioning, and your own body use, also contribute to a client's perception of pain. Chapter 3 will give you many tips and directions to make your work deep, effective, and comfortable for your client and for you.

Maintaining an awareness of your client's pleasure/pain level assures that the intended relaxation response builds during your session. You won't stimulate counterproductive sympathetic arousal in either the mother or the fetus. Remember that pain activates adrenal production of the hormones that elevate blood pressure, heart rate, and respiratory rate and that lower immune function and blood flow to the uterus. Because these hormonal signals diffuse into fetal circulation through the placenta, the fetus is similarly negatively impacted (Ricci 2009).

If you work energetically but not painfully, your clients will learn more from your work with them. Forceful and abrupt movements activate the client's defensive withdrawal reflexes, which trigger increased muscular tension rather than relaxation. At high pain levels, the entire body may push away from the source of pain. Remember, it is only in a receptive state that clients can readily explore and learn new behaviors, such as correct breathing, relaxation, and postural alignment (Juhan 1998). If the pregnant client is to realize the maximum relaxation and educational benefits of somatic therapies, then perform even the deepest work gently.

REMINDER: *Avoiding extremely painful techniques increases the stress-relieving and educational goals of prenatal massage therapy.*

Emotional Expression Precautions

Strong feelings of anger, fear, or sadness also release stress hormones into both maternal and fetal circulations. Most expectant women inevitably will tap into one or all of these emotions, and on your table, she may feel safe and supported to explore and express them. As soft tissues yield tension, so can the heart and the mind. You will want to allow for this type of stress reduction in most cases. Support as complete an expression as your client pursues. Allow for her outbursts, and be sensitive to not encourage her feelings to the point that

Table 2.2 Color Method of Labeling Pressure/Pain Level

Color	Client's Sensation	Therapist's Response
Green	Completely pleasurable	Keep on going
Yellow	Pleasure tinged with mild discomfort but still feels good	Proceed with caution
Red	More pain than pleasure	Stop

they overwhelm her for extended periods. Restrict intense emotional processing to when issues naturally surface. See Chapters 4 and 7 and online resources for more guidance in supporting your clients emotionally.

Remember that psychological dynamics are outside of the massage therapist's scope of practice and expertise. Investigate and establish a reliable network of professionals knowledgeable and experienced in working with maternity mental health.

Cautionary and Contraindicated Body Areas

The need for a solid grounding in physiology, indications, and contraindications is particularly important when working with pregnant clients. Clear understanding of normal and abnormal prenatal developments, along with our good intentions and skillful techniques, will be a tremendous reassurance to these women.

● ABDOMINAL MASSAGE

Several misconceptions about massaging the pregnant abdomen persist in the profession (see previous Points of View feature). Some teachers warn students to never massage the belly for fear of provoking miscarriage. Only one small study, described below, supports the miscarriage belief, but that was of deep abdominal massage. However, it seems reasonably cautious to advise students who don't receive a comprehensive education in prenatal massage to avoid working on the pregnant abdomen. It is critical that all bodyworkers follow certain guidelines when massaging the abdomen to ensure the safety of the client and the baby.

Safe Abdominal Massage Guidelines

With a client's permission, superficial abdominal massage is safe and often soothes nausea through parasympathetic stimulation. It can help reduce stress, a possible contributor to miscarriages, premature labor, and other physiological complications, when performed within certain parameters. It can help women to connect emotionally with their unborn child, reinforcing prenatal bonding (Nichols and Humenick 2000) (Fig. 2.5).

Take care to never increase intrauterine pressure, decrease uterine blood flow with inadequate or inappropriate positioning, or press deeply or pointedly into the abdomen. Ensure the safety of both the mother and the fetus by doing the following:

- Effectively positioning and supporting her, as detailed earlier in this chapter and in Chapter 3.
- Touching the pregnant abdomen no deeper than the skin and superficial fascia level. Remember that the rectus abdominis eventually separates, leaving only the skin, adipose, and fascia between your hand and the uterus; thus, only a very thin layer of tissue can separate your hand from the uterus.
- Being superficial on the lateral abdomen, anterior of the quadratus lumborum, and the entire area between the distal edge of the ribcage and the pubic bone, as well as directly on the anterior belly.
- Using the entire flat, relaxed palm of your hand for broad, superficial effleurage strokes. For smaller strokes, such as superficial fanning, use only the broad edges of your thumbs, and avoid pointed pressure.
- Completely "molding" your hand to the belly contours so that there is no space between your hand and the belly. This creates full, relaxed contact that is soothing, without being ticklish or too deep. (See Chapter 4 technique manual for specific techniques.)

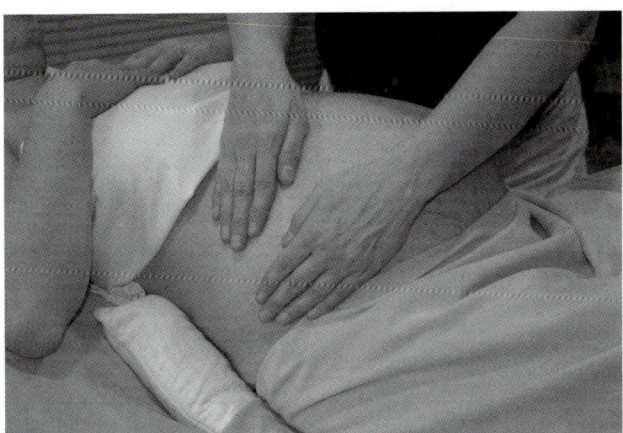
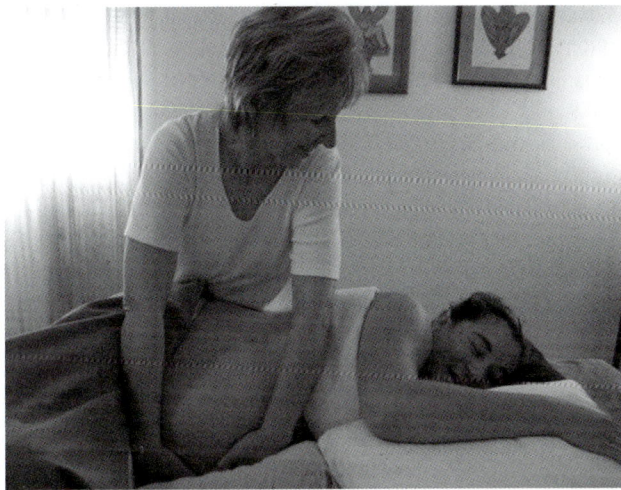

FIGURE 2.5 Abdominal massage. Both sidelying and semireclined positions allow for gentle but connected superficial strokes to soothe the mom and to help connect her and her baby.

- Considering the borders of the pregnant abdomen to be the pubic bone, inguinal ligaments, xiphoid process, and the quadratus lumborum, and observe all precautions within those boundaries.

As mentioned above, the only study of abdominal massage techniques during pregnancy looked at the traditional abdominal massage practices of southern Nigeria. This regional type of abdominal massage consists of stroking and kneading of the anterior abdominal muscles and gentle lifting of the soft tissue over the abdomen. It also may involve kneading of the thighs, which, separate from the abdominal work, could be problematic as well due to risks of thrombi. Of the 284 pregnant women in this study, 15% had this type of abdominal massage. The maternal mortality rate of the massaged women was almost 5%, and the infants' was 14.3%. Unfortunately, researchers included no comparison to a nonmassaged group of Kenyan women, and this was a small sample size. Nevertheless, the researchers recommended that women stop receiving this type of abdominal massage (Ugboma and Akani 2004).

Although no studies have specifically examined the effects of superficial abdominal massage, light, full-handed pressure avoids any possibility of abdominal trauma such as that examined above. It seems reasonable to theorize that deep or pointed pressure into the pregnant uterus could disturb the placenta, particularly if the attachment is tenuous. The uterine ligaments suspend the uterus in place, and they also carry the blood vessels serving it. Sustaining deep pressure into the anterior iliac region compresses into the fascial attachments of the broad ligament.

This precaution applies to any method of somatic practices including deep tissue, trigger point, and acupressure. To be safest, also find alternatives to deep abdominal work aimed to improve sluggish elimination. In the second or third trimester, the uterus is between your touch and the intestines that you seek to affect with these techniques anyway, rendering them mostly ineffective. You will have more success using reflexive techniques, such as zones on the feet and hands. When you are addressing iliopsoas tension and inactivity, avoid mechanical pressure anywhere along these muscles and their attachments. Try stretching, passive movement, and other awareness and educational techniques. (See online Points of View: What Is Safe Abdominal Massage? for further discussion on deep abdominal work and Chapter 4 technique manual for safe and effective abdominal techniques.)

Take some clues from physicians and midwives who commonly qualify their approval of massage therapy for a patient by contraindicating abdominal massage, especially if there is some increased concern about miscarriage or early labor occurring. Of course, you will follow those directions when issued.

Before touching her abdomen, it is just as important to get the client's permission. For many reasons, some women prefer to skip abdominal techniques entirely. Others might be eager to learn how she and her partner can massage her belly, enjoying that intimate, bonding time with their baby on their own.

> **REMINDER:** *Superficial strokes on the belly are usually soothing and safe.*

When to Avoid Abdominal Massage and Why

Although gentle abdominal massage can be performed safely on most pregnant clients, some therapists prefer to avoid entirely touching a woman's abdomen until after the first trimester to ensure that neither they nor their clients ever question the safety of their work. In addition, in cases in which clients are at high risk for miscarriage or preterm labor, you may prefer, for liability reasons, to avoid the abdomen throughout the pregnancy (Box 2.2). If women show signs of these complications (see Box 2.4), you should consult with her maternity healthcare provider before proceeding.

Miscarriage is a natural termination of pregnancy before the fetus has reached viability, generally before 20 weeks of gestation, with the fetus weighing less than 350 g, and most commonly occurring in the first trimester. It is the most common complication of pregnancy, occurring in at least 15% of clinically identified pregnancies. Preembryonic (conception to 5 weeks) and embryonic (6 to 9 weeks) miscarriages

---

Box 2.2

Liability Considerations

Some sobering facts of American maternity care are very relevant to massage and other somatic therapists: more than 75% of obstetricians and gynecologists are sued, more than 33% of them are sued more than three times, and nurses and other perinatal healthcare providers are more and more frequently being included in these lawsuits (Gilbert and Harmon 2003). Be aware of this litigious atmosphere in childbearing; at the same time, there is no need for alarm. Since 1980, only a handful of therapists have actually been sued, and, to the author's knowledge, none have been convicted of any fault in a pregnancy loss. The chances are especially small that you would have legal repercussions if you do the following:

- Follow the safety recommendations of this text and of clients' healthcare providers.
- Ask each client to complete a written health history form at the first appointment and make thorough progress notes that document each appointment. (See Chapter 8 for more guidance.)
- Practice conservatively, ethically, and conscientiously, staying within the scope of your profession.
- Pursue a comprehensive, prenatal and perinatal massage therapy hands-on education.

occurring before pregnancy are confirmed, probably bringing the total rate of miscarriage closer to 40% of conceptions. Preterm labor jeopardizes the health and lives of the mother and the fetus in 12.5% of American pregnancies. Preterm labor involves regular contractions that dilate the cervix after 20 weeks and before the end of 37 weeks of gestation (Gibbs et al. 2008).

> **REMINDER:** *Determine whether risks or conditions indicative of miscarriage or preterm labor make it more prudent to eliminate abdominal massage with some clients.*

Here's how to recognize these potential problems with the length of gestation. One of the most common symptoms of premature labor and miscarriage is low back, thigh, and/or pelvic pain, referred from the contracting uterus. However, there are *usually* other identifying symptoms, such as bleeding, amniotic fluid leakage, abdominal cramping, or regular uterine contractions. Ask the client's physician to rule out miscarriage, labor, or other possible causes of back pain, such as urinary tract infection, other organ and neurological dysfunctions, or prior, unresolved injuries before beginning or continuing massage therapy. Remember that musculoskeletal back pain is usually relieved with a change in position or activity, whereas referred organ pain is not. Take full prenatal and medical histories, and evaluate your client's progress thoroughly at each massage therapy session. (See Chapter 8 and online resources for materials to use.)

Certain maternal conditions, high-risk factors, and complications of pregnancy may increase the occurrence of miscarriage or premature labor. When your client has had or experiences any of the following, be particularly alert for the warning signs listed above.

- History of previous miscarriage or preterm labor
- Fetal genetic abnormalities
- Drug abuse, including illicit drugs, over-the-counter and prescription medications
- Altered nutrition leading to low maternal weight gain
- Smoking and alcohol use
- Low socioeconomic status
- Stress, both acute and chronic
- Heavy work load at home or on the job
- Domestic violence
- Decreased blood flow to the uterus caused by the following:
  - **Placental abruption, placenta previa**, diabetes, renal disease, cardiovascular disease, anemia, systemic lupus, and other autoimmune factors
  - **Preeclampsia**
  - Overdistension of the uterus in multiple gestations and excess amniotic fluid (**polyhydramnios**)
- Abdominal trauma or surgery

My Story

Regardless of the fact that I had uterine abnormalities, my doctor had no concerns that massage therapy would in any way interfere. Not only did the massage not interfere but it also was a tremendous physical and emotional support during this pregnancy, which was at risk of delivering early or miscarrying altogether. It was very helpful to go to my therapist, not only for the reduction in stress, but also for the emotional support that I was given. It was very important to stay relaxed and calm through this pregnancy, for the baby as well as myself.

—*Jennifer*

- **Premature rupture of membranes (PROM)** and low amniotic fluid (**oligohydramnios**)
- **Cervical insufficiency** and other uterine anomalies, such as fibroids, short cervical length, or congenital malformations
- Infection of the urinary tract or vaginal or uterine diseases such as **endometriosis**
- Fever and infectious diseases such as **rubella, cytomegalovirus,** active **genital herpes,** or **toxoplasmosis**
- Maternal age under 16 and over 40
- Extreme hypothermia
- African-American ethnicity (doubles the risk) (Ricci 2009)

● LEG MASSAGE

Novice therapists and uninformed women often are unnecessarily apprehensive about abdominal massage. On the contrary, they are often unaware of the potentially more critical implications of massaging pregnant women's legs. Certainly, expectant women's legs are subject to a variety of aches and pains, prompting them to seek leg massage. As a caring, responsive therapist, you want to meet their needs, but you must respect the physiological limitations to safely massaging pregnant women's legs.

Repeating certain types of techniques, particularly to the medial side of the leg, potentially carries enough risk that many Swedish massage texts before 1985 considered pregnancy a total contraindication to massage of any body part. Most of these books gave little or no rationale for such strict contraindications. With a solid understanding of prenatal circulatory system changes, however, massage therapists can safely perform some leg massage on most women.

Remember to perform all Swedish strokes working the most proximal areas of the extremities first. This will help improve the draining potential of effleurage, pétrissage, and other circulatory techniques. In addition, the direction of these strokes from distal to proximal is just as important, as possible relief from uncomfortable swelling is often the intention of this work. When your primary intention is to move excess fluid from the legs, work superficially throughout the leg before increasing pressure into the muscular level. (See Chapter 7 Points of View on types of edema and leg massage.) Above all, though, you will need to modify your leg work for blood clots, varicose and spider veins, and reflex points that are potentially unsafe before a woman's due date.

Blood Clots

Normal circulatory system adaptations result in several problematic maternal changes. Increased blood and interstitial fluid volume, combined with uterine restriction of the iliac vessels, results in an expected increase in femoral venous pressure. Because the elevated progesterone level relaxes the smooth muscular walls of these vessels, they are more prone to developing varicose veins and accumulating more stagnant blood. These areas are more likely to develop blood clots that are not readily dissolved due to the decrease in clot-dissolving factors (see Chapter 1).

Clot formation can occur in any vein during pregnancy; however, **thrombophlebitis** and **deep vein thrombosis (DVT)** are greatest and most dangerous in the veins where blood is most stagnant. The veins most likely to harbor clots during pregnancy are the deep iliac, femoral, and both superficial and deep saphenous veins, and, to a lesser extent the popliteal and posterior tibial veins (Fig. 2.6) (Walton 2011). When clots accumulate in these vessels, they may create some discomfort, but they pose no major threat, unless inflammation is severe and/or infection develops. DVTs in the larger, deeper veins are more serious because they can be of sufficient size to occlude smaller vessels in the lungs (pulmonary embolism) if they dislodge, moving into circulation. These types of **thromboembolisms** occur six times more frequently in pregnant than in nonpregnant women, and they can be fatal (Callahan and Caughey 2007).

Because a major contributing factor to DVT is high levels of estrogen and progesterone, most women will develop clots. In addition, the more sedentary a woman is, the higher the likelihood of thrombi. Women on bed rest are especially prone to clot production, as are smokers and women over 30, and those who have recently used birth control pills, are obese, have lupus, or are expecting their fourth baby or more babies. Separation of the placenta from the inner uterine wall (**placental abruption**), preeclampsia/eclampsia, and intrauterine fetal death all increase clot formation, sometimes leading to a further serious complication involving generalized activation of the coagulation process (**disseminated intravascular coagulopathy**) (Callahan and Caughey 2007).

The characteristic symptoms of leg thrombi include increased edema in the foot and/or leg (often unilaterally), localized swelling, heat, redness, and painful, achy legs that can be tender with palpable, ropy thrombi. Although these symptoms may indicate the presence of thrombi, swollen and achy legs unrelated to thrombosis are common in pregnancy. These symptoms are particularly worrisome if they increase when she walks. A clear determination of the presence of clots is also difficult because often thrombi are asymptomatic (Callahan and Caughey 2007).

Given the increased tendency of blood to coagulate in pregnancy and the potential harm of freely circulating clots, treating all pregnant women as though there were clots in their legs seems prudent. To be totally safe, eliminate massage procedures that have the potential to flush thrombi from their likely harbors in the leg veins. To do that, follow these guidelines:

- Do not press deeply or for a sustained time into the lower pelvis or inguinal area, where the iliac vein crosses the pelvis.
- Use only superficial, whole-hand pressure throughout the medial surface of the legs, where problematic veins traverse, specifically for several inches along and posterior to the sartorius muscles, distal to the medial knees, and along the medial tibial borders.
- Perform no deep, pointed, or stationary pressure sufficiently sustained to restrict localized blood flow (ischemic pressure) in these areas, regardless of the type of technique and its otherwise potential benefits. The flush of blood propelled when you release your pressure can potentially move clots more proximally. Use cross-fiber friction, trigger point therapy, deep tissue, acupressure, and any other deep pressure only on the lateral leg, on the anterior and posterior leg if pressure vector is *not* laterally directed, and on other, safer body parts.
- Eliminate tapotement (percussion) from Swedish leg work and any technique that creates a jiggling of leg tissues, such as rolling or wringing. Be gentle and slow with all of your leg strokes and movements of the hips, knees, and ankles to avoid shaking clots loose from leg vessels. Monitor the jostling effect to the legs of your work on other body parts, as well.
- Eliminate leg work, except for stationary, energy work, or the most superficial strokes (just to spread lubricant on the skin), when a client is on bed rest or if other conditions increasing clot risks occur. If you work under direct medical supervision, you may be able to safely do more with these women's legs. Seek and follow any physician guidelines given. (See Chapter 7 for bed rest leg guidelines.)
- Massage therapists without hands-on verification by an instructor of appropriate techniques for the legs would be wise to not work with high-risk women and those with more complicated pregnancies, in which thrombosis formation is higher (Fig. 2.6).

Varicose and Spider Veins

Following the guidelines above will also protect vascular areas weakened by progesterone, including spider veins and varicose veins. These reddish, broken superficial capillaries that look like multilegged spiders indicate capillary fragility. Squiggly, bulging varicose veins often develop in the same blood vessels as blood clots. They are more noticeable when the more superficial veins become varicose, but varicosities

Chapter 2 General Prenatal Guidelines, Precautions, and Contraindications   37

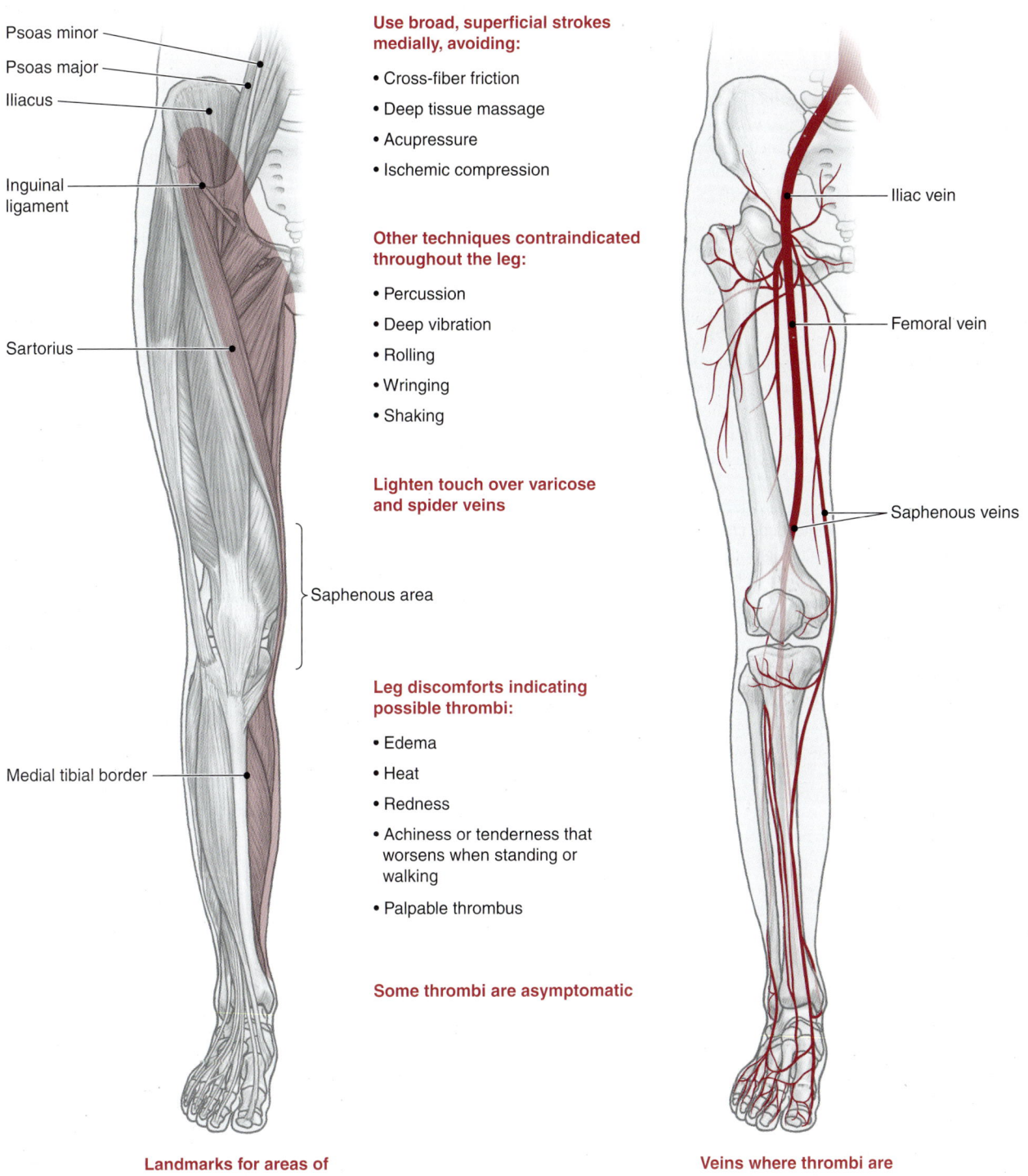

Landmarks for areas of greatest precaution

Veins where thrombi are most likely to form

FIGURE 2.6 Leg precautions summary.

in deep veins will not necessarily be visible. In any areas of varicose or spider veins, additionally modify massage therapy techniques according to the severity of the condition. With severe varicosities that are palpable, raised, very convoluted, and discolored, use only featherlight touch and energetic, that is, noncontact, modalities (Werner 2008).

Regardless of varicose vein severity, use other procedures described in Chapter 4 to help relieve pelvic congestion. If thrombi have been confirmed in any vein, do not massage that leg without direct medical supervision, and consult with her physician or midwife regarding the advisability of massage on the other, unaffected leg. If there are lesions,

Points of View: What Adaptations to Leg Massage Are Critical During Pregnancy?

Most contemporary authors and instructors think that totally contraindicating leg massage during a normal pregnancy is unnecessarily conservative and outdated. However, there is considerable discrepancy on how to determine normalcy and how to safely massage the legs (Jordan 2001, Stager 2010; Stillerman 2008; Yates 2010).

Several experts recommend testing for thrombi to determine the safety of proceeding. Testing includes feeling the semireclined woman's outstretched leg for heat or tenderness. Then, holding the knee extended against the table, flex her ankle toward her knee. If she has pain with that, this is considered a positive indication that she has a clot (Stillerman 2008). The obvious problem with this test, known as Homans sign, is that there are many other reasons for leg pain with this maneuver, making a solid assessment difficult. For this reason, it is no longer a recommended test (Ricci 2009).

Regarding safe strokes for leg massage, deep, long strokes on the legs often are not recommended. This is unnecessarily restrictive, particularly on the lateral leg, where the long bones offer considerable protection from the possible vein-stripping effects of such work. As your hands work more medially, lightening up and shortening your strokes make good sense. Similarly, your caution should increase as clot risk factors increase or systemic edema occurs so that your pressure for any technique on the legs should decrease to the point of extreme superficiality.

ulcerations, inflammation (phlebitis), or infection, do not massage directly over these areas. Gentle drainage proximal of the area can be effective and safe.

● REFLEX AND ACUPRESSURE POINTS

Reflexologists and reflex zone therapists claim that deep pressure to areas of the feet and hands stimulates relaxation, facilitates metabolic functions that support pregnancy, and helps to reduce common prenatal discomforts. Although they claim these generalized positive results, most authorities also warn about several reflexive cautions during pregnancy (Enzer 2000).

Feet, Legs, and Hands

Widely circulating anecdotal evidence suggests that deep, bone-to-bone pressure to the uterus and ovary zones can potentially initiate labor or strengthen weak labor contractions. Because there is little to no data to confirm or dismiss these claims, any ischemic compression or pressure to the center of the medial or lateral calcaneus would be ill advised during pregnancy. Be particularly cautious of these areas in the first trimester and with clients more prone to miscarriage or premature labor (Enzer 2000).

Without comprehensive training in reflexive zone therapy, be cautious in performing extensive reflexive work on the feet of women with complications such as threatened miscarriage, preterm labor, or preeclampsia and when deep vein thrombosis is more likely. Additionally, limit the stimulation of the endocrine gland points to allow the hormonal orchestration of pregnancy to proceed undisturbed (Fig. 2.7).

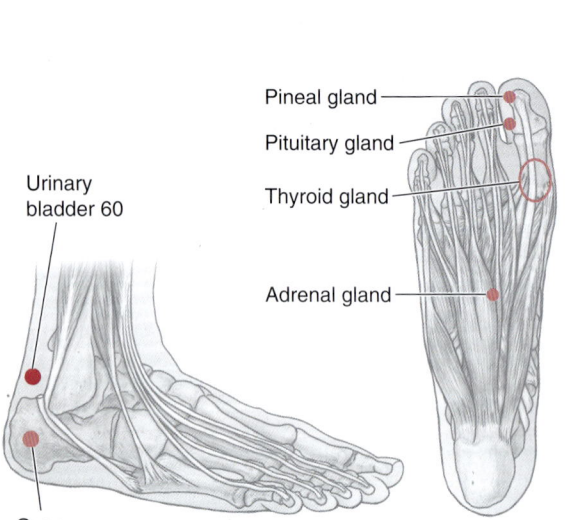
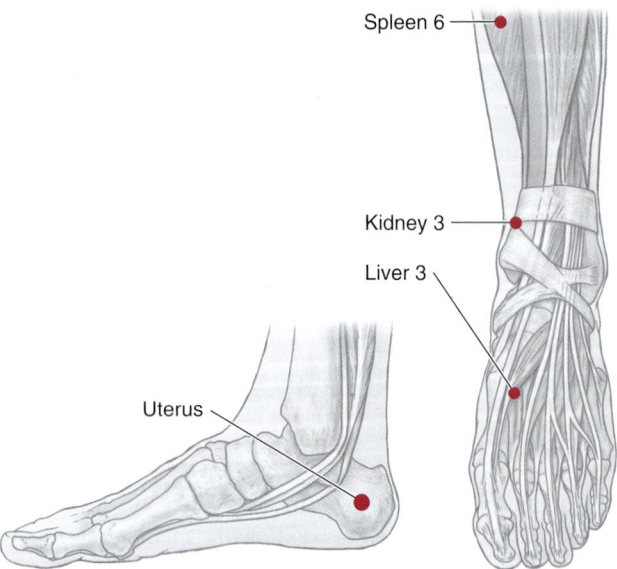

FIGURE 2.7 Lower leg and foot contraindicated and precautionary zones. Areas to avoid deep, bone-on-bone pressure include reflex zones (*labeled lighter*) and acupuncture/acupressure points (*labeled darker*).

Be cautious in using reflexology with substance abusers and others whose lifestyles or general health may predispose them to higher stored metabolic waste levels, as these are believed to be released into general circulation with zone therapy (Lett 2000).

Therapists trained in Asian Bodywork Therapies rooted in Chinese medicine and the philosophy of Qi, such as shiatsu and acupressure, learn many protocols to enhance women's pregnancies (Ferguson 1995; Jin 1998). They also learn where to withhold their energy-focused pressure. There are varying opinions on their potency, but it is wisest to avoid deep, pointed pressure to the acupuncture points traditionally needled to promote uterine contractions (Figs. 2.7 and 2.8) (Jin 1998). These include:

- Spleen 6 (four client-fingerwidths proximal to the malleolus, along the medial tibial border)
- Kidney 3 (on the superior border and just posterior to the medial malleolus)
- Urinary bladder 60 (behind the ankle joint, in the depression between the prominence of the lateral malleolus and the Achilles tendon)
- Urinary bladder 67 (on the dorsal aspect of the little toe, at the junction of lines drawn along the lateral border of the nail and the base of the nail, just beside the corner of the nail)
- Liver 3 (at the proximal border of the first and second metatarsal bones)
- The complementary Hoku hand point, Large Intestine 4 (at the junction of the thumb and index finger)

If you observe the precautions concerning clots described in the section above, you will never activate most of these leg points.

Torso

Though reflex points in the torso are generally regarded as less potent, address soft tissue needs in the following areas with broad, general pressure (Fig. 2.8):

- On the sacrum, particularly at each sacral sulcus (Urinary bladder 31–34)
- Halfway between the nape of the neck and the acromion at the trapezius apex (Gall bladder 21) (Deadman and Al-Khafaji 2001)

Be precise in your application of deep, pointed pressure in nearby structures so that you avoid inadvertently interacting reflexively with all of these contraction stimulative points.

Some clients may tell you that they've heard that they should never allow any massage of their ankles or feet. This misconception has unfortunately spread via books written

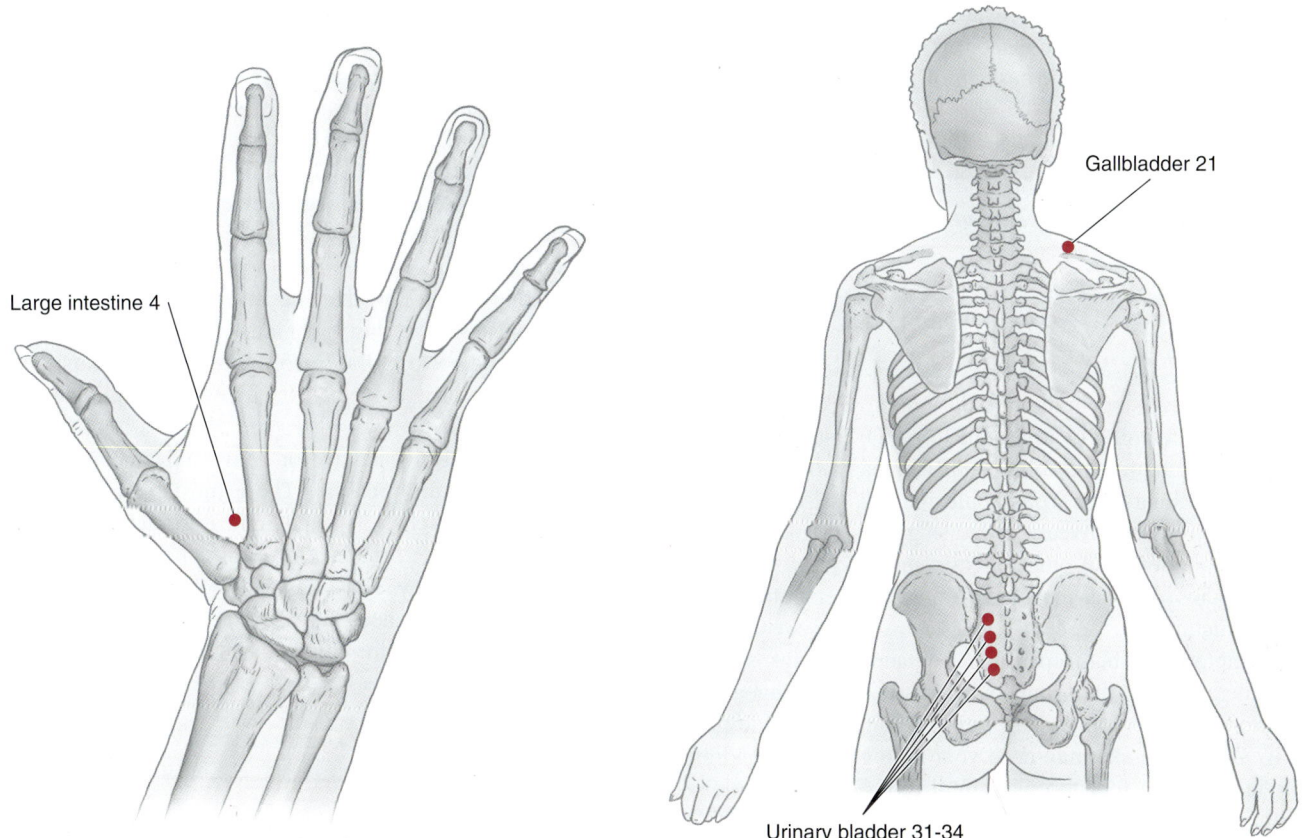

FIGURE 2.8 Other points contraindicated. Before a woman's due date, use broadly applied techniques over these acupressure points on the hand and torso.

What Would You Do?

As you spread oil in preparation to massage the feet of a new pregnant client, her eyes suddenly pop open in alarm, and she exclaims, "I heard that it wasn't safe to have my feet massaged when pregnant, that it could cause a miscarriage." How will you respond to her concerns, ease her worry, and proceed with an appropriate session?

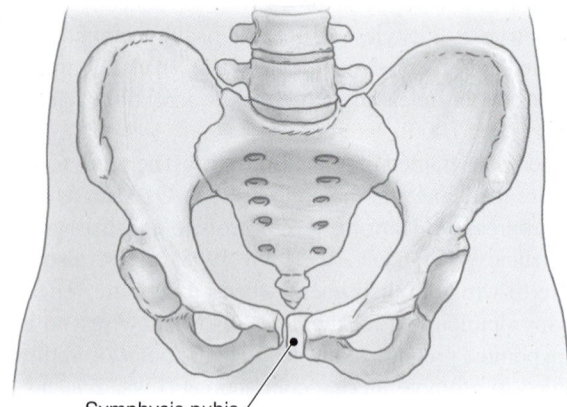

FIGURE 2.9 Symphysis pubis dysfunction. When hormonally softened, this anterior pelvic joint can painfully spread horizontally, or shear on the vertical plane, creating considerable pelvic instability and pain.

by authors who aren't trained in acupuncture/acupressure or reflexive zone therapy. Their understandable concern is to protect the pregnancy, but the level of warning is excessive. Only bone-to-bone, energy-focused pressure to these exact reflex areas will possibly create these negative prenatal effects. Misconstruing this precaution as a total contraindication to touching the heels or the feet of pregnant women deprives them of the soothing relief and grounding possible from other ways of massaging in these areas.

Although these areas do have labor-stimulating potential, they only reach their full potency when a woman is in labor or on the verge of it, when all points are methodically and repeatedly stimulated, and under the hands of one trained in interacting with energetic pathways. If you compress broadly or sweep over these points, you will not create unwanted reflexive responses. (See online box for an acupuncturist's further discussion of accupoints contraindicated in pregnancy.)

> **REMINDER:** Modify work on the legs for risks related to blood clots, varicose veins, and reflexive points.

JOINT PRECAUTIONS AND PASSIVE MOVEMENTS

As relaxin levels begin to build during the second trimester, avoid overstretching of joint structures. Overstretched ligaments result in joint instability and can mean more pain, prenatally and long-term. You should modify assisted-resisted stretches, positional release, Swedish gymnastic movements, range of motion, and other passive and active movements, such as those in Thai massage, to prevent overstretching of joint structures.

Symphysis pubis separation demands several special considerations in choosing and performing massage therapy to avoid provoking sharp, midline anterior pelvic pain (Fig. 2.9). First, she may need your help getting on and off the table, and a footstool is helpful too. Consider working with the client only in the semireclining position or working only one side each session. Because rolling over is painful with this condition, minimize position changes during your sessions. If she does turn, help her to keep her legs together with her thighs even when she rolls over from side to side (see Fig. 3-2c). Try elbows and knees rollover rather than having her go supine to roll over.

Also, firm, reliable bolsters and other supports are essential in all positions to prevent extended tugging on the joint. Be sure that you have evenly aligned and securely supported her pelvis and legs. Some women will be more comfortable on their side with pillows between their knees. Finally, eliminate any techniques that intentionally or inadvertently create traction on the pelvic and hip joints or that compress the pelvis unilaterally. Examples are grasping one foot and lower leg to extend the knee and hip joint or deep tissue work on the anterior pelvic attachments. The pain invoked at the symphysis pubis from these types of movements overshadows any possible benefits (see Fig. 4-6).

Women suffering nausea may not appreciate any rhythmic, rocking movements that can worsen morning sickness. Be sure to use gentle, slow techniques, even on the extremities, and avoid rocking the torso. Once nausea has passed, perform all passive movements with small amplitude and slow, rhythmic frequency.

Take care that any passive or active movements do not increase intrauterine pressure. Those most likely to do so would be knee-to-chest leg and lumbar stretches, hip circumduction, ribcage mobilizations, torso flexion, and similar maneuvers. Many Thai massage techniques and range of motion maneuvers need considerable modification to not press dangerously into the enlarged abdomen.

Oils and Lotions

When techniques require lubrication, use only unscented oils, or those with fragrances that she finds appealing. The best are pure seed oils such as apricot kernel or grapeseed. You may want to use a single ingredient to minimize the risk of allergic reaction; in the rare case where there is an allergic reaction, you will know exactly what it is—the one ingredient! Most lotions or creams, even natural creams, contain preservatives and a large number of potentially skin-irritating ingredients. Natural vitamin E oil as well as cocoa butter and shea butter in their pure form are helpful in relieving itchy, stretched skin. Shea butter, cocoa butter, and extra virgin coconut oil all contain substantial amounts of hyaluronic acid, which stimulates new skin cell regeneration and moisturizes deeply below the top layer of the epidermis (Leduc 1993). These lubricants may be effective in minimizing stretch marks.

There are many varying opinions as to which **essential oils** are safe and effective for the mother and the baby. Unless you are a highly trained **aromatherapist** or work with one to create specific oils for your practice, you should avoid using these powerful plant essences. (See online box for further discussion of essential oils during pregnancy and resources for high-quality essential oils.)

Other Skin Products and Spa Treatments

Be sure that any products that you use for spa treatments are safe for pregnant women. This can be difficult if you have no or limited education in the chemistry of emollients, essential oils, and other components of products. A few suggestions are as follows: Seek the masters or originators of spa treatments, and consult with the manufacturers of the products that you use to confirm their use prenatally. Research the actions and precautions of essential oils during pregnancy with a reliable source (see online resources listing at http://thePoint.lww.com/Osborne-Pregnancy2e). Another option is to use only simple, pure unscented oil as a lubricant.

Before applying any product, check the aroma to determine whether it is pleasing to her, especially those women with sensitive noses or queasy stomachs. Therapists customarily perform many spa services incorporating such products while a client is prone or supine on a table. Remember the safety and comfort positioning guidelines detailed above, and adapt your wraps, facials, and other treatments accordingly.

When using spa treatments or other modalities involving heat, modify the duration and extent of applications. Prolonged heat exposure over large body areas can increase maternal core temperatures. In the first 20 weeks, this can interfere with fetal development or even cause fetal death. Saunas, steam cabinets, hot tubs, and other heat immersion treatments are generally contraindicated prenatally. If women do use these, they should carefully monitor their body temperature and keep exposure to around 10 minutes (Simkin et al. 2010).

No studies have yet confirmed the appropriate amount of time for local heat application, but common sense suggests that you limit your use of hot wraps, hot packs, heat lamps, hot stones, and other heat modalities to local area applications of less than 20 minutes. If a pregnant client becomes uncomfortably hot or if her oral temperature rises 1° or more (Fahrenheit), discontinue heat treatment. No modifications in use of cold are required prenatally or perinatally.

Other Precautions

Specific techniques sometimes require specific safety and comfort adaptations. The detailed instructions for techniques throughout the book include these individual precautions. There are many somatic methodologies that can be adapted for prenatal and perinatal use. Some particular considerations for adaptations you should contemplate are included in Box 2.3. Detailed maternity applications for every possible somatic therapy cannot be adequately explored in this text. When you want to use polarity therapy, Thai massage, Watsu, or any other system not covered in these pages, study with a master practitioner and/or instructor of those systems prior to working with expectant women. Always observe pertinent,

Box 2.3

Is This a Safe Technique During Pregnancy?

Once you understand the rationale for the guidelines and contraindications included in this chapter, you can safely expand your repertoire of prenatal techniques. Ask yourself these questions before using any somatic practice with a pregnant woman.

1. Do I need to adapt the customary client position for this technique to meet prenatal positioning requirements?
2. Do I need to adapt the customary speed or pain level of this technique to avoid sympathetic arousal?
3. Do I need to adapt the emotional intensity of this technique to avoid sympathetic arousal?
4. Do I need to adapt this technique to avoid ischemic compression on the iliac vein and other medial leg veins, or vigor that could dislodge blood clots in the legs?
5. Do I need to adapt this technique to avoid pressure over weakened veins and capillaries?
6. Do I need to adapt this technique to avoid increased intrauterine pressure or other irritants to the uterine muscles?
7. Do I need to adapt this technique to avoid bone-to-bone contact on the reflex points that are contraindicated before a woman's due date?
8. Do I need to adapt this technique to protect vulnerable joint structures?
9. Do I need to adapt this technique due to a prenatal complication or a higher risk of complications?
10. Do I need to adapt this technique or protocol to avoid increasing core body temperature?

general contraindications, as well as any restrictions issued by a client's prenatal healthcare provider. The precautions, guidelines, and contraindications covered so far in this chapter apply to those with healthy, low-risk pregnancies. Check the section below and Chapter 7 for other contraindications and guidelines for women with high-risk factors and complications in pregnancy.

When Pregnancy Is Not Normal

Pregnancy induces extensive but normal systemic changes and typical aches and pains, as described in Chapters 1 and 4. The vast majority of women's pregnancies progress in these ways and without medical complications. For others, unhealthy changes in sugar and protein metabolism and blood pressure can develop. Fetal growth might slow or terminate, and the pregnancy might end prematurely in a miscarriage or an early labor. Physical, emotional, and environmental factors can make it more likely that these conditions might develop. Twenty to twenty-five percent of North American women's pregnancies deviate from the expected physiological adaptations or are at higher risk of these types of complications (Ricci 2009).

Most of this one quarter of pregnant women can still benefit from maternity massage therapy, but their needs can be unique. As such, Chapter 7 covers care of these clients. In this section, you will learn to recognize when a pregnancy isn't proceeding normally. When her doctor or midwife identifies the particular "special need," you can refer to Chapter 7, where you will find guidance for how to make appropriate adaptations. Your sessions with complicated and high-risk pregnancies have the potential to improve a woman's chances for a positive outcome, provide some stress reduction, and support her if her or her baby's condition deteriorates. Your work with such women can be highly rewarding (Fig. 2.10).

> *REMINDER:* Collect information about your client at each session to alert you to any prenatal complications or high-risk factors.

● RECOGNIZING PRENATAL COMPLICATIONS

At each session, and especially your first time, thoroughly assess your client's general state of health and pregnancy. Palpate and observe for edema, tenderness, and varicose veins. Ask if any prenatal testing has been abnormal or if she is experiencing any of the following signs that a complication might have developed.

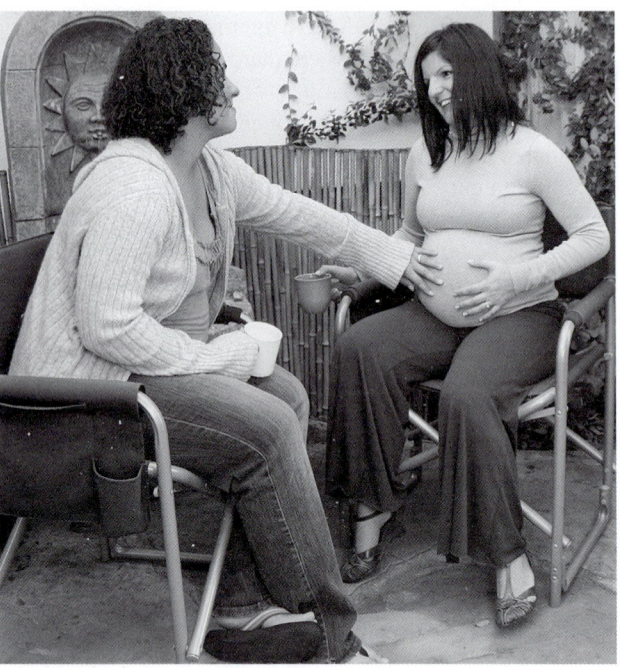

FIGURE 2.10 Support during high-risk pregnancies. Along with her healthcare providers, friends, and family, massage therapists can offer much appreciated support when a pregnancy isn't proceeding as anticipated.

- Vaginal bleeding (spotting or more profuse) or a gush or leakage of vaginal fluids
- Pelvic or abdominal pain or cramping
- Lower back or medial thigh pressure or pain, unaffected by positional or activity changes
- Regular uterine contractions before 37 weeks
- High blood pressure
- Swelling of hands or face
- Swelling of legs in the 1st or 2nd trimester
- Pitting, systemic edema, and/or sudden, rapid weight gain
- Abnormal lab tests indicating protein in urine
- Persistent and severe midback pain, especially on the right side and shoulder, unaffected by positional or activity changes
- Severe nausea or vomiting
- Severe headaches, blurry vision, or chest (epigastric) pain
- Convulsions
- Excessive hunger and thirst
- Abnormal lab tests indicating sugar in the urine
- Swelling, pain, and/or heat or redness in the leg
- Severely bulging veins, discolored and painful, or unilateral leg pain or swelling
- Cessation or reduction of fetal movement
- Abnormal fetal heartbeat
- Concern about the fetus's size or weight (Ricci 2009)

When a client has any of these symptoms, you need to carefully and appropriately respond. A good next question is,

"What does your doctor/midwife have to say about this?" When a diagnosis has been given, follow the caregiver's level of concern about the symptom and condition. You may want to ask your client to seek her caregiver's advice or to secure a written release before proceeding with a massage therapy session. (See Chapter 7 for more suggestions on how to handle this situation without alarming your client.)

In some settings, health history intake forms are not routinely completed by clients. Owners and staff should carefully consider the safety and quality of care consequences of these practices with their pregnancy clientele. At least the following basic screening questions are necessary: How far along are you? Are you having any conditions that your doctor/midwife is concerned about? What are you hoping to gain from your prenatal massage session today?

What Would You Do?

A prospective client calls you for an appointment. She is 33 weeks into her first pregnancy and has been having back pain this past week, primarily in her lumbar and sacral areas. Her prenatal exercise teacher has referred her to you for this and to help her with her very tight thigh muscles, especially her inner thigh muscles. She's also beginning to notice her shoes are very tight and her ankles swell in the afternoon and evenings. What additional information would you need from asking or observing her to make knowledgeable decisions about her care? Is it likely that she has any complications? What precautions in techniques should you take in addressing her edema and her medial thigh tension?

● RECOGNIZING HIGH-RISK FACTORS

The obstetrical profession has identified a number of conditions that they consider are more likely to result in prenatal complications developing. In some cases, the likelihood is very small; in others, more than 50% of women develop prenatal problems. Because these conditions jeopardize the health of the mother, her fetus, or both, Chapter 7 covers specific guidelines for massage therapy with these groups of women. The major categories of high risk include the following:

- Mother's age under 20 and over 35 (some sources list 15 and 40)
- A previous problem pregnancy
- Multiple pregnancies (twins, triplets, etc.)
- The following maternal illnesses:
  - Diabetes mellitus
  - Cardiac, liver, or renal/bladder disorders
  - Chronic hypertension
- Asthma or other pulmonary disorders, history of DVTs, and connective tissue and collagen diseases
- **Rh-negative** mother or maternal genetic problems, including **diethylstilbestrol (DES)** exposure and other uterine anomalies
- Drug or other hazardous materials exposure
- Risk of fetal genetic disorders (Ricci 2009)

● OTHER CAUTIONARY CONDITIONS

You should also be cautious when you work with clients in other situations. Often these risks are the result of cultural preferences or racial or socioeconomic injustices, but they are very relevant nonetheless:

- No prenatal care
- Risky lifestyle habits: smoking, drinking, drug use, poor nutrition, caffeine, or multiple sexual partners
- Childhood sexual abuse
- Spousal abuse
- Inadequate support system and/or high stress levels
- Sexually transmitted diseases (STD), including HIV and AIDS
- Low weight gain, obesity, or an eating disorder
- Severe anemia
- Convulsive disorders
- Overdue (fetal postmaturity)
- Genetic and acquired dysfunctions of platelets, coagulation, and other clotting factors
- Nonwhite ethnicity (Ricci 2009)

Remember that most of these women do have healthy pregnancies, even though the risk of higher morbidity and mortality is real.

CHAPTER SUMMARY

Following this chapter's precautions and contraindications (summarized in Box 2.4), you and your clients can know that prenatal massage therapy is safe in most pregnancies. As you create sessions using a variety of somatic methods, be sure that you make conservative decisions following this chapter's guidance on when and when not to massage and what positions to use. Remember these recommendations to modify depth, speed, and intensity of techniques, paying particular attention to your work in the abdomen and the legs, with joints, and on reflex points. Throughout your client's pregnancy, be alert for deviations from normal physiology and any factors that could foster a pregnancy complication. Within these safety parameters, you can expect your clients to benefit greatly and your work to promote healthy outcomes for women and their babies.

Box 2.4

Summary of General Methodological Precautions and Contraindications by Trimester

Abdominal Massage (any method)

First trimester:
- Consider eliminating as a liability precaution.

Second and third trimesters:
- Superficial effleurage and gentle rocking only

First through third trimesters:
- Liability precaution with hypertensive disorders, premature labor, miscarriage, or placental dysfunction symptoms or risks

Swedish Massage (all trimesters)

General directions:
- Direct strokes toward heart. Drain proximal areas first. Work superficially, then more deeply.
- Use procedures that help relieve pelvic congestion.

Precautions for varicose veins:

Mild (visible/ropy) and/or spider veins: Use only appropriate Swedish and lymphatic drainage strokes at moderate pressure.
Moderate (palpable/raised, ropy): Use only appropriate Swedish and lymphatic drainage strokes using a light touch.
Severe (palpable/raised, purplish/bruised surrounding tissue): Use only featherlight touch and energetic work.

Precautions for clot (thrombi) danger zones:
- Use soft, whole-hand pressure on the medial thigh.
- Avoid deep or pointed pressure on the medial border of the tibia, on the saphenous area of the knee, along or posterior to the sartorius muscle, and at the inguinal area.
- Avoid percussion (tapotement), wringing, brisk rocking or other movements, and vibration on or that travels to the legs.

Leg Massage of Any Methodology (all trimesters)
- See Swedish precautions above for legs.
- Also, avoid acupressure, cross-fiber friction, deep tissue, trigger points, or other deep ischemic pressure into the medial leg.
- Circulatory leg massage is contraindicated for clients on bed rest and those with increased clot risks, except with direct medical supervision.

Reflexive Therapies (all trimesters)
- Reflexology: Contraindicated to uterus and ovaries; use precaution with endocrine gland points; use caution with substance abusers, those with unhealthy lifestyles, and those with certain complications.
- Acupressure: Avoid stimulation of Spleen 6, Kidney 3, Bladder 60 and 67 and 31 to 34, Liver 3, Large Intestine 4, Gall bladder 21.

Deep Tissue (all trimesters)
- Avoid in abdomen; use only on structures chronically stressed by pregnancy; observe precautions for varicose veins and clots as above for Swedish and legs.

Passive and Active Movements

First trimester:
- Rocking movements contraindicated with nausea

Second and third trimesters:
- Rocking movements are contraindicated with nausea; use caution on hips and legs with symphysis pubis separation.

All trimesters:
- Avoid hyperextension of joints.

Consult master teachers of other somatic practices prior to applying techniques prenatally and perinatally. Modify for complications and high risks as described in Chapter 7. Observe any restrictions issued by the prenatal healthcare provider.

Test Yourself

For answers, visit the website at http://thePoint.LWW.com/Osborne-Pregnancy2e!

1. What are the advantages to using the sidelying position during prenatal massage therapy?

2. What adaptation of supine positioning will help prevent supine hypotensive syndrome in weeks 14 to 22, and what position is recommended after week 22?

3. When performing a technique, why should you maintain a depth and a speed that are no more intense than pleasure on the borderline of pain?

4. What are three main parameters for safe massage of the pregnant abdomen?

5. Describe the type of pressure and touch that can be problematic on certain reflex zones and points, particularly on the feet and before a woman's due date.

6. Describe the physiological reasons for thrombi development in expectant women's legs.

7. What adaptations to Swedish massage of the pregnant woman's legs help to prevent thrombolytic embolism in pregnant women's lungs?

8. What two lab results are indicative of the most common prenatal physiological imbalances?

9. What signs can help you to distinguish normal prenatal back and pelvic pain from that associated with miscarriage, preterm labor, or other visceral imbalances?

10. List five of the maternal health issues that put a woman at higher risk for developing gestational complications.

REFERENCES

American College of Obstetricians and Gynecologists. You and your baby: Prenatal care available at http://www.acog.org/publications/patienteducation/ab005.cfm. Accessed April 5, 2009.

Callahan T, Caughey A. Obstetrics and Gynecology. Baltimore: Lippincott Williams & Wilkins, 2007.

Deadman P, Al-Khafaji M. A Manual of Acupuncture. Acupuncture: A Comprehensive Text. East Sussex, England, 2001.

Enzer S. Reflexology: A Tool for Midwives. New South Wales, Australia: Enzer, 2000.

Ferguson P. The Self-Shiatsu Handbook. New York: Berkley Publishing Group, 1995.

Gilbert E and Harmon J. Manual of High Risk Pregnancy and Delivery. Third Edition. St. Louis: Mosby, 2003.

Gibbs R, Karlan B, Haney A, et al. Danforth's Obstetrics and Gynecology. 10th Ed. Baltimore: Lippincott Williams & Wilkins, 2008.

Jin Y. Handbook of Obstetrics and Gynecology in Chinese Medicine. Seattle: Eastland Press, 1998.

Jones C. Mind Over Labor. New York: Penguin Books, 1987.

Jordan K. What About Varicose Veins? First published in Massage Today May, 2001. Available at www.katejordanseminars.com/Article.aspx?a=16&l=2. Accessed Oct. 27, 2010.

Juhan D. Job's Body: A Handbook for Bodywork. New York: Station Hill Press, Expanded Edition, 1998.

Leduc M. Stretch marks: striae gravidarum. In: Encyclopedia of Childbearing: Critical Perspectives. Rothman BK, ed. Phoenix: Oryx Press, 1993.

Lett A. Reflex Zone Therapy for Health Professionals. London: Churchill Livingstone, 2000.

Nichols R, Humenick S. Childbirth Education: Practice, Research and Theory. 2nd Ed. Philadelphia: WB Saunders Co., 2000.

Noble E. Essential Exercises for the Childbearing Year. 4th Ed. Harwich: New Life Images, 1995.

Osborne C. Pre-and Perinatal Massage Therapy: Survey of Massage Therapists, 2009. www.bodytherapyassociates.com. Accessed May, 2010.

Pirie A, Herman H. How to Raise Children Without Breaking your Back. Cambridge: IBIS Publications, 2003.

Ricci S. Essentials of Maternity, Newborn, and Women's Health Nursing. Baltimore: Lippincott Williams & Wilkins, 2009.

Simkin P, Whalley J, Keppler A. Pregnancy, Childbirth, and the Newborn. Fourth Edition. New York: Meadowbrook Press, 2010.

Stager L. Nurturing Massage for Pregnancy. Baltimore: Lippincott, Williams and Wilkins, 2010.

Stillerman E. Prenatal Massage. St. Louis: Mosby/Elsevier, 2008.

Ugboma H, Akani C. Abdominal massage: another cause of maternal mortality. Niger J Med 2004;13(3):249–262.

Walton T. Medical Conditions and Massage Therapy. Baltimore: Lippincott, Williams, and Wilkins, 2011.

Werner R. A Massage Therapist's Guide to Pathology. 4th Ed. Baltimore: Lippincott Williams & Wilkins, 2008.

Yates, S. Pregnancy and Childbirth. Edinburgh: Churchhill Livingstone/Elsevier, 2010.

For additional resources, please visit http://thePoint.LWW.com/Osborne-Pregnancy2e!

Client Positioning, Draping, Body Mechanics, and Other Practical Considerations

Learning Objectives

After study of this chapter, you should be able to:

1. Establish and maintain an appropriate environment for maternity massage therapy.
2. Choose and adjust your massage table to a comfortable and effective height for sidelying and semireclined client positioning.
3. Arrange and maintain pillows and other supports on your table to safely and comfortably work with your prenatal clients in a variety of positions.
4. Modestly and smoothly drape and undrape clients' body areas as you massage.
5. Provide assistance for pregnant clients to get on, off, and shift positions on your table.
6. Practice proper body mechanics at your table for ease and effectiveness of your work.

In previous chapters, you have learned why prenatal and perinatal massage therapy is beneficial. You know when to and when not to massage and generally how to modify various methodologies for prenatal clients with normal pregnancies. In this chapter, we move into the massage therapy room for the physical practicalities of your work. This is a how-to chapter that forms the foundation for making your work effective for your client and comfortable for you both.

Nurturing the birth of a mother and her baby starts with the environment and equipment you choose. You will learn what tables, pillows, other support systems, skin products, and linens can enhance or detract from your session intentions. Using examples from actual therapists' work environments, you will see how to choose and arrange your equipment.

Variations in client positioning creates more and unique access to problematic areas. Some clients are more comfortable in one position than another, and others' health conditions limit how they receive a massage. Some therapists, especially those who are accustomed only to prone and supine work, initially find client positioning daunting. With clear, step-by-step instructions, you will soon find that the nuances of comfortable, safe, and secure client positioning will come easily for you, and you will drape modestly and easily. You will also learn how to help your client as she moves on and off and turns over on your table.

Sidelying positioning quickly becomes a favorite for perinatal massage therapists, even for their nonpregnant clients; however, this only happens when you embody the unique principles of body mechanics for this position. You will need to adjust your stance, weight shift, and alignment, and modify again when your client is semireclined. Using tai chi principles as a basis for these mechanics, you have maximum efficiency, fluidity, and adaptability and the least strain as you work.

General Practical Considerations

If you work in a spa or another healthcare provider's office, your employer usually assigns you a room, with or without consideration for its readiness for prenatal massage clients. Knowing a few priorities regarding supports and space can make a significant improvement even in the most difficult therapy room. On the other hand, you might be a part of developing that facility's prenatal services, giving detailed input regarding how the therapy rooms are set up. In private practice, all decisions are yours, like it or not. In any case, here's what to think about and plan for in your physical space.

● ENVIRONMENT

To help reduce stress in your clients, gear every aspect of your therapy room toward parasympathetic stimulation (Fig. 3.1). Although a small, dimly lit room can be womb-like, a cramped, confined feeling in your room will detract from relaxation. Pregnant women are often larger, sometimes feel clumsy, and generally can't see their feet as they walk in the last few months. They need room to maneuver and clear spaces with nothing to trip on. You should also allow space for postpartum clients' babies and their accessories if they need to bring their little one. Look for a room with at least 10' × 16' of usable space for interacting with your client, both on and off of the table (Box 3.1).

Check that outside noise and voices will not disturb your ambiance and that outsiders cannot readily hear your clients. Be particularly attentive to whether strong odors drift into your room. Use soothing color combinations on walls, furniture, equipment, and accessories.

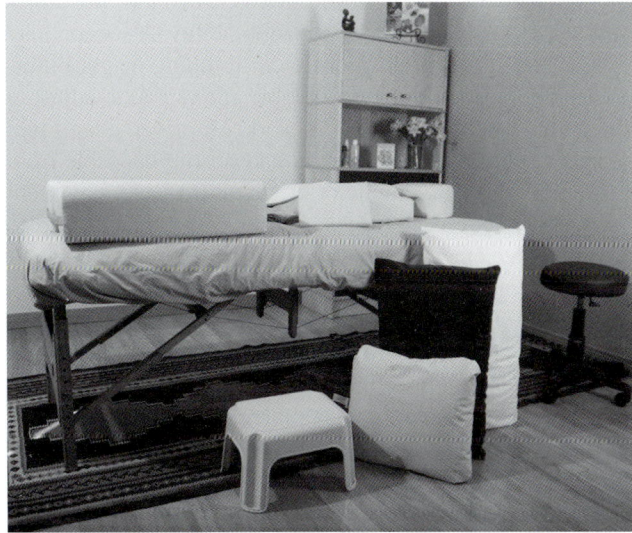

FIGURE 3.1 Prenatal massage therapy room. A spacious, well-equipped, and professional therapy room supports the benefits of prenatal massage therapy.

> **Box 3.1**
>
> **Environmental Qualities Conducive to Maternity Massage Therapy**
> - Encourages parasympathetic stimulation
> - Adequate size for you and the client
> - No distracting noise or odors
> - Decorative and educational décor
> - Easy to access, sturdy furniture, and adapted for maternity needs
> - Restroom in an adjacent or nearby room

Some therapists like to decorate in ways that convey the fluidity of pregnancy, pregnant and laboring women's power and grace, or the inspiration of cuddly, happy babies. Like many midwives and obstetricians, therapists collect many photographs of "their babies" often assembled into a wall collage. On the other hand, be sensitive that photos of healthy babies may emotionally trigger your clients with unexpected outcomes. Also, you may not want to overwhelm your non-pregnant clients with too much "baby stuff," particularly if you have a diverse clientele.

Don't forget educational items in your room decor by including charts, models, and books. You will repeatedly use replications of joints, muscles, the uterus, and the pelvis to explain and reinforce your postural guidance and teach her and her partner techniques they can use. Childbirth education supply stores can be good sources for this equipment (see online resources list at http://thePoint.lww.com/Osborne-Pregnancy2e).

Also, consider how easy it is to access your room. Is parking close enough for a third trimester woman to arrive at your room without being out of breath and overheated? Even a few steps can be challenging for some expectant women, and a full flight or two impossible; an elevator option is ideal when you are not on ground level. Be sure that chairs and tables provided for clients are sturdy, not too low, and adaptable for women coping with larger bellies, ligamental laxity, round ligament strain, and other physical discomforts.

You should also consider where the nearest restroom is. Remember that your client usually will need to use the toilet immediately before and after a session, and sometimes in the middle of it. Ideally, access to the restroom should be private so that she does not have to be fully dressed to get there. Changing and cleaning her baby is easier with a convenient restroom, too.

● EQUIPMENT AND SUPPLIES REQUIREMENTS

Below are the essential items you will need for an effective prenatal and perinatal massage therapy office setup:

- Professional massage therapy table (see details below on features to prioritize)

- Sturdy, wide, step stool, ideally with a hand support to help with balance on and off the table
- A wedge pillow for supporting the abdomen and under the right hip (see online resources)
- Six to eight firm pillows of various sizes and densities plus a foam wedge or other foundation for semireclining support (see positioning instructions below for various options), including one very firm king-sized pillow, several of standard size and firmness, and one or two thin, pliable ones
- A **Sidelying Positioning System** or a bodyCushion™ (see online resources list), plus four firm pillows of various sizes and densities, is a very desirable alternative to the pillows above to increase stability and comfort of most clients
- A 4- to 6-ft long strip of nonslip shelf lining to secure your pillows
- Twin-sized sheets, including fitted bottom sheets
- Breast drapes (king-sized pillowcases)
- Enough pillowcases to allow for hygienic laundering of all of your pillowcases after their use
- Unscented natural oil or lotion (see Chapter 2 for precautions on lubricants)
- At least one reference book, chart, or anatomical model that includes anatomical drawings of pregnancy and relevant musculoskeletal structures

● EQUIPMENT AND SUPPLIES RECOMMENDATIONS

Although it is difficult to work without a table and pillows, you can get by without some of the items recommended below. However, having most of these can really take your maternity work to a higher level.

- A lightweight blanket for those extra chilly days
- One or two double- or queen-sized cover sheets, so that you can modestly drape all sizes
- Two to three hospital gowns to easily drape when assisting women on or off the table or for seated massage
- A robe for when a client needs to use the bathroom during your session
- A height-adjustable rolling stool for you
- A reference library of books, DVDs, and other educational materials (see online resource list). Many maternity massage therapists make this a lending library.
- Models of the pelvis and uterus
- A secluded waiting area for nursing mothers who prefer more privacy
- Ottomans or other structures in your waiting area for elevating clients' legs
- Childcare provider so that new moms and those with older children can more readily schedule sessions
- Retail products that you use in your practice that women might find useful at home such as oils, abdominal wedge pillows, CDs

> **REMINDER:** *Develop an environment that promotes parasympathetic stimulation, increased self-awareness, and the other educational benefits of prenatal massage therapy.*

Massage Table Particulars

When choosing a massage table with maternity work in mind, you will need to consider the model type, width, height adjustability, and padding and covering.

● WIDTH, HEIGHT, AND MODEL

Your massage table should be about 30 inches wide to accommodate sidelying belly and supports; 27 inches is the absolute narrowest table width to consider. Sidelying, the position most commonly used with pregnant clients, requires a table at a higher height than that needed for prone and supine positions. For this reason, you need a table that features adjustable height. To measure your ideal working height, stand up straight next to a table with your arms at your sides; the table top should be level with your wrist. Be sure that any table you are considering using adjusts up to this height.

Using the body mechanics suggested later in this chapter, you will need to have your table at this height, especially when your client is sidelying. This will facilitate the more horizontal weight transfer that sidelying clients require. When your client is semireclined, you may want the table a couple of inches lower than this. This will give you leverage when working on her upper body and more gravitational lean toward the table for leg work.

In addition to width and height, be sure to choose the appropriate table model for your needs. Of course, **lift tables** offer the ultimate in table height adjustability. A session may include two different positions, with resulting height differences required, and this type of table allows you to adjust to an optimal height for all of your work. Moreover, clients will appreciate the ease of getting on and off of your table from a lower height. A hydraulic or electrical lift table may seem financially out of reach for you, but remember that it will also accommodate other clients with special needs, possibly qualifying your purchase of this table for considerable tax credits under the Americans with Disabilities Act (ADA).

Another table model to investigate is one with the **tilt-top** feature. Because you can lift one end to a variety of angles, they make sturdy and secure semireclined positioning very easy to achieve with less supports. Of course, a lift table with this tilt-top feature would be ideal.

There are tables on the market labeled as prenatal massage tables. Usually featuring a cutout section for the abdomen to hang into while prone, they may also have a supportive sling under that hole and/or two additional cutouts for the breasts.

> **My Story**
>
> *I like my table higher for my prenatal clients so that my alignment is better, and I can use my stool more. I use 4 × 4 blocks (custom made to my height by a friend) so that it saves time and wear and tear on the table knobs and my back when changing the height. I often have prenatal clients as well as regular clients scheduled during a single day, and it has been helpful.*
>
> —Nanci Newton, Hadley, MA

Despite their well-intended features, these tables are problematic for all of the reasons detailed in Chapter 2 on prone positioning.

• PADDING AND COVERINGS

Manufacturers usually do not design their standard massage tables with the sidelying or semireclining client in mind. In the sidelying position, the client's body has problematic pressure points at the shoulder joint (especially for those with edema, carpal tunnel syndrome, thoracic outlet syndrome) and the hip joint (especially for those with piriformis syndrome); in the semireclined position, pressure points are located on the client's sit bones (especially for those with sciaticlike sensations). If the table foam is inadequate, these areas will uncomfortably press against the wooden foundation beneath the padding. Look for a table with at least 3 inches of triple-density foam or with Aero-cell™ padding. Another option is to add thick, padded covers to your table to significantly reduce discomfort at these pressure points. A likely advantage to positioning systems and cushions is some relief at these achy spots.

Most vinyl and other materials for table coverings are satisfactory for perinatal applications. Although many joke about "waters breaking" at the most inopportune times, rarely does that happen, so you need not be concerned about excessive fluids soiling your table. You will want your table to have a covering that allows you to sanitize it to prevent bacteria or odor buildup. Most covering materials are odorless after an initial break-in period, but be sure that the vinyl is not emitting smells that your sensitive prenatal clients might find offensive or detrimental.

• HELPING THE CLIENT ONTO THE TABLE

Most pregnant women are accustomed to moving about without undue difficulty. These women can get onto your massage table unassisted. Tell her clearly or demonstrate where you want her to be on the table. Provide a sturdy step stool, particularly if you are taller than she is. You may leave the room while she undresses and then gets settled on the table.

If your client appears particularly uncomfortable with normal movements or if she has signs of pelvic instability, symphysis pubis dysfunction, or diastasis recti, ask if she would like your help. Place your footstool at the side of the table that you want her back to face (if in the sidelying position), approximately where her pelvis will be when she lies down. To brace or support her, plant yourself firmly on the floor, with at least a shoulder width between your feet. A hand or your forearm under hers will give her secure support to step onto the stool. Next, have her sit on the table. Have her keep her thighs mostly parallel and ask her to bring her legs onto the table on the side on which you want her to lie. She should use her arms to gradually bring her torso down onto that side (Fig. 3.2).

If you must be in the room with her as she gets on the table, it can be useful to have a hospital gown or some garment that opens in the back for her to wear. After she is settled, you can open the gown and have her slip it off each arm as you work on that side. She'll be able to reposition it to modestly get off of the table. A robe, opened at her back, can work too.

> **REMINDER:** *Assess and ask your client whether she needs your assistance getting on or off of your table.*

Client Positioning

Here are essential guidelines for positioning your client in the prone, supine, sidelying, semireclining, and seated positions. Box 3.2 summarizes the main points related to each position in several checklists.

• PRONE

If you or your client prefers to use the prone position for first trimester sessions, remember that you must make an individual assessment to determine the safety of it for her (see Chapter 2 regarding positioning safety). If her size, supported by your equipment, will keep from compressing her abdomen into the table and she is otherwise comfortable when you are working on her back, this will be an acceptable position to work in for the first trimester.

Suggested Supports and Their Placement

To help prevent increasing intrauterine pressure, use two pillows providing 3 to 5 inches of lift or a four-part body-Cushion™ to support her pelvis at both anterior superior iliac spines. You will also need a high ankle bolster or other such support, taking care to avoid deep plantarflexion of her ankle joints that can induce calf cramps.

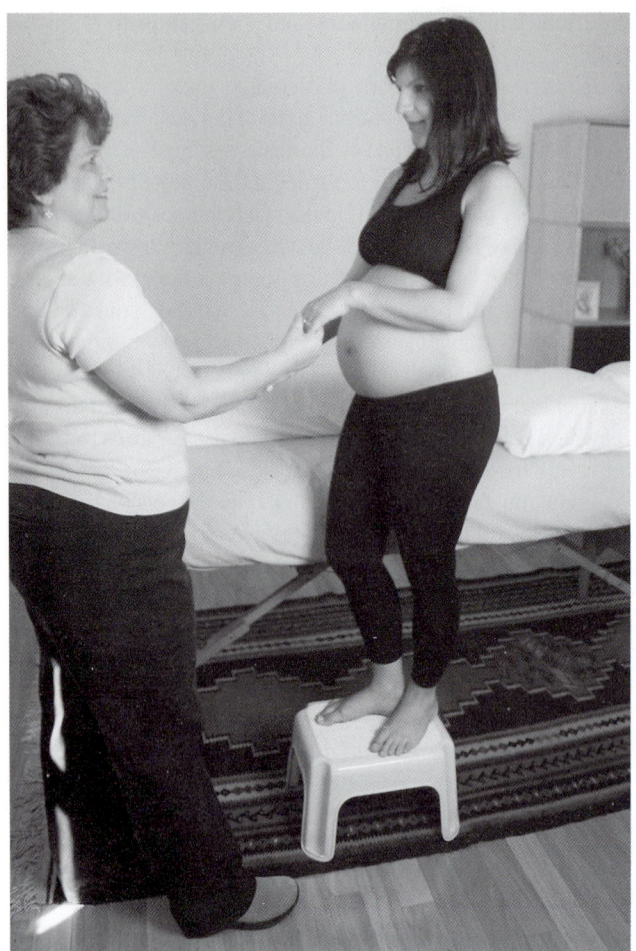
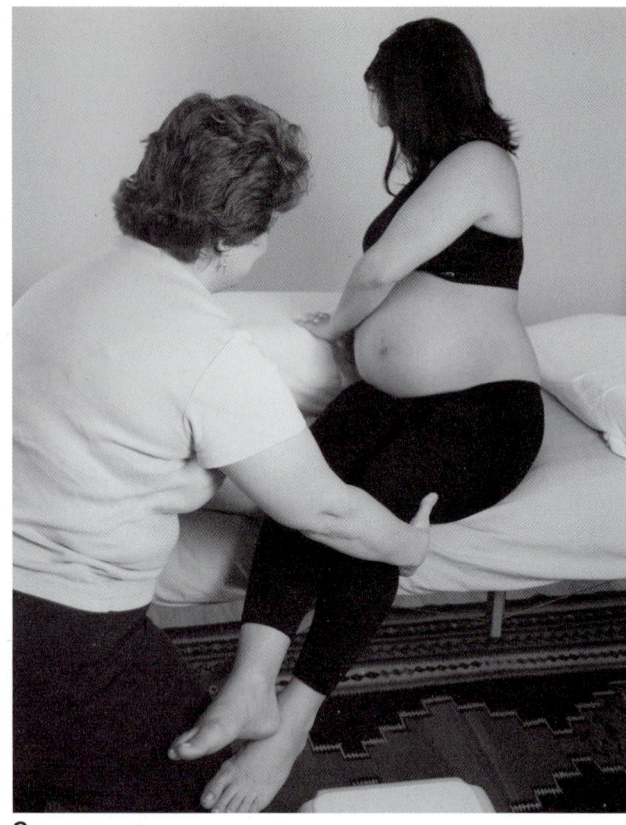
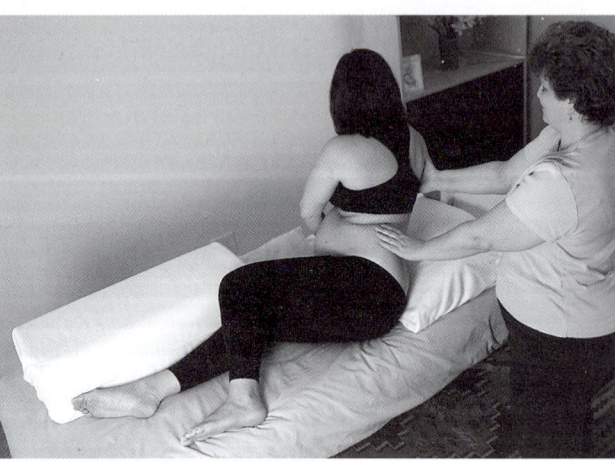

FIGURE 3.2 When a client needs help onto the table, **(A)** provide balancing support as your client mounts the step stool, **(B)** coach her to roll to her side using her arms for support, and **(C)** sometimes, you will need to help hold her thighs parallel to prevent pelvic pain. Reverse these steps when she gets off the table.

Other Safety and Comfort Tips

Some women also like a third pillow or rolled towel or blanket under their clavicles to help take some pressure off of their sensitive breasts. Be sure to adjust the face cradle to a comfortable height. Use this position for the shortest possible time to reduce the potential for undesired effects.

● SUPINE

You will reach the head, neck, and anterior of your client's body most easily when she is supine. Most women are comfortable for an extended period on their backs, but be sure to shift her uterine weight off the vena cava in weeks 14 to 22

Chapter 3 Client Positioning, Draping, Body Mechanics, and Other Practical Considerations 51

> **Box 3.2**
>
> ### Positioning Checklists
>
> **Prone**
> - Support for pelvis at anterior superior iliac spines
> - Support under chest or breast recesses, if tender breasts
> - High bolster under ankles
>
> **Supine**
> - Additional supports for weeks 14 to 22: 2- to 4-inch thick, small wedge pillow under right side from lower rib cage to hip joint
> - High bolster under knees, adding a pillow under calves and feet
> - Pillow under head, if desired
> - Soft surface to prevent sacroiliac pain
>
> **Semireclining**
> - 45 to 75 degrees head-to-hip joint elevation
> - Sufficient lumbar and cervical support
> - High bolster or pillow under knees
> - Additional pillow under calves and feet
>
> **Sidelying**
> - Firm supports to prevent rolling onto abdomen
> - 2- to 4-inch foam wedge under abdomen
> - Entire ceiling-side leg supported anterior of other leg with firm bolster and pillows; maintain horizontal line between hip, knee, and ankle; hip flexed at 55 to 80 degree angle to torso and knee flexed
> - Table-side leg directly on table, slightly flexed
> - Horizontal and slightly flexed spinal alignment
> - Appropriate-height head pillows to avoid cervical hyperextension or sidebending and acromioclavicular compression
> - Possible additional supports: under top arm, lumbar spine, ribcage and/or greater trochanter
> - Sidelying Positioning System or bodyCushion™ highly recommended

if she is supine for more than 3 to 5 minutes (see Chapter 2 for rationale).

Suggested Supports and Their Placement

This position requires no extra equipment in the first trimester; just use a knee bolster sufficiently high enough to help flatten her lumbar spine to the table. Offer her a head pillow if she prefers one. At 14 weeks, begin using an 8- to a 10-inch square wedge or pillow that is 2 to 4 inches thick. Cover it with a clean case, and place it directly onto the bottom sheet. Position it under her right side, with the narrowest side of the wedge tucked at her spine and sloping laterally to her right side (Fig. 3.3). Elevating her right side from the lower rib cage to the hip joint in this manner usually will prevent supine hypotensive syndrome.

Other Safety and Comfort Tips

Occasionally a woman will feel that the left tilt of her lower torso propped as above creates an uncomfortable spinal or pelvic twist. If so, you can add additional pillows under the rest of her right side so that her entire body is canted slightly off to her left but still aligned. Some therapists use the bodyCushion™ with the wedge placed under the right side for improved supine comfort. Regardless of your other equipment, lift her calves and feet level with her knees by adding a pillow under them. Use additional padding on your table if your supine client experiences sacroiliac pain (see Chapter 2 for description).

● SEMIRECLINING

Remember to shift to a semireclined position rather than the supine position after week 22 in most pregnancies, if client has heartburn, or whenever she has multiple gestations or feels dizzy, light-headed, or uncomfortable when supine (Fig. 3.4).

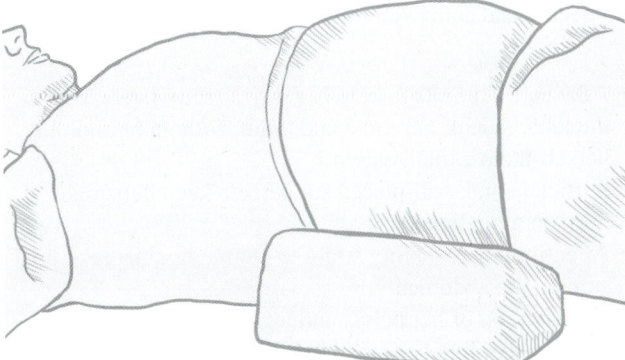

FIGURE 3.3 Supine positioning: weeks 14 to 22. Use a small wedge-shaped pillow under the right pelvis to shift weight off of the vena cava.

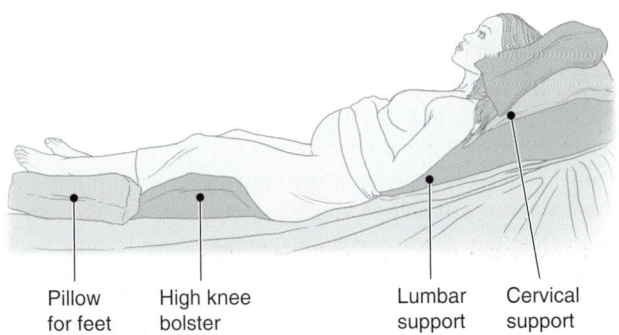

Pillow for feet | High knee bolster | Lumbar support | Cervical support

FIGURE 3.4 Semireclining positioning: weeks 23–term. Use props to elevate the client's torso from the hip to head at 45 to 75 degrees, and add additional knee bolster and foot pillow too.

Suggested Supports and Their Placement

The goal of semireclined position is to get her abdominal weight shifted toward her pelvic floor rather than posteriorly onto her vena cava. Do this by elevating her torso 45 to 75 degrees above the level of the table, from her hip joint to her head. You will need equipment to create a firm, steady, and secure foundation for propping your client to this height (Fig. 3.4). Some of these choices accomplish this with fewer additional elements needed (Fig. 3.5A–E). If you only have pillows available, use three of your firmest, biggest ones for this foundation, and you'll need another three to five pillows as well.

Place your foundation support at the head end of the table and cover it. Next, begin stacking any additional pillows you need onto the covered foundation. They will be more secure if you alternate placing them lengthwise and then widthwise on the stack. If you have accurately estimated the height of pillows needed for her torso length and width, you may only need to make small adjustments after she settles onto the table.

Those adjustments might include sufficient supports under her lumbar area to accommodate her back, regardless of lumbar lordosis depth. Assure that her head and neck are neither hyperflexed nor extended, and adjust as needed. Use a high, firm knee bolster to help hold her in this position. For added comfort, circulation, and edema relief, elevate her lower leg with a pillow under her calves and feet. You will not need the pillow under her right pelvis if you have positioned her correctly (Fig. 3.4).

If you use a tilt-top table, you will probably only need additional bolsters or small pillows to provide both the lumbar spine and the cervical spine with essential support.

Other Safety and Comfort Tips

Here are a few ideas for helping to secure your supporting wedge when the client leans back. The Side Lying Positioning System has a strap to secure it. If you have an adjustable-tilt face cradle, position it so that the cradle faces the foot end of the table, at a 90-degree angle from the table top. Do be judicious in using your face cradle in this way as manufacturers only test them to support a client's head, not the torso. Some therapists prefer to back their table up against a wall for the ultimate in solidity behind their supports. If you take this option, you will need to reach her upper body from each side of the table rather than from behind her.

If your table has a smooth, slippery covering, you may want to put a 4- to 6-ft long strip of nonslip vinyl shelving material between it and your foundation supports. Even with a no-slip surface, weaving this strip between your pillows as you add them will help to hold them together, too. For added safety, test the security of your foundation by leaning back against it yourself before your client does.

Direct her sitting on the table so that she brings her buttocks completely against the supports and is able to lean directly against, rather than having to scoot back against them. Should she slump so that her abdomen is actually flat on the table, help her to reposition, adding any additional pillows needed so that she can truly be upright from her hip to her head. Monitor her position throughout your session to be sure that she hasn't slid down, risking supine hypotension.

Your supports need to be secure enough that she doesn't feel as though she will push them off the table when she rests back against them. They also must have enough side-to-side stability that she isn't tilted to the left or right. "Weaving" a few larger pillows rather than stacking oodles of smaller ones will help with this.

You can also help stabilize her as you work on her upper body, particularly her arms and torso. Use some traction with one hand on her shoulder to counter any pressure moving her to the opposite side. Taking the time to rearrange when you see her slumping or tilting won't distract from your session; it will increase her relaxation because she feels more secure.

You may need to fine-tune her head and neck position for comfort. Try a small wedge pillow, your face cradle cushion, or a cervical roll to support her cervical spine correctly. With a wide enough table, you can also place matching bolsters or rolled pillows or towels under each forearm and hand, and she will feel like the "queen mom."

> **REMINDER:** Monitor your semireclined client's position and maintain it so that her entire torso from hip to head is elevated from 45 to 75 degrees.

● SIDELYING

You may be surprised at how quickly you become both proficient and enthusiastic about the sidelying position. With an understanding of your goals, the proper equipment collection, an efficient order to maneuvering pillows, and some practice, you will soon spend very little additional time managing your supports. In explaining this position, "**ceiling-side**" will refer to the side of your client's body that is available to work with, and "**table-side**" the side that she is lying on.

Secure and comfortable sidelying positioning requires the following:

- Adequate supports to help her stay directly lateral on the table-side of her torso and thigh, without her holding herself there while you work
- Sufficient and well-placed supports to keep her spine horizontally aligned
- Attention to preventing strain to uterine ligaments or pressure on the abdomen
- Stabilization of her pelvis and legs with high bolsters to effortlessly align her ceiling-side hip, knee, and ankle horizontally
- Minimization of painful pressure on her table-side hip and shoulder and both breasts

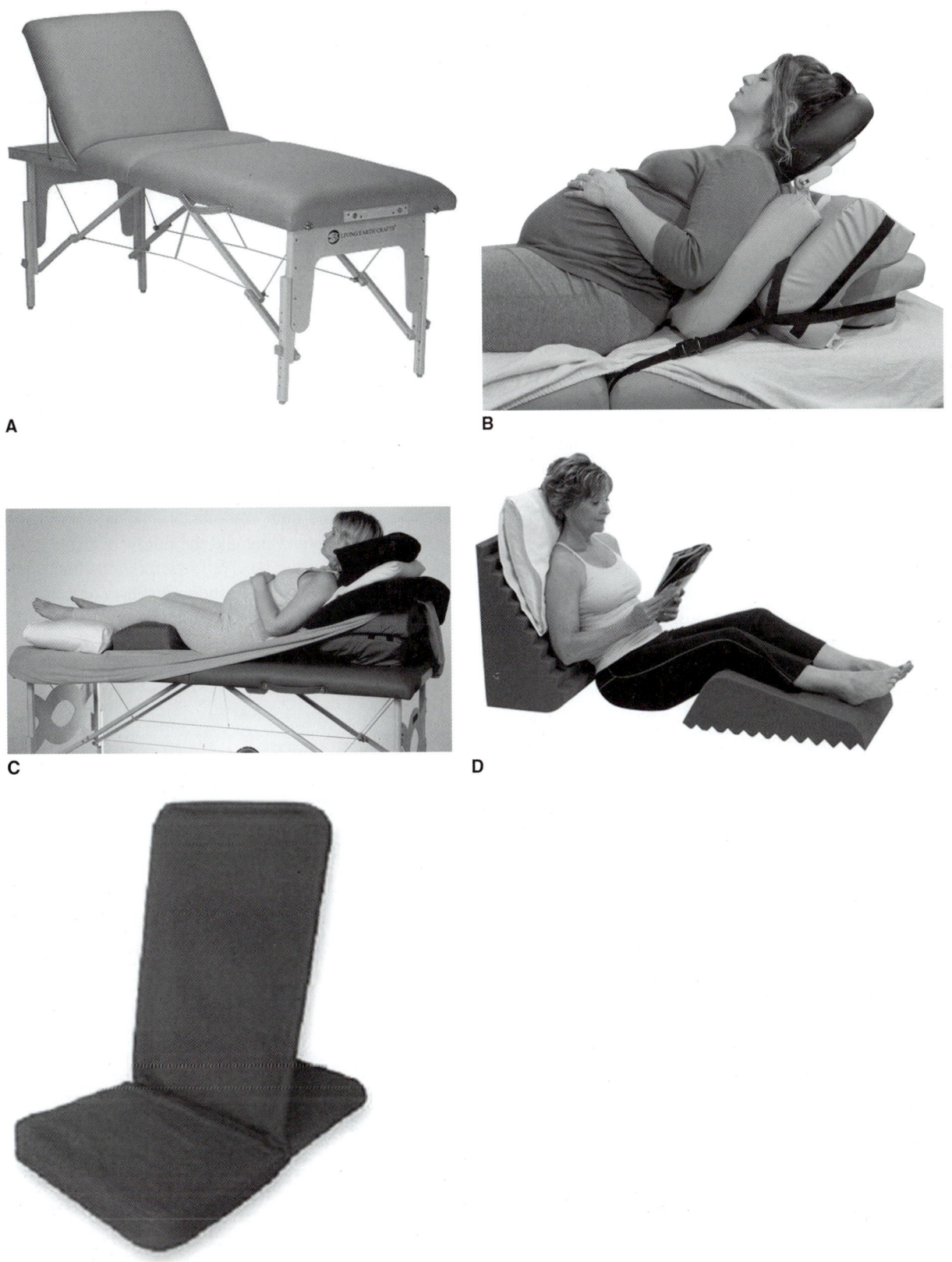

FIGURE 3.5 Prop options for semireclined positioning. **A.** Tilt-top table. **B.** Sidelying Positioning System reconfigured for semireclining. **C.** bodyCushion™. **D.** Large wedges. **E.** Back-jack. With each of these options, you usually will need additional pillows to achieve the alignment shown in Figure 3.4. You may need to adjust your face cradle upright or use the wall to provide a supportive barrier for your props. Weave a strip of nonslip shelf-liner between items to help secure them together.

Suggested Supports and Their Placement

There are three equipment sets to choose from to achieve the sidelying positioning pictured in Figure 3.6: the Side Lying Positioning System, the bodyCushion™, and pillows. (see online resources for these products). Each has advantages and disadvantages. Experiment to find what works best for you and your clients. Whichever one you use, position your supports off the table midline so that your client will be as close to the back edge of the table as possible; help her to align her entire torso an inch or two from this edge when she first settles onto the table. Refer to Figure 3.6 as you read the directions below on how to fine-tune your supports. Watch the online video too.

Gently check that there is no space between the supports and her belly, adding more under her belly if it is insufficiently cradled. Don't use so big a belly pillow that she feels as though she is rolling backwards off of the table.

It is easier to stabilize her leg and pelvis if she extends the table-side leg, positioning it posterior of the other leg that is flexed from 55 to 80 degrees. With this arrangement, you need bolsters and/or pillows for the ceiling-side leg of sufficient height and density to maintain a horizontal line between this hip, knee, and ankle, with a moderately flexed hip and knee. Pillows between the legs are usually not as stable, forcing clients to tense to maintain their position; however, this might be more comfortable if she has signs of symphysis pubis dysfunction.

Visually assess the alignment of her ceiling-side leg. If her knee medially rotates so that it is lower than her hip, check to see if the pillows need to be further under her thigh and knee. One corner should be near the groin with 2 to 3 inches of pillow anterior of her thigh. Align the pillows lengthwise with the table rather than skewed at an angle. If her knee still slumps down, you may need to add an additional pillow or two. Getting the knee and ankle level may require another pillow or two placed under her foot, particularly with taller women.

All of this attention to the supports under her leg will prevent strain on the sacroiliac joints and the lumbar spine, and anterior rolling onto her belly. Proper leg height also mechanically assists in the reduction of leg edema and can provide relief from painful varicose veins. Leveling the ceiling-side leg is usually the most important part of sidelying propping.

Let's look at her torso now. Both the systems in Figure 3.6A and B have a great advantage over pillows in that they lift some of the torso weight off of the table-side shoulder and hip. These supports should accommodate the space between the acromioclavicular joint and the head, aligning her cervical spine with her torso, without hyperextending or sidebending her neck and head. Snug the supports up completely under her neck so that it is well supported. A full pillow and a relatively flat one placed with a small gap for the shoulder to rest between can sometimes work instead. If her lumbar spine sags toward the table, then put a very small pillow or rolled towel or sheet between her ribcage and iliac crest to lift and support her lumbar spine to horizontal with the thoracic spine.

Finally, give her a pillow of sufficient height and firmness for under her ceiling-side arm to lift it off of her breast, help to prevent anterior rotation of her body, and open the anterior pectoral region for circulation. If her hands are swollen, you may want to use another pillow to level her hand with her shoulder too. If this pillow is outside of her covering drape, it also will help to hold that drape in place over her breasts.

The Oakworks Side Lying Positioning System (Fig. 3.6A) was specially designed to help you achieve these parameters, supporting most women comfortably and securely. Another option may be to use the head, torso, and leg pieces of the bodyCushion™ (Fig. 3.6B). Some therapists prefer to use pillows: one or two head pillows, the abdominal wedge pillow, and dense king-sized ones for under her ceiling-side leg (Fig. 3.6C). A long body pillow can form a foundation of support, but you will still need other pillows to add to get the appropriate alignment (see online video at http://thePoint.lww.com/Osborne-Pregnancy2e for additional pointers for refining sidelying supports).

Most therapists find that they can set their table up for the client to get on and then come back into the room to fine-tune the client's positioning and the pillow placement. Put a foundation down for her: head pillows, torso cushion, abdominal pillow, and one or two leg supports. Show or tell her how you want her to use these, and then let her get undressed and

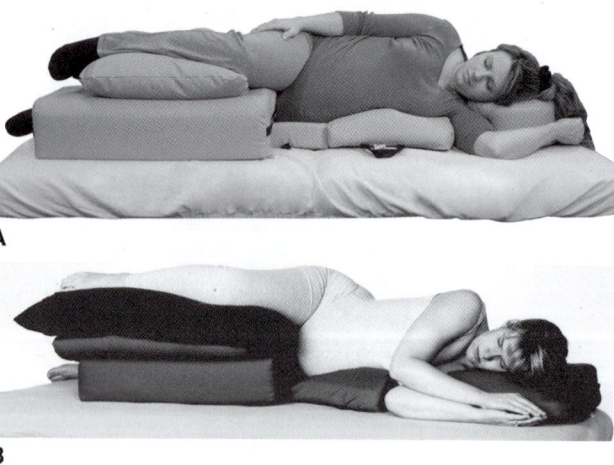

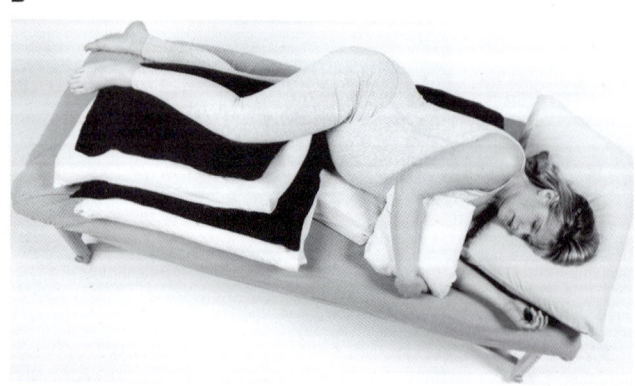

FIGURE 3.6 Prop options for sidelying positioning. **A.** Sidelying Positioning System. **B.** bodyCushion™. **C.** Pillows.

> ### My Story
>
> *The correct positioning is not only important for certain techniques on the low back, sacrum, pelvic, and hip areas to be effective. Good positioning and supports do half your work for you. Almost all of my clients, upon being effectively supported in the sidelying position, say, "I haven't felt this comfortable in weeks!" Before I have kneaded, or rocked, or gently stretched any of their areas of discomfort, my clients already feel significantly better.*
>
> —Anne Gilbert, Boston, MA

on the table. If she needs your assistance, remain in the room to help as above.

Other Safety and Comfort Tips

As mentioned previously, uncomfortable pressure at the shoulder and hip joints can occur if your table padding is inadequate. Either of the two positioning systems will help prevent this. Without this equipment, you could try laying down a thin pillow or two under her shoulder and hip for more cushioning. A specialized cushion for under the hip joint is available as another alternative (see online resources list). Some therapists choose their pillows carefully, placing one under the ribcage just below the armpit to reduce pressure on the shoulder.

If she wants to shift off of her acromion, help her to reach her table-side arm further in front of her rather than putting her arm behind her back; that will shift her upper torso posteriorly and not roll her weight more onto her belly into a half prone position.

As pillows compress and the woman relaxes under your touch, you may find that you periodically need to adjust your supports. Depending on the relaxin levels and her ligamental laxity, you may find her loose skeleton hard to keep stabilized. Monitor her alignment, adding and subtracting supports so that she stays comfortable and stable throughout your session. If you move supports about gracefully and calmly, supporting her well will not detract from your session. Instead, she will feel attended to and cared for by your detailed attention to her comfort.

Often women remark that this is what they need to sleep more comfortably. Point out to her the essential elements of your setup that she can provide for herself: a belly pillow, level hip, knee and foot alignment, and adequate head pillows.

> **REMINDER:** *Leveling the ceiling-side leg is the most important part of sidelying propping for a safe and comfortable position.*

● SEATED

When there is no table available or the client can't get comfortable in any other position, you can still do a partial session with her seated. Women who might be more comfortable seated include extremely obese clients, those carrying twins or triplets, or those with severe symphysis pubis pain, all of whom might have trouble getting onto a table even using a step stool and your help; clients with severe gastric reflux; and clients who are fearful about lying down and feel more control when seated.

If you use a household chair, try to get one that is relatively firm and that won't compress excessively under your pressure. A lower back will make access to her neck and shoulders easier. Prop her legs up on an ottoman or another chair to help reduce edema. If she can comfortably spread her legs to sit backwards in a kitchen or dining room chair, you can work on her back. Use a firm pillow or cushions between her body and the chair back. You will need to be very superficial in your posterior work so as to avoid increasing intrauterine pressure, but this is a viable alternative. If you place the chair back at a table, you might also stack enough pillows or cushions on the table so that she can rest her head, too.

Use an **on-site massage chair** in an unorthodox manner to achieve a semireclined position (Fig. 3.7). If she

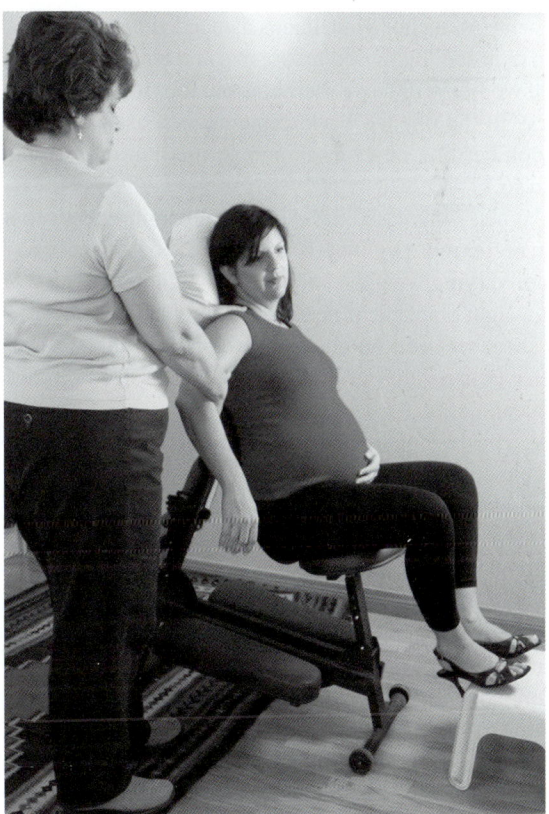

FIGURE 3.7 On-site massage chair for prenatal sessions. Using your step stool under a client's feet will allow her to comfortably lean back, semireclined against the chest rest and face cradle of an on-site chair.

leans forward, as these chairs are typically used, you will risk creating uterine ligament strain or intrauterine pressure. Instead, adjust the angle of the chair to between 45 and 75 degrees, and then have her sit backward on it. Place a stool for her feet, and then she can lean back against the chair into a semireclined position. Most women like to rest their arms on their swelling bellies while you can easily work on most of the body, including the lower back.

Draping

Your use of covering linens has the same purpose in prenatal massage as in all therapeutic massage: keeping the client modestly and comfortably covered and warm while allowing you the maximum access to structures. There are a few more unique considerations in prenatal draping.

Some women feel more modest, even shameful, about their increased size. Others are comfortable, even proud and flamboyant, about their "baby bump" and their rounder body shape. You need skill in professionally draping women along all points of the modesty spectrum. Due to increased vaginal secretions, many women will leave their underpants on for massage. Be prepared to drape such women, using these garments to anchor your linens as needed and never leaving them exposed. Increased breast size and tenderness can mean some women will leave their bras on, too. If you need further access to the client's back, remember to ask permission to unhook her bra, never assuming permission or coercing her to do so.

Women's increased basal body temperature tends to make them prefer more lightweight sheets. It is best to have a selection of varying weights, and your heavy flannels can work as lightweight blankets, if needed. Be sure that you confirm that any sheet sets you purchase include a covering sheet that is at least twin-sized. For breast drapes, king-sized pillowcases are ideal.

As a professional massage therapist, you are already comfortable with draping prone and supine clients. Your semireclined and sidelying draping should be just as graceful and not distract from your session focus. There are some draping differences, though. For instance, in the semireclined position, it is easier for drapes to slip down from the breast area. In the sidelying position, the buttocks and even the genital area can feel more exposed, even when drapes are completely covering. For these reasons, it is important that you ensure that you not only adequately place your drapes, but also securely tuck them rather than leave them loose. Your client needs to be able to feel these intimate areas covered so that she can more completely relax. Remember to re-cover each body segment as you complete it before uncovering another. Let's look at how to efficiently drape for these two positions.

● SEMIRECLINING

In many ways, semireclined draping is very similar to supine draping. Your biggest challenge will be in anchoring the cover sheet and/or breast drape over her chest and swollen abdomen. A twin-sized cover sheet will be wide enough for you to center it on your client and cover her completely, with a foot or more on each side left over to tuck under her if necessary. Tuck down her torso to her upper thigh, or just tuck at chest level. Of course, you should only secure the drapes, not make them constrictive, especially over her abdomen.

When you need to work on the ribcage or abdomen, first tell your client about the draping changes about to occur. Add a breast drape and maneuver it as you are accustomed to with a supine client. Gently slide the sheet inferior of her abdomen, and then anchor it under her buttocks on each side.

If her breasts cover the lower ribcage or upper abdominal area where you need to work, ask her to hold the top of the breast drape. Use the lower edge of the breast drape to lift her breasts away from the area. Do this by holding both sides of the drape near her sides, pressing it against her lower ribs while scooping under her breasts, and lifting them toward her clavicles. Keep your tension on the fabric as you tuck each end under her, near her armpits. She should then be able to release the drape, comfortably letting her arms and hands rest where she prefers (Fig. 3.8A).

To re-cover her, just bring the sheet back over the breast drape. You can remove the breast drape then, when she changes position, or just leave it in place until you are finished with your session.

● SIDELYING

To keep the abdomen and chest covered while you work on your client's back and lateral hip and thigh, you need to shift more of the covering sheet to her ventral side. With the sheet lengthwise on her body, line the long edge up with the edge of the back side of the table. This will distribute more sheet to the larger side of her body. The propping of the leg in the sidelying position can make some women feel exposed even when they aren't. For this reason, always tuck a few inches of the covering sheet between the table and her gluteals and upper thigh (Figs. 3.9 and 3.10E). Depending on where you want to work, follow one of the following sequences.

Undraping the Back

1. Stand behind your client at pelvis level, facing her head.
2. Hold a fistful of sheet between the table and the table-side buttocks while your other hand slides across her sacral area, gathering the sheet to the other side of her pelvis.
3. Roll the sheet into the waist of her panties or just superior of the gluteal cleft.

Chapter 3 Client Positioning, Draping, Body Mechanics, and Other Practical Considerations 57

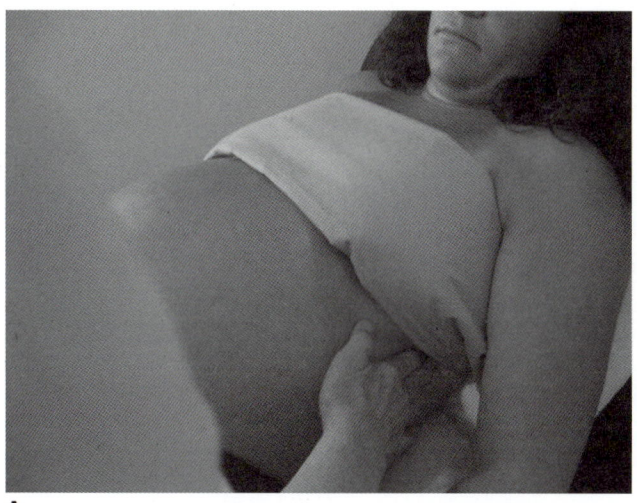

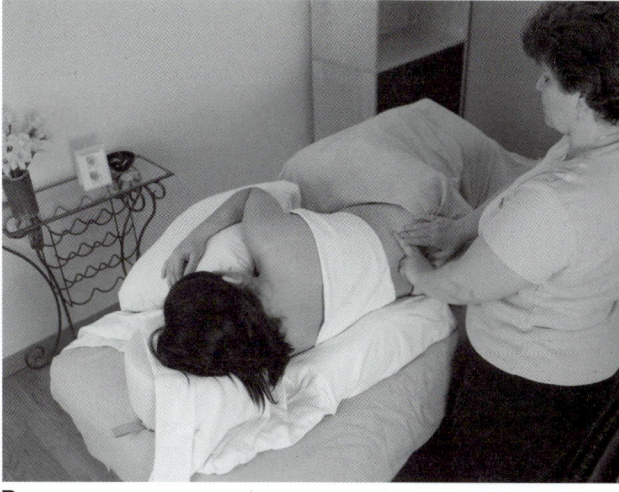

FIGURE 3.8 Draping the breasts. **A.** Semireclined: Tuck the ends of the drape under the client's torso to secure it. **B.** Sidelying: Secure the breast drape by tucking it posteriorly under the table-side ribcage and with the arm pillow.

4. Collect the remaining sheet off her back, rolling and pressing it firmly against her ribcage. The drape will now be shaped like a backward letter "L."
5. Finish securing the drape by tucking several inches between the table and her buttocks and thigh (Fig. 3.9).

Undraping the Ceiling-Side Hip and Leg

As you make the following maneuvers, monitor the sheet section covering her abdomen and genital region. You may need to tighten and rearrange as you go to avoid gaps in her coverage there but don't poke or tuck in the genital region.

1. Again, stand behind her at pelvic level, but facing her feet. Reach across the table taking only a fistful of the far corner into your outside hand (Fig. 3.10A).

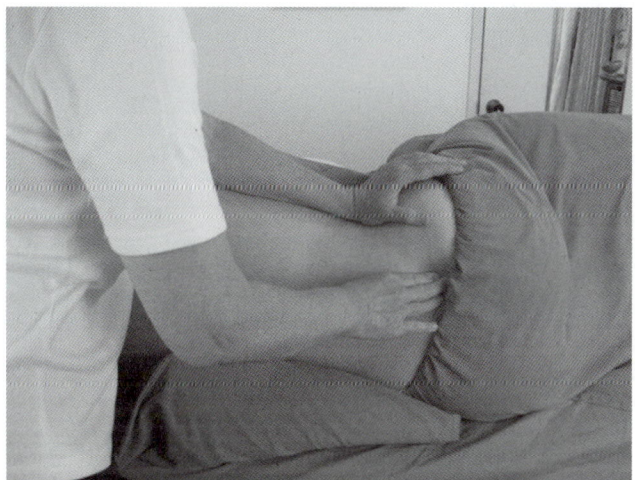

FIGURE 3.9 Undraping the back. Gain access to the entire back to just superior of the gluteal cleft with a tucked and secure L-shaped drape configuration. Remember to also tuck under the tableside gluteals and thigh.

2. Thread that past the crease of her bent knee, moving from posterior to anterior (Fig. 3.10B).
3. Switch hands pulling only a fistful to the anterior side of her knee. Use the outside hand to shape a deep U in the sheet on her lateral thigh. Pull a bit more sheet with each hand until you have formed a deep U at the level of her gluteal crease (Fig. 3.10C).
4. If her underwear will allow for it, ask if she would be comfortable with your shifting the sheet to bikini-height. If she says no, then tuck the corner of the sheet under the most anterior portion of the U. If she okays a higher drape, continue on alternating your pull with each hand until the entire ceiling-side gluteal area is accessible, and then tuck the end near her lateral iliac crest (Fig. 3.10D).
5. Remember to keep the drape taut throughout so that neither her gluteal cleft nor her abdomen is exposed.
6. Finish securing the drape between the table and her buttocks and upper thigh (Fig. 3.10E).

When you no longer need the ceiling-side lateral hip and leg exposed, unfurl the sheet.

When moving her legs for passive moves and stretches, you will probably find it easiest to keep the drape loosely over her, only opening the section that you need to grasp and secure her leg for the movements. This is especially important if you are moving in more than a few degrees of motion, particularly with circumduction of the hip and other hip movements.

> **REMINDER:** Ensure that your sidelying draping is not only adequately placed but also securely tucked rather than loose around her legs and buttocks.

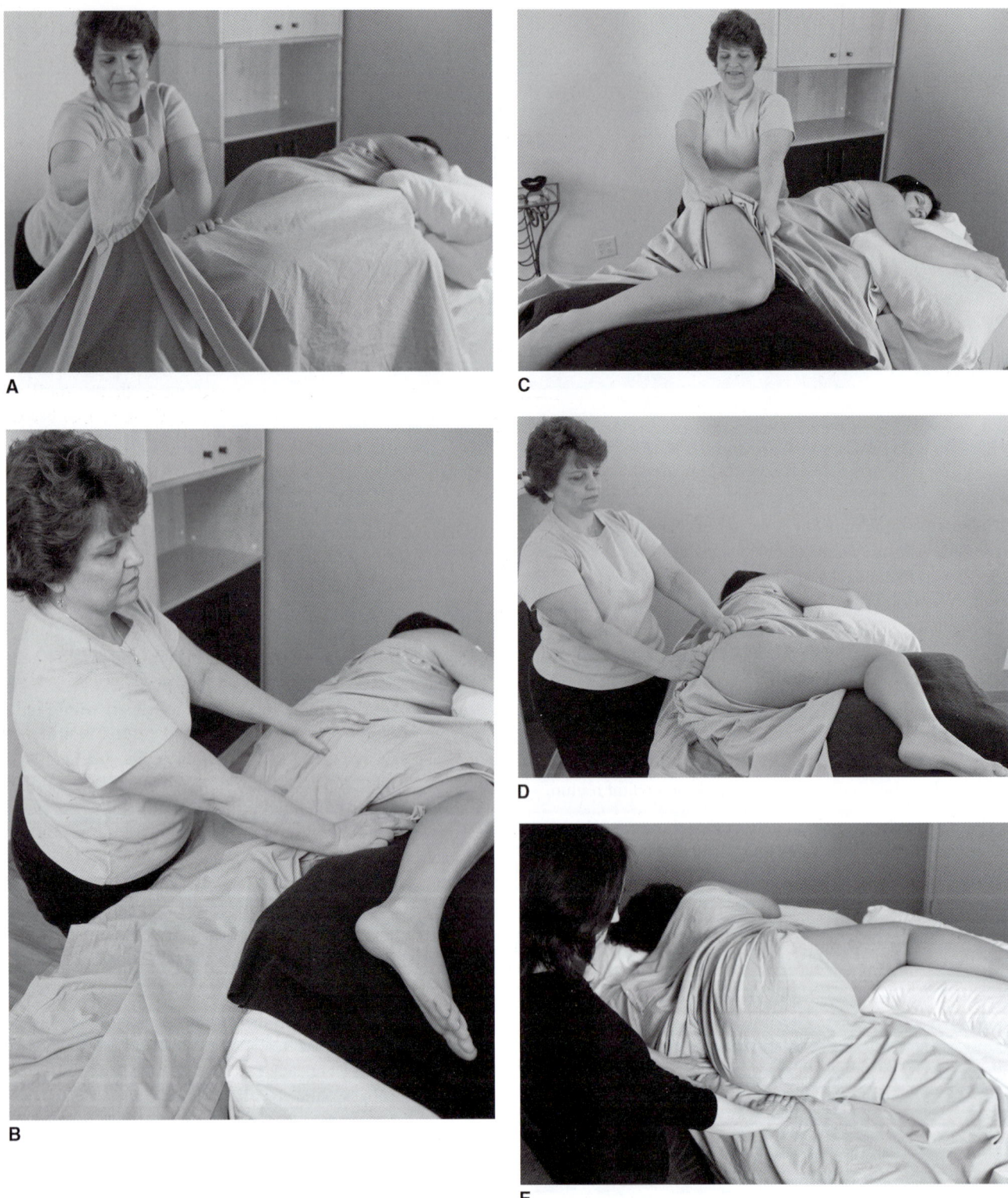

FIGURE 3.10 Sidelying draping for the ceiling-side hip and leg. The sequence for sidelying draping for work on the lateral flank proceeds from **(A)** reaching across the table for the opposite corner of the cover sheet, **(B)** slipping that corner between the ceiling-side knee and its supports, **(C)** alternating pulling a U-shape up the lateral thigh while sliding the sheet along the medial thigh, **(D)** tucking the end of the sheet around the lateral pelvis, and **(E)** tucking drape under gluteals and thigh to help her perceive that she is modestly covered.

Chapter 3 Client Positioning, Draping, Body Mechanics, and Other Practical Considerations   59

What Would You Do?

Your 38-week pregnant client comes into your office breathing heavily, red-faced, and sweaty from the 90 degrees heat outside. You notice that her feet and ankles are very swollen, but all else seems normal with her pregnancy. When you return to the room, she's on the table, wearing only her panties; all supports except her head pillow and the cover sheet are pushed aside. She comments gratefully about cooling off. How will you handle positioning and draping this client for her session?

Undraping the Table-Side Leg

1. Begin at her foot and shift the sheet off of her medial foot and leg, tucking it between the table and the leg supports for the other leg.
2. Keep tucking until midthigh. Be sure that it feels secure to her. To redrape, simply pull the sheet from under the supports and over her down-side leg (see Fig. 4-29).

Undraping the Ribcage and Abdomen

1. Remove her arm support as she shifts her flexed arm. Add a folded pillowcase across her breasts all the way down to the table. Ask her to tuck it under the table-side arm if possible (Fig. 3.8B).
2. Scoop it under her breasts as you sweep it across her lateral torso to tuck it between her back and the table.
3. Tuck the sheet diagonally across her back or straight across it between her ilium and the table.

● SEATED

Many therapists find seated massage easiest with the client clothed, or with a sports bra and loose or spandex pants. This is a very viable option, although it limits your work to those techniques that do not require lubricant. Another option is to use your cover sheet evenly arranged widthwise around your client at armpit level. Bring each end completely around her shoulders from front to back to front, and tie it securely at her upper chest. Keep her breasts and gluteal area covered, leaving her upper back and chest accessible. You also could use a hospital gown.

Making Transition Changes

In a typical 50- to 60-minute prenatal massage session, you will likely need one change in position on the table. More than that can be disruptive of the session's serenity. Of course, you may have situations in which comfort or safety reasons suggest more repositioning or limit you to only one position. Sometimes you might want to concentrate on one area, and a position change isn't necessary.

When it is time for your client to assume a different position on your table, just a bit of organization and direction goes a long way. Clearly tell her where and when you want her to move. Encourage women with symphysis pubis discomforts to keep their knees together whenever possible, and often they do best rolling to hands and knees. When you manage your equipment properly, she will usually manage herself just fine in these transitions.

● SUPINE/PRONE SWITCHES

Supine to prone or reverse switches of your expectant clients are almost exactly like with nonpregnant clients. You'll only need to remove or position the small wedge under her right hip. Remember to have her push up to a seated position with her arms and to stabilize and align her knees if she has symphysis pubis pain.

● SUPINE OR SEMIRECLINING/ SIDELYING SWITCHES

A supine to sidelying transition proceeds similarly as above until it is time for placement of the supports. If she is transitioning to sidelying, first place her head and belly pillows only while she pauses seated. If using either support cushion system, place the system with the edge lined up along the side where her back will be. After she settles down onto those, you can then place her leg supports and any others needed to make her content.

Occasionally, you will need to transition from a supine to a semireclined position due to dizziness or heartburn developing. If so, ask her to push up to a seated position while you gather the drape around her upper torso and ask her to hold it. Take your time to build a sturdy, sufficient support. Ask her to scoot back, using her arms to avoid straining the abdominal muscles as she leans back fully.

● SIDE-TO-SIDE TURN OVERS

One of your most common transition changes will be from one side to the other (Fig. 3.11). This goes smoothly if you first loosen any tucked areas and arrange the sheet evenly over her. Ask her to stay on her side while you get some of the pillows out of her way. Remove the pillows in the opposite order that you placed them: arm, leg, and then belly, leaving the head pillow in place. Put these pillows near the side of the table where you will be replacing them. Standing on the side of the table at her back with the sheet pressed between the tableside and your thighs, hold space for her, and ask her to turn over.

Most women will roll to the back and then to the other side. If that is the direction of her momentum, ask her to

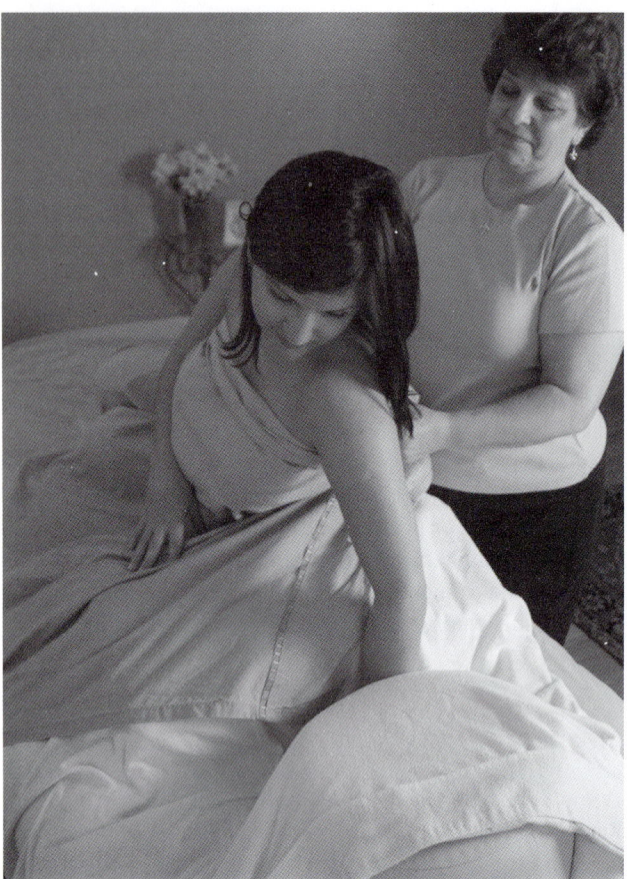

FIGURE 3.11 Turning from side to side. Help your client to turn over by giving clear, simple directions; moving supports efficiently; and managing the covering drape.

pause on her back while you move to the other side of the table. You will be in position to ensure that she safely moves to that edge of the table. Then you will replace the supports, first belly and then legs, arm, and other fine-tuning items. If she turns toward her abdomen, direct her to push up onto her hands and knees and then to pause while you shift to the other side of the table, and proceed as above.

The procedure varies and is a bit more simple when using either the Sidelying Positioning System or the bodyCushion™. Remove the arm and leg supports. Have her push up to a seated position with her arms while you keep her covered. Simply slide the torso and head cushions to align with the other side of the table and then move to that side so that she can turn and settle into it. Replace the other pillows then.

Helping the Client Off the Table

First you need to determine whether she would like your help getting off the table. If not, then you can remove all of the pillows except anything that is beneath her. Remind her where the edge of the table is and to roll from her side to sit up, pausing with her legs dangling for 30 to 60 seconds. Alert her to the position of the footstool that you have moved out to the tableside, and then leave her to rise on her own. If she prefers assistance, help her to push up from her side as when turning over, regardless of what position she was last in for her massage.

If she needs more help up from the semireclined position, stand at her side interlocking arms closest together, forearm to upper arm. Place the palm of your hand over her scapula, and ask her to do likewise on you. Shift your weight toward the head end of the table, and then tell her to sit up. At her initial movement, immediately shift your weight back, and you will easily help her to sit up without any engagement of her abdominal muscles. She can sit for a few moments before easing down to the footstool, with you bracing her at the forearm if necessary.

Therapist's Body Mechanics

To effectively use your body as a tool for therapeutic bodywork, you must understand some key concepts related to **body mechanics** (Fig. 3.12). Body mechanics involves how you align and coordinate yourself while generating pressure, power, and sensitivity to your client. Coupled with a keen **kinesthetic awareness**, good body mechanics means your work will be less effortful, your touch more readily received, and your outcomes more satisfying for your client and you. Developing an internal awareness of your body use can help to protect you from injury and to improve both your sensitivity and your ability to stay present in each moment of your session.

The foundations of the concepts in this section are rooted in the ancient martial art of **tai chi chuan** (Cheng 1999) and the twentieth century structural integration modality of Rolfing, as taught by Edward Maupin (2005). Tai chi offers insight into alignment principles, weight direction and transfer, and "rooting" and "generating" of body energy. Centered around a vertical and a horizontal polarity concept, Maupin's approach lends space and grace to organization at the table. Synthesized from these two systems, with over 35 years of bodywork practice to experiment with and refine their application, the principles below can direct you to more gratifying and less effortful tablework.

You probably have already developed your body mechanics for working with prone and supine clients. If you hurt or feel depleted when you work, the guidance below might give you some insight as to how to change your prone and supine work, too. Because you will work most extensively with your expectant clients on their sides, this section focuses on applying these principles for sidelying sessions. This position usually involves directing the force of your touch horizontally and diagonally into your client and less down through the client toward the table. Many therapists struggle with their body use with sidelying clients because they don't modify their approach for this fundamental difference.

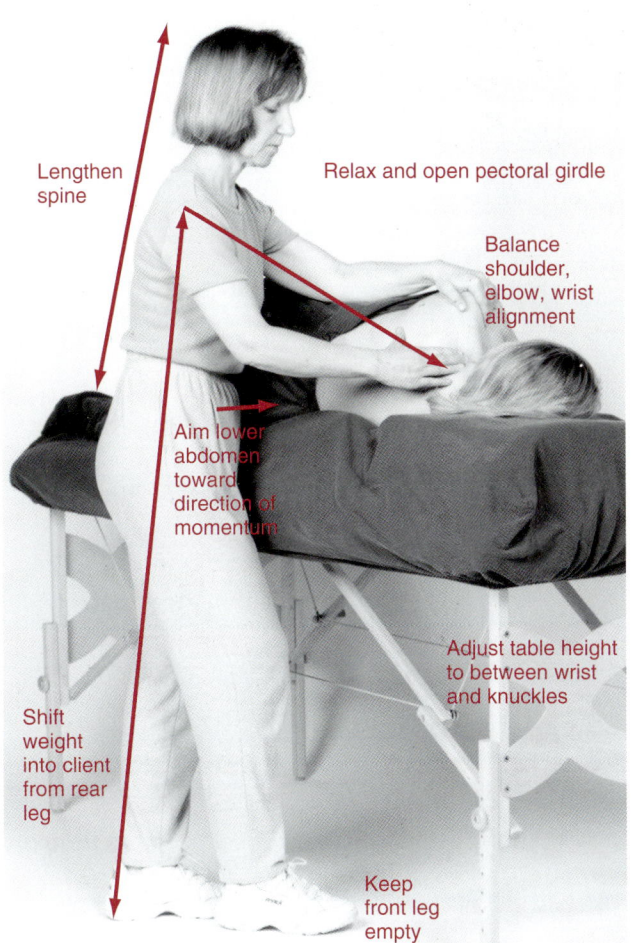

FIGURE 3.12 Summary of body mechanics in the modified tee stance. Effective, less effortful use of your body requires vertical and horizontal expansion, clear weight shifts, and a relaxed, stable alignment.

● BASIC PRINCIPLES OF ALIGNMENT

Imagine a vertical line from the crown of your head dropping directly down to your feet. See the subtle curvatures of each spinal segment softening that line. Visualize your ear, shoulder joint, hip joint, knee, and ankle bisected by that vertical line. Now imagine a horizontal ring of structure at your shoulder joint, diaphragm, and pelvis. Imagine any lateral movement at these rings reaching out from your core, into the related joints and structures. You now have a simplified vision of a dynamic way of being in your body. This **"expansional balance"** concept balances the polarity of up and down and expands the thrust of your movement (Fig. 3.13) (Maupin 2005).

There is a bit more symbolism in how tai chi principles illuminate similar alignment concepts: Imagine a string from the crown of your head extending up to the heavens above. Imagine another string on your coccyx with a 1,000-lb weight attached and stretching down into the earth. Relax, opening your joints by allowing your body energy to move freely through them like a silk thread through a string of pearls (Cheng 1999). These metaphors create a stable and dynamic structure for palpating, compressing, expanding, moving, oscillating, and gliding types of touch. Using your body with these images in mind physically fosters some of the other skills of therapeutic touch. These include breathing, engaging your mind, and directing your energy (Burman and Friedland 2006). Taking this to the table for specifics, you can organize your body with each of these principles in mind.

● STANCES, SHIFTING WEIGHT, AND ALIGNMENT

There are three basic stances in most styles of tai chi: bow, horse riding, and "tee." Many therapists have learned to use some version of the **bow stance** with good results. Often called a lunge or one-foot-forward stance, this usually features one foot positioned 2 to 3 foot lengths forward of the rear foot with a shoulder's width between feet, and the knees and hips are flexed. In this stance, weight shifts from foot to foot and into the working tool while the spine stays lifted and aligned as when doing an effleurage-type stroke (Frye 2010).

In a **horse-riding stance** or parallel stance, the feet are a shoulder's width apart but aligned with each other directly under the flexed ankle, knee, and hip joints. This stance works well as a stationary stance or when alternating hand motions such as in petrissage techniques. Weight can easily slide from foot to foot to power the momentum and pressure of the hands (Fig. 3.14C).

In this section, we focus on modifying the less frequently used tee stance for your sidelying work. The **tee stance,** or "white crane" stance, makes a very effective base for most forms of massage and bodywork (Fig. 3.12). In this stance, point one foot in the direction of your work's movement. Place the other foot a shoulder's width away, but with the toes even with the heel of the front foot. Allow your rear leg to externally rotate slightly, to no more than 15 to 20 degrees, so that the rear hip joint is freer for movement. (This is the main modification of the tai chi tee stance, where the rear foot is externally rotated 45 to 90 degrees.)

Rather than distribute your weight between your feet, as in the lunge or parallel stances, gather all of your weight into your rear leg, sinking down into your slightly flexed knee and hip. This empties weight from your front foot and leg but allows the weight of the leg itself to rest on the floor with no tension in it: thus the image of a white crane standing effortlessly in balance on one leg.

Continue with these directions as though you were using your fist to compress into a tight muscle. Imagine standing at the head end of the table and placing your fist on a sidelying client's midtrapezius, for example. Initiate and maintain pressure by pushing into the ground with the rear leg, but do not lock that knee in doing so. Lean forward while allowing your body weight to transfer through your pelvis, spine, and

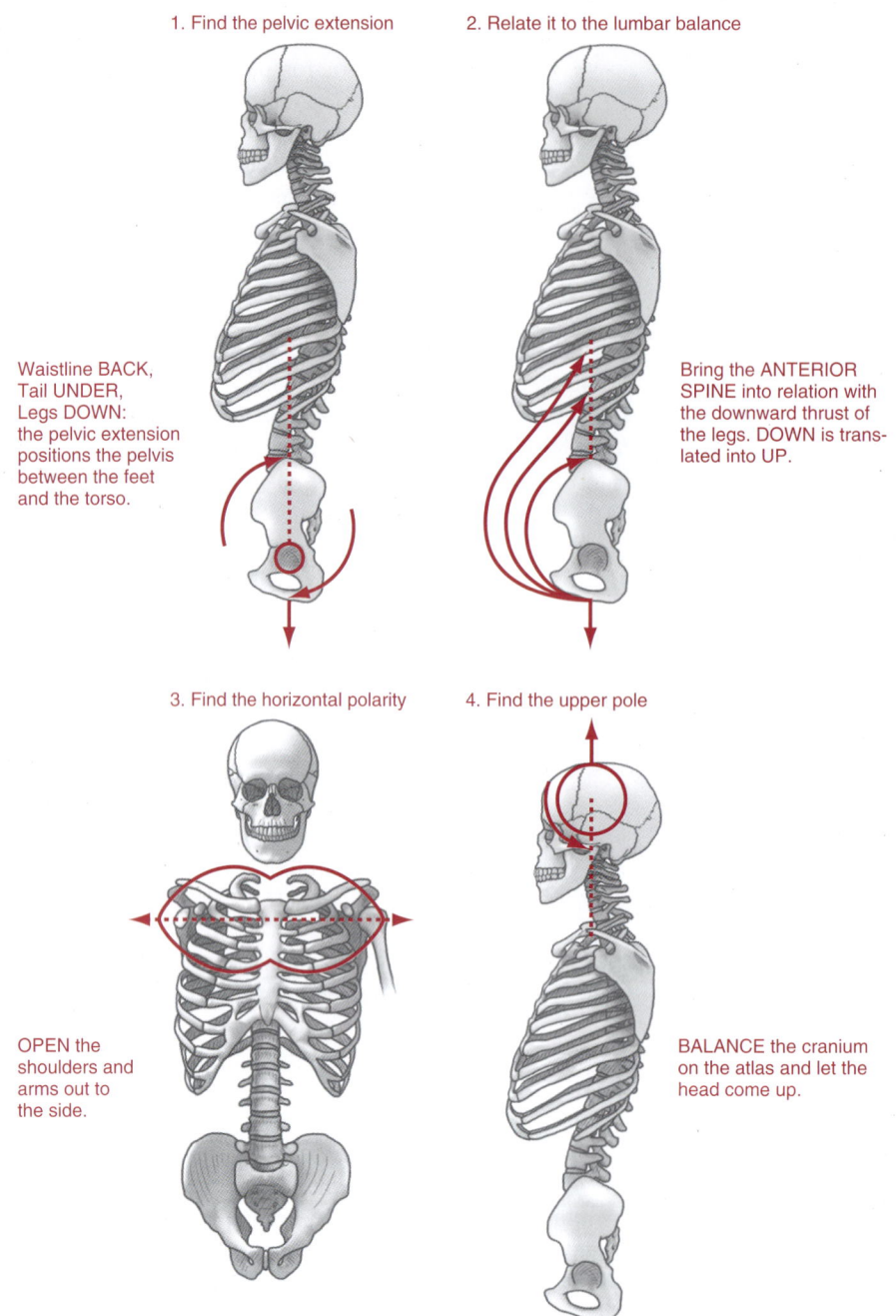

FIGURE 3.13 Expansional balance. Keep these concepts in mind while you work with your clients, aligning yourself from the ground up, following the steps numbered in these diagrams. (Used with permission of Maupin E. A Dynamic Relation to Gravity, vol 1. San Diego: Dawn Eve Press, 2005:34, 35.)

shoulder girdle into your fist. Direct your weight into your working tool, and avoid loading your front leg, which should remain empty, relaxed, and free to step if needed. Your center of gravity will then be somewhere between you and your client as you lean into her. With these dynamics, you should be able to lift your front leg from the floor without any weight adjustments. Increase your pressure by pressing into the ground and leaning more heavily onto your fist; lighten it by subtly shifting back into the rear leg.

Remember those expansional polarities and open joints discussed above? As you lean from your rear leg, let your spine extend downward and upward, your head centered over your spine. Notice and correct any collapse or sidebending of your head or torso (Fig. 3.14A). Look downward when you need to locate structures and monitor client reaction. Then, realign your head on your spine, reestablishing a gentle cervical curvature, with your chin gently tucked in (Figs. 3.12 and 3.14).

> **REMINDER:** Lift the crown of your head and your sternum, extend your lower spine downward, and balance each joint.

Relax all unnecessary contraction of the pectoral girdle muscles so that your shoulders remain down and relaxed, balanced horizontally on the torso. Avoid hunching and anterior rounding of the shoulders by allowing your sternum to lift rather than collapse between your ribs. Pay particular attention to releasing excess tension in your trapezius, levator scapulae, supraspinatus, and rhomboids. You won't overuse your deltoids, pectoralis major, biceps, triceps, latissimus dorsi, and trapezius if you use your body weight efficiently to create pressure rather than muscling in with these muscles.

To stabilize your shoulder and scapulothoracic joints as you shift your weight into your client's body, balance the functions of the serratus anterior/rhomboids and the latissimus dorsi/upper trapezius, along with the humeral stabilizers, that is, teres minor, infraspinatus, and subscapularis. Allow your pectoral girdle to relax downward and open horizontally throughout your work. This type of proper care of your shoulder and scapulothoracic joints while working helps to avoid injuries such as rotator cuff syndrome, shoulder bursitis, muscular strain, and kyphosis.

If you are not near or far enough from the table for a slight flexion in your elbow but a straight wrist, then correct your distance. You must protect the integrity of your fingers, wrists, and elbows. Whatever technique you apply, perform it with as much open, balanced alignment of these joints as possible. If you repeatedly hyperextend your wrist, you put yourself at higher risk of carpal tunnel syndrome, tendonitis, and/or ligament strain in the wrist. Excessive pressure on your fingertips, particularly on the thumbs, can hyperextend or hyperflex the metacarpal-phalangeal joint. The resulting ligament strain and stretching can cause pain, swelling, and instability in the affected joints.

Avoid these problems by bracing or supporting your fingers and hands to create additional protection for the joints sustaining the greatest pressures. Use smaller tools such as these for thin and small muscles and specific sites of tissue disorganization. Broader tools, such as your forearm and loosely fisted hand, deliver more generalized, broader effect to larger areas of tissue. Not only they tend to be less penetrating and painful but also their structure better supports heavier pressure without risking damage to your body (Osborne 2002). Like a silk thread through pearls, let your weight and energy slide out your hand (Barrett 2006). Release your pressure by regathering your weight into your rear leg.

What Would You Do?

Fifteen minutes or so into a session, you feel your back and neck tiring and beginning to ache. You realize that your client's upper body, where you need to work, is not lined up with the back of the table; instead, it is at an angle such that you need to reach one third of the way across the table to work in her midback. Your client seems almost asleep. What measures can you take to attend to your body mechanics with the minimum disturbance to your client?

For this to be a light, easy posture rather than an effortful stance, adjust your table so that the top is level with your wrist when you are standing in this modified tee stance. Otherwise, the deep hip and knee flexion will be more demanding than most can manage. With the right table height, and following a few other guiding principles, therapists who switch to working in this manner often become enthusiastic about its benefits and have fewer occupational injuries and more satisfied clients. Others will continue to find the bow stance works for them so they keep their tables lower, and they are hopefully very attentive to not bending their torso or twisting their neck.

● POSITIONING AND STABILIZING YOURSELF WHEN WORKING WITH A SIDELYING CLIENT

In tai chi, it is said that energy and its movement begins in the legs, finds direction through the lower abdomen and pelvis, and completes its expression through the arms and hands (Barrett 2006). Here's how to direct your weight and energy in this way. Think about how you use a flashlight when you walk in darkness: pointed in the direction that you want to see so that you know better where to step. Now, imagine that your lower abdomen is like a flashlight, shining with your vital energy. Direct that light toward your work by facing your abdomen and torso in the direction you want to shift your weight (Fig. 3.12). This will guide the direction of your feet, too, and your weight will easily rise and "fall" into your client as you lean into her. Then, your work can originate in your physical center and flow into your relaxed torso through your heart center and into your hands.

One common tendency of therapists unaccustomed to sidelying work is to sidebend the head and upper body rather than stay upright (Fig. 3.14A). Perhaps this occurs in an effort to align the eyes with the spine so that things look "normal," as when the client is prone. Sustained sidebending quickly becomes tiring and damaging, and you can't as readily focus your weight and energy into your hands. Remember to stay

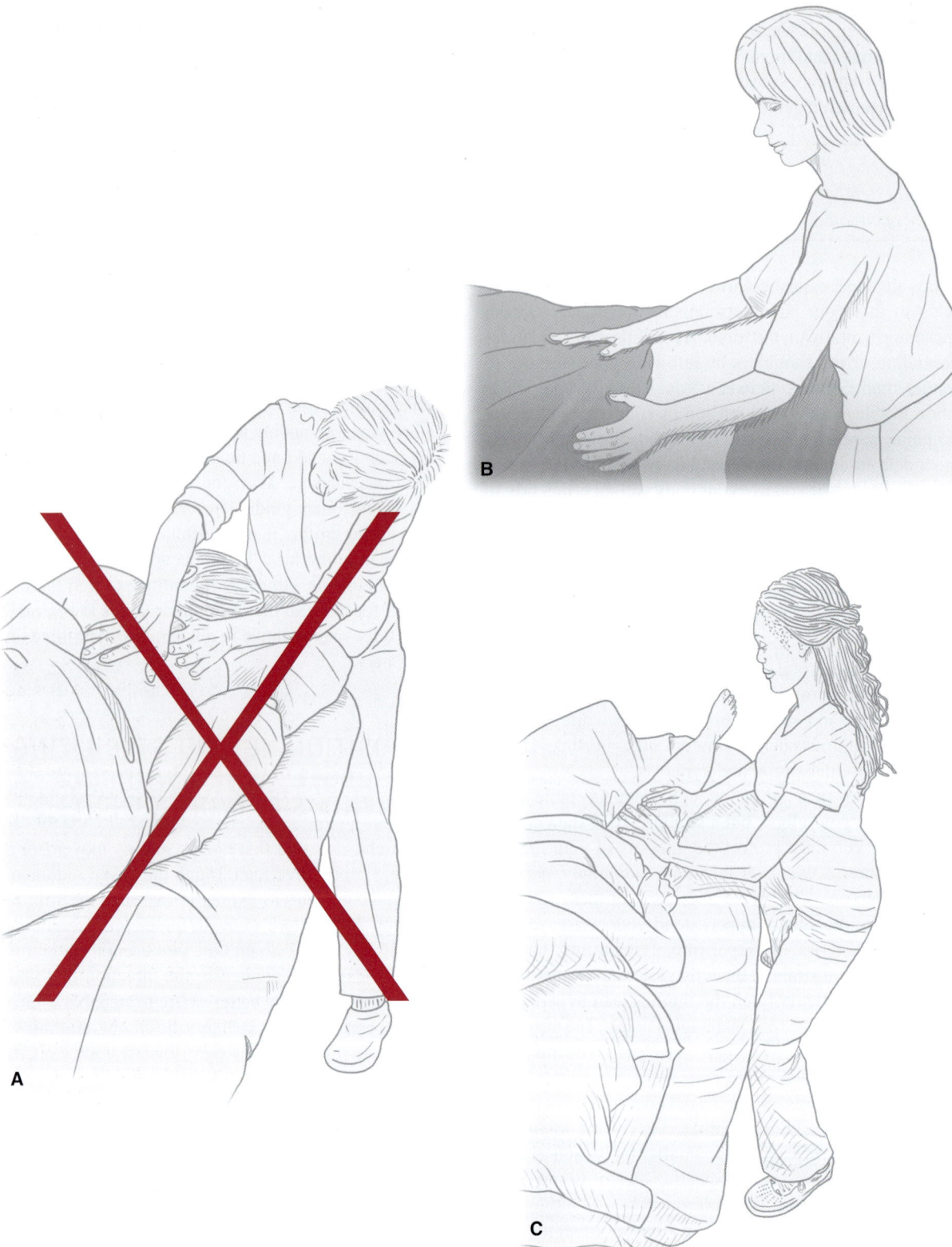

FIGURE 3.14 Body mechanics pointers. Compare the strain experienced by **(A)** the therapist who sidebends and slumps to **(B)** one who is upright and aligned. **(C)** Note the relaxed shoulders, use of the legs for power and momentum, and the vertical alignment of the pelvis with the rest of the spine in horse-riding stance.

Box 3.3

Principles for Body Mechanics

- Relax and expand into each joint.
- Guide direction of application of weight by pointing the lower abdomen in the direction of work.
- When in modified tee stance, gently flex the ankle, knee, and hip. Shift weight from the rear leg into the client. The front leg remains "empty" (reverse for traction).
- When in horse-riding stance, shift weight from foot to foot.
- When in bow stance, fluidly shift weight from leg to leg, beginning at your feet.
- Align spine and lengthen downward and upward with no excessive spinal curvatures.
- Lift the head at occiput to tuck the chin in.
- Lift sternum anterior and superior without overinflating the chest.
- Maintain balanced and horizontal pectoral girdle through engagement of serratus anterior.
- Maintain open and balanced shoulder, elbow, wrist, and finger joints.
- Breathe fully from deep in the abdomen, expanding/compressing in all directions on each breath cycle.

upright as you work. Move your eyes rather than your head and neck. Bend at your hips or knees and not at your waist or lateral ribcage if you need to get lower (Fig. 3.14B).

From this modified tee stance, you can accomplish movements away from the client's body, too, such as many traction stretches and return effleurage. Just start with your weight in your front foot instead. Gradually shift weight from your front foot to back foot, again emptying your front foot. To get a fuller traction, bend deeper into your hip and knee joints to leverage more of your weight.

OTHER BODY MECHANICS POINTERS

The horizontal direction of your work on the sidelying client means that you will sometimes need to modify techniques so that she remains safely and comfortably aligned. For example, when effleuraging the lateral thigh, anchor her knee with one hand exerting a slight traction toward you. This will counterbalance the force of your other hand, which is pushing her leg and pelvis toward the back of the table. Another common stabilizing hand placement would be to gently mold your hand around the ceiling-side ilium to prevent the pelvis rotating toward the table when you work along the gluteal and lateral rotator attachments along the sacrum.

You will sometimes do procedures that require you to squarely face the side of the table, such as petrissage. This is when the horse-riding stance is more efficient. With the table higher for sidelying, you will not need to sink low into your knees and hips as when at a lower table. In this stance, vertical polarity and expansional balance principles still apply, as does the flashlight concept, discussed above. Shift your weight between your feet to power your arms for techniques. Allow your torso to rotate around your lower abdomen, much like a washing machine agitator would move (Fig. 3.14C).

This position is often best when you need to lift an arm or leg for passive movements. Remember to use your legs rather than your back to lift. Bend into your knees, encircle the thigh or arm, and then straighten your knees to lift. Even the strength of your leg muscles might not be sufficient to comfortably lift and maneuver a very large woman's leg. When your client's size is too large for you to safely lift, eliminate these types of techniques and address her needs with techniques that will not be risky for you (Frye 2010).

Particularly when working on the table-side of the back, working seated can be efficient. Use an adjustable stool so that you can get your hands level with your work without elevating your pectoral girdle. Plant your feet firmly on the floor, even though most of the actual weight shifts must result from your ischial tuberosities pressing into the stool, thereby functioning as the feet do when standing. Of course, always maintain expansional balance and spinal alignment with the head erect, too.

Your own self-care is as critical to your body mechanics as how you actually organize yourself at the table. Maintain your flexibility and strength with regular stretching and exercise. Replenish your energy with rest, healthy nutrition, recreation, and other activities that bring you peace and rejuvenation.

Body mechanics are about the efficient organization and use of your body's energy and structure to perform your work. It is not a static posture, but rather the dynamic flow of how you use pressure, speed, strength, direction, subtlety, and energy. It involves not just what you are doing to the client but what you are feeling from the client and your sensitivity in responding to those signals. Equipment, stance, weight shift, and alignment are critical but useless if you forget to do one other thing, breathe! Engage your diaphragm fully for maximum oxygen and waste exchange. Your breathing will be less effortful and your upper body more relaxed, which, in turn, translate into softer, more powerful touch. Fuller breathing means more rhythm and dynamic in your work, more parasympathetic effect that you can transmit to your client, and more energy for you (Osborne 2002).

CHAPTER SUMMARY

A cozy, well-equipped room; a safely and comfortably positioned, draped client; and a dynamic, focused therapist: this chapter has equipped you to achieve all of these and has moved you from theory to practicalities. You are now ready to make your way through the trimesters of pregnancy and learn specific techniques to meet your clients' maternity needs.

Test Yourself

For answers, visit the website at http://thePoint.LWW.com/Osborne-Pregnancy2e!

1. List five primary considerations for establishing a good environment for prenatal and perinatal massage therapy.

2. List five features of a desirable prenatal massage table.

3. List five pieces of equipment, besides a table, that are essential for a maternity massage therapy practice.

4. What are the degree of angle and the section of the body that must be elevated in semireclined position to ensure that the vena cava is not compressed?

5. List the most efficient sequence of pillow and support placement for sidelying positioning.

6. What is the recommended size for a covering sheet and for breast drapes?

7. When a client lies down or gets up from your table, how should she do this to best protect her abdominal muscles from strain at the linea alba?

8. What piece of equipment will make ascending and descending from your table safer?

9. In the modified tee stance, what parts of your body are weight bearing when you are doing a technique?

10. What is the general principle for aligning your torso for the most direct line of weight shift?

REFERENCES

Barrett R. Taijiquan: Through the Western Gate. Berkeley: Blue Snake Books, 2006.

Burman I, Friedland S. TouchAbilities: Essential Connections. Clifton Park: Thomson/Delmar Learning, 2006.

Cheng M. Master Cheng's New Method of T'aichi Ch'uan Self-Cultivation. Berkeley: Blue Snake Books, 1999.

Frye B. Body Mechanics for Manual Therapists. 3rd Ed. Baltimore: Lippincott Williams & Wilkins, 2010.

Maupin E. A Dynamic Relation to Gravity, vol 1. San Diego: Dawn Eve Press, 2005.

Osborne, C. Deep Tissue Sculpting. 2nd Ed. San Diego: Body Therapy Associates, 2002.

For additional resources, please visit http://thePoint.LWW.com/Osborne-Pregnancy2e!

Trimester Recommendations

Learning Objectives

After study of this chapter, you should be able to:

1. List two to five major maternal physiological changes that typically occur during each of the three trimesters.
2. List two to five major maternal structural or functional changes that typically occur during each of the three trimesters.
3. List two to five typical emotional concerns that develop during pregnancy.
4. List safe positioning options for massage therapy in each trimester.
5. Adapt your therapy sessions for the general concerns of each trimester and for the unique, individual needs of your client.
6. Perform massage and therapeutic bodywork techniques that address typical prenatal discomforts.

Every woman's pregnancy is a unique experience that follows predictable developmental stages. Most pregnant women share typical changes in each 3-month trimester. A pregnant woman's body adapts exquisitely toward the goal of fostering a healthy pregnancy. Initiated hormonally and manifested functionally, these adaptations usually ensure a healthy and normal pregnancy, with no medical emergencies involved. Regardless of their normalcy, some stages and changes create pain, discomforts, and concerns that challenge a woman's physical and emotional resiliency.

About 80% of babies stay in the womb long enough and grow big enough, and their moms' bodies support that process without illness, a fact that should give confidence to all prenatal and perinatal massage therapists (Gibbs et al. 2008). As a facilitator of health, well-being, and physical and emotional comfort, you are uniquely positioned to support this "normal" model of pregnancy. Your words, information, body language, and massage therapy sessions can exude this confidence and strength when you are knowledgeable about each trimester's adaptations.

To respond appropriately to both her individualized and characteristic needs, you must understand and respect these changes. Each trimester requires specific considerations for positioning and safety protocols. As her needs fluctuate and grow with her maturing fetus, you will need to select appropriate, effective, and safe techniques to include in your sessions with her. This chapter is your theoretical and technique handbook for nurturing the births of mothers and their babies.

You can adapt virtually all therapeutic massage and bodywork methods for maternity work if you understand the necessary modifications. You'll find a variety of general suggestions for effective therapeutic somatic activities appropriate for each trimester. Additionally, you will learn, one by one, powerful and nurturing individual techniques to specifically address your client's issues of concern, areas of discomfort, and perhaps pain. You'll find video segments in the online resources at http://thePoint.lww.com/Osborne-Pregnancy2e to further refine your understanding and performance of these procedures. Of course, qualified hands-on instruction in these methods will be the final step in bringing them to the childbearing women in your practice. (See online resources for a list of certification programs available.)

First Trimester (Weeks 1 to 13)

Watching the pregnancy test stick indicate "positive," a woman confirms what her tender, swollen breasts and her queasy stomach have been telling her for the 2 weeks since her menstrual period was due. She's pregnant! From two cells uniting, the embryo will grow to a recognizable human shape during these first 13 weeks, and her body and her emotions will begin to reflect that growth. This section will guide you in tailoring your work to this early gestational period (Fig. 4.1).

See Box 4.1 for a summary of maternal developments during this trimester.

● MATERNAL AND FETAL DEVELOPMENT

An intricate sequence of hormonal communications immediately begins preparing the newly pregnant body for the 9 months of creative activity ahead (Fig. 4.2). Human chorionic gonadotrophin (hCG), a hormone detected in home urine pregnancy tests, ensures adequate first trimester hormonal levels. The fertilized egg itself manages the pregnancy for the first few days before the placenta takes over, an example of how well the body works to ensure a viable pregnancy.

The mother's endocrine glands and ovaries enlarge and accelerate hormonal production that causes extensive maternal physiological adaptations. In its functions as an endocrine organ, the placenta produces additional estrogen and progesterone and other pregnancy-specific hormones (see online resources for more about the placenta). These powerful chemicals stimulate positive changes that increase fuel and vitamin and mineral supplies, ensuring sufficient maternal energy levels and robust fetal growth. These changes include increased energy storage in the form of fat in the thighs, buttocks, and abdomen.

Progesterone also relaxes smooth muscle linings of the following: (1) the digestive tract, thus maximizing intestinal absorption time and uptake of iron, calcium, and other nutrients; (2) the uterine muscles, to prevent excessive, premature contractions; and (3) the vascular walls, to maintain a healthy, low blood pressure. The hormone relaxin, working

> **Box 4.1**
>
> **First Trimester Common Maternal Developments**
> - Enlarged, tender breasts
> - Emotional and hormonal adjustments
> - Fatigue
> - Frequent urination
> - Morning sickness or all day nausea and/or vomiting

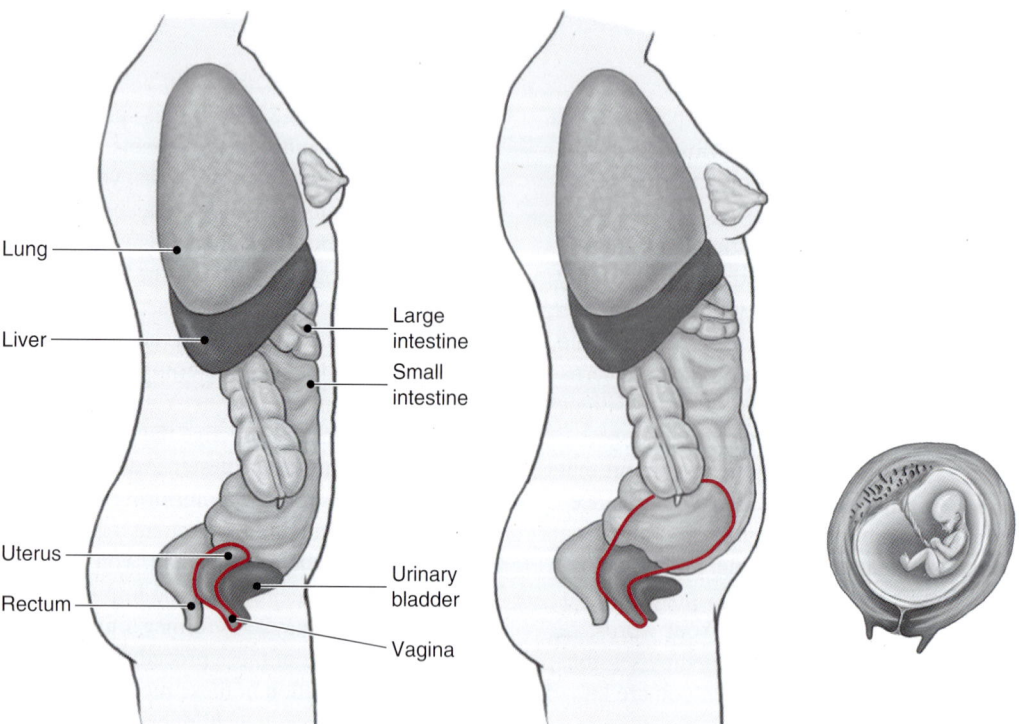

FIGURE 4.1 First trimester of pregnancy. From its non-pregnant size (left), the uterus grows until it can usually be felt halfway up to the maternal umbilicus (right). Inside (inset), the fertilized egg grows through an embryonic stage into a fetus with all body systems functioning. It floats in a sac of amniotic fluid, nourished through the placenta attached in the thickened uterine muscle walls. The fetus is protected from outside bacterial invasion by a mucous plug that seals the now-softened and more vascularized cervical opening.

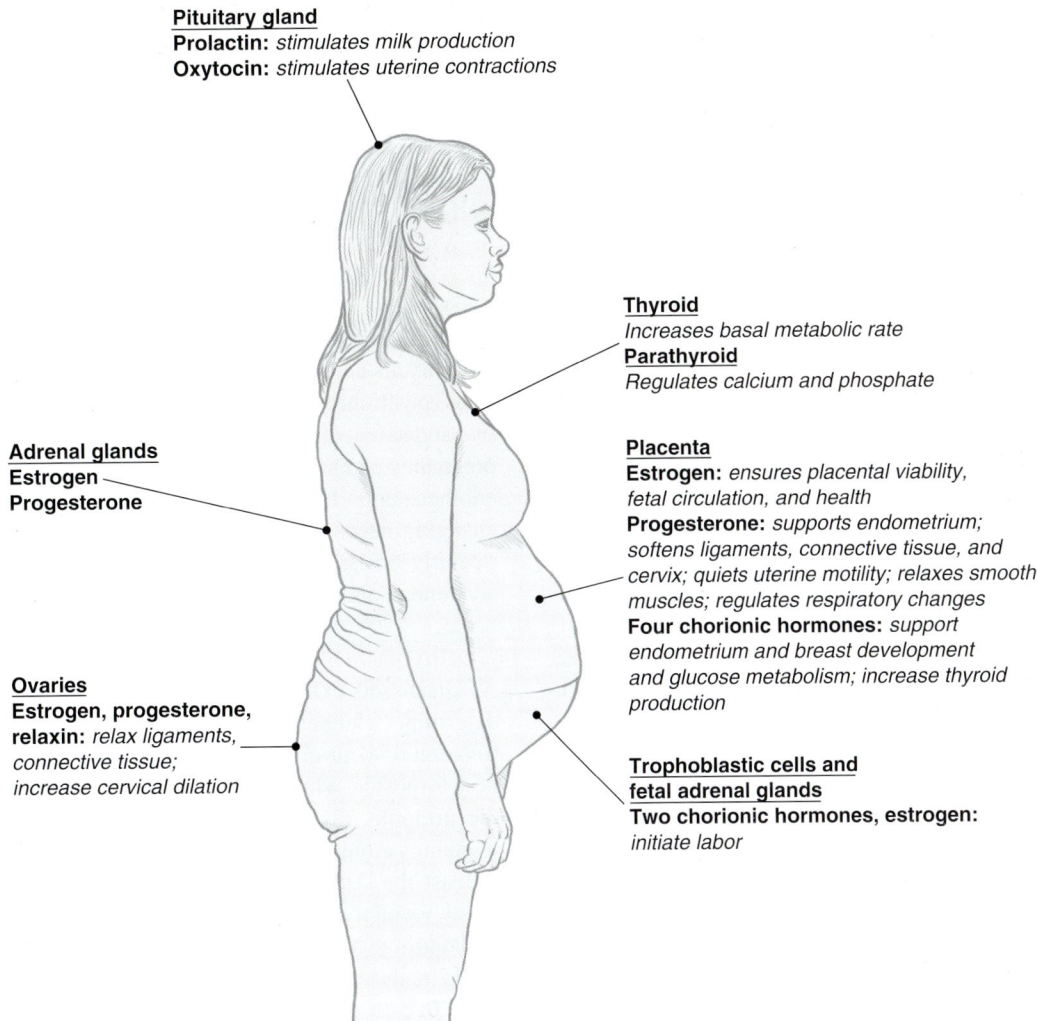

FIGURE 4.2 Prenatal endocrine activity. Beginning in the first trimester and throughout pregnancy, many maternal organs (underlined and bold) produce pregnancy-related hormones (bold) that have far-ranging effects on both mother and fetus (italic). Note that multiple production sites are necessary to produce adequate levels of some hormones.

with progesterone, softens connective tissue so that joints and soft tissues accommodate the new growth, peaking in the 14th week and again at labor's onset. Another of progesterone's effects is increased respiratory efficiency characterized by greater tidal volume in the lungs and faster respiratory rate to handle increased cardiac output.

Meanwhile, estrogen stimulates the following: (1) uterine growth and blood supply; (2) balanced salt, water, and insulin levels; (3) and increased metabolic efficiency in sugar and carbohydrate use. These vital hormonal adaptations are evidence of the body's "wisdom" in sustaining a healthy pregnancy. They are also responsible, in part, for the mother's initial 3 months of exhaustion, urinary frequency, and, often, morning sickness.

In this most developmentally critical trimester, the embryo grows from a microscopic fertilized egg into a 3-inch fetus weighing 1 oz. It has a developing body, including eyes, ears, and a beating heart. As the fetus grows, so does the supportive placenta, usually firmly implanted on the upper (**fundus**), posterior uterine wall. Vascularly intertwined with the uterine blood vessels, it is the fetal conduit for nourishment and oxygen, as well as its waste removal system. Infused with estrogen, the uterus itself grows to one third larger than normal, from plum to grapefruit size.

Though her abdomen may not look identifiably pregnant in this first trimester, the newly pregnant woman's waistline widens. Her sensitive breasts continue to swell, and pressure on them is often painful. In these early weeks, the expectant woman may feel unusually tired. After one or two naps each day, she may collapse early in the evening for 9 or 10 hours of sleep; however, frequent urination brought on by hormonal influences and the enlarged uterus pressing on her bladder will probably interrupt this much-needed sleep (Gibbs et al. 2008).

Some women experience no nausea; however, 60% to 80% have a very queasy stomach in the morning or early evening, and many are hypersensitive to smells (Gibbs et al. 2008). Some women may even suffer nausea and vomiting all day during this time. Although unpleasant for the mother, one evolutionary biologist, Margie Profet, has theorized from her work with plant toxins that this may offer some evolutionary benefit. Morning sickness may prevent women from ingesting toxins that cause fetal malformations in this critical first trimester. She suggests that women follow their instincts toward blander foods to ease morning sickness (Profet 1995).

Structural stresses to the newly pregnant woman's body are minimal in these first 13 weeks. Increased breast size initiates an inevitable postural and functional shift in her structural organization. The thoracic spine and rib cage may begin to collapse with the weight of the breasts and as a protective posture for sore breasts and upset stomach. The pectoral girdle may tend to rotate anteriorly, further compressing the rib cage. Her head shifts forward with her chin more lifted. As her body makes these postural adjustments, a woman whose prepregnant posture is swaybacked may begin tilting her pelvis even farther forward into lordosis.

Although a woman in her first trimester is usually overjoyed, even the most desired pregnancy may prompt fear, worry, regret, or sometimes anger or a fatalistic feeling. She is embarking on a transformative journey that will leave no part of her unchanged. Especially in the first trimester, fear of miscarriage or debate about **abortion** may distract her, as well as guilt about prior drug use, lifestyle choices, or health issues. Even this early, typical worries about the actual birth might begin to percolate. Other women have supreme trust in their body's natural wisdom and power to grow and birth their baby. They seldom fret or become anxious and glide through their pregnancies in a gestational euphoria. Be alert and aware that some childbearing women may want your empathetic ear to explore these issues.

Many women's partners are happy and anticipatory of their baby's birth. Remember that they might also need support and nurturing, particularly if they sometimes feel isolated, trapped, jealous, angry, disconnected, or fearful. Some partners are worried about failure, financial stresses, rejection, and older children, and their own memories of life issues and traumas can begin to stir (Simkin et al. 2010).

● CONSIDERATIONS AND GUIDELINES FOR PRACTITIONERS

Your safe practice of first trimester prenatal massage therapy requires an understanding of precautions and contraindications, positioning for massage sessions, and selecting effective and safe techniques. Working with a woman early in her pregnancy can help launch her into the process. You become another support person, one who carefully responds to her changing needs and who can be a reassuring authority, particularly on issues of stress reduction, comfort, kinesthetic awareness, and functional activities.

Contraindications and Precautions

As discussed extensively in Chapter 2, you will need to determine whether massage therapy is advisable and safe for each of your clients. This is of particular concern in the first trimester, when more pregnancy losses occur. Review the previous discussion of this topic carefully. Unless a woman is already a client of yours, she will likely wait until at least the second trimester to schedule massage therapy. Many women are so fatigued that making time for massage is daunting. Many would rather just rest. If she is excessively nauseated, she may not feel well enough for a session. In any of these cases, postponing sessions until the second trimester is often wise. If you do decide to proceed, schedule massage sessions at the time of day when the

Points of View: Sacral and Lumbar Work

Yet another area of discrepancy among pregnancy massage instructors (Stager 2010; Stillerman 2008; Yates 2010) involves work to the sacrum and lumbar areas, particularly in the first trimester and up to 18 to 20 weeks. Some instructors teach that deep massage in these areas can cause miscarriage. One argument made is that deep stimulation of the sacral nerves might affect the uterus negatively. This seems unfounded as these nerves are deep to the sacrum. Another argument centers around misconstrued prohibitions related to creating a "downbearing" effect through gliding over acupuncture and acupressure points below the first lumbar vertebra (similar fears are perpetrated about foot and lower leg points).

A less alarmist precaution that avoids deeply focused, pointed pressure into Bladder 31 and 32 points associated with the sacral sulcuses protects those women whose pregnancies and general health might make them more vulnerable to strong stimuli of these points (particularly in first trimester). Broader pressure to the sacrum is not only safe but often indicated for all expectant clients, depending on their posture, activity, gait, and injuries.

One instructor cautions against quadratus lumborum and piriformis work particularly in the first 8 weeks due to the proximity of these muscles to the now-enlarged uterus. This seems unfounded as the uterus begins to outgrow the full protection of the pelvis only after the first trimester, the rule of thumb being at approximately 20 weeks the fundus is usually at umbilical height. It doesn't fill the abdomen laterally to the QL until 20 to 26 weeks. Certainly after that point, you must be precise in locating the QL posterior of the midline of the torso and compressing into it without also directly compressing the lateral side of the uterus.

Excessive caution about "forbidden areas" conveys fragility in the pregnant body that is unfounded and that may contribute to fear the woman may already have as she begins her pregnancy—that the pregnancy is so vulnerable and that she is a miscarriage waiting to happen.

pregnant woman is most comfortable and least tired and/or nauseated.

Because of the statistically higher incidence of pregnancy losses, you must take great care in the first trimester when massaging the abdomen and points that can potentially stimulate uterine contractions (see Chapter 2 for detailed precautions). This added precaution will seldom compromise women's needs, as you can reflexively address any abdominal organs needing attention.

Remember to observe all contraindications and precautions detailed in Chapter 2, especially the following:

- Avoid altogether or carefully consider abdominal touching (legal precaution).
- Avoid reflexive pressure to points on the lower legs, feet, hands, sacrum, and upper back.
- Avoid rhythmic rocking movements when she's nauseated.
- Although compromise of femoral veins is usually minimal in the first trimester, begin to limit techniques on the medial leg and inguinal area to soft, whole-hand pressure.
- Use a gentle, yet firm touch with all techniques moderated to an experience of pleasure on the borderline of pain as maximum depth.

Positioning

Most positions are safe for first trimester massage therapy: supine, prone, sidelying, semireclining, or seated. Only minor adaptations are necessary for safety and comfort. In particular, if using the prone position, assess whether her abdomen is still small enough for the anterior superior iliac spines to entirely protect the uterus from an increase in internal pressure. Remember that your pressure on her back results in her abdomen pressing against the table; be sure that the bony arches of the pelvis provide the needed protection. Some women's breasts will be too tender for her to lie face down, even with additional support. Remember to use pillow or bolster support under the knees to reduce lumbar curvature when in supine position (see Chapter 3 for details).

> **REMINDER:** *Listen openly and objectively to the full spectrum of emotional responses that a newly expectant woman usually has.*

Selecting Effective Techniques

In the early weeks of pregnancy, focus massage therapy on relief for fatigue, nausea, and other physiological adjustments (Fig. 4.3). When techniques require lubrication, remember the guidelines in Chapter 2, being particularly careful to not increase nausea with strong scents. Suggest that she empty her bladder immediately prior to her session, and accommodate her urinary frequency at midpoint in the session, if necessary.

Expect the newly pregnant woman to have a high need for relaxation and empathetic listening; self-care information; reading recommendations and guidance in preparing for

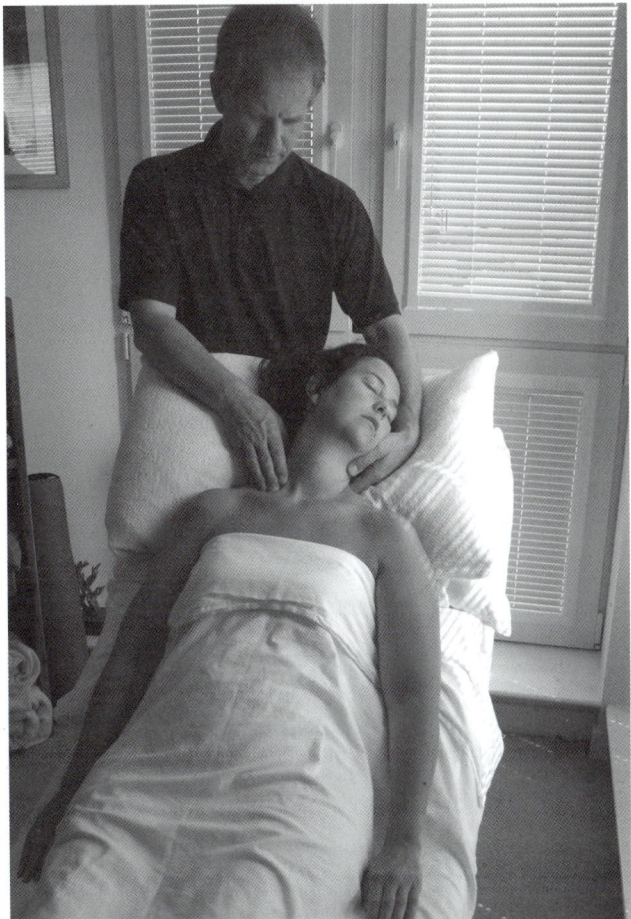

FIGURE 4.3 As breasts double in size and stress builds, upper body strain is more likely. Include therapeutic massage of pectoral and neck structures and look to relieve any nausea. (Follow this client's prenatal growth and sessions in Figs. 4.5 and 4.9, and online.)

the months ahead. (See online resources for a recommended reading list and websites.) Encourage her to consult with her healthcare provider and begin appropriate exercises for pelvic floor and abdominal strengthening and for stretching of tight muscles (Calais-Germain 2003; Mayo Clinic 2010).

● SUMMARY OF RECOMMENDED BODYWORK

Women in their first trimester will benefit most from the following therapeutic somatic activities:

- Body-use education in diaphragmatic breathing, pelvic positioning, iliopsoas development, and other postural alignment and structural balancing; awareness of and appropriate strengthening of abdominal and pelvic floor muscles
- Experiences of deep relaxation, internal focus, and awareness, through touch, visualizations, and other relaxation techniques
- Cross-fiber friction, deep tissue, trigger point, and joint mobilizations techniques to reduce strain to the joints

What Would You Do?

An established, very athletic client of yours comes in for her quarterly massage and happily announces that she is 9 weeks pregnant! She usually enjoys a very deep, cleansing Swedish and deep tissue massage, particularly addressing her tendency toward constipation and an extreme lumbar lordosis. She has also recently increased her preparation for a 5K race next month that she still intends to run, as long as her fairly intense nausea eases up by then. This is the third pregnancy for this 28-year-old woman. She has no high risk factors and has had no problems with her previous pregnancies. Her midwife expects this to also be a low-risk, uncomplicated pregnancy.

What changes in your usual positioning and techniques to address her constipation and lumbar lordosis are advisable? Staying within your scope of practice, what might you teach her and what techniques might be effective in helping her be more comfortable with her pregnancy-related discomforts?

and soft tissue of the upper spine and pectoral girdle, especially the cervical, scapulothoracic, and rib cage joints and the following muscles: trapezius, rhomboidei, erector spinae, levator scapulae, supraspinatus, scalenes, suboccipitals, and pectoralis major and minor
- Nurturing, gentle touch to reduce stress, create a supportive, caring experience, and to help illuminate for the mother her body's amazing adaptations
- Nonjudgmental, **active listening** and other somatoemotional processing to assist her in assimilating feelings

My Story

My work with Ashley actually began in the 18 months prior to her first successful pregnancy. She had just miscarried after 10 years of trying to get pregnant, including extensive fertility treatments. How sad and angry she was! A "caretaker" and hard worker, she wanted to clear her feelings, become more in tune with herself and her true goals, and be more receptive to her natural fertility.

Over the course of our bimonthly sessions, with committed lifestyle changes, and after a session when she yielded to her image of her nurturing grandmother, she conceived again. We evolved, together, a visualization of her breath holding this baby protectively inside her. We focused on relaxation, particularly in her legs, pelvis, and computer-cramped neck and upper back. What an achievement and joy for her to deliver her naturally conceived daughter later that year!

—Carole Osborne, San Diego, CA

and emotional issues that she may be experiencing. Provide appropriate referrals to other professionals, as needed.
- Circulatory, craniosacral, and reflexive techniques to assist relaxation, reduce stress and fatigue, relieve nausea and other digestive disturbances, and support the normal and unfolding general prenatal physiological processes

These general guidelines and foci will help you identify techniques you already know that may be adaptable for your first trimester clients. You will find numerous specific techniques from some of these somatic therapies detailed in this chapter's technique manual that follows. (See sequential first trimester session sample online.)

Second Trimester (weeks 14 to 26)

Most pregnant women usually enjoy weeks 14 through 26. Many women feel as though their pregnancies, especially these 3 months, are the most vibrant and vital times of their lives. By this point, she has adjusted hormonally and usually has adapted her nutrition, exercise, and daily routines to nurture her pregnancy. She has an identifiably pregnant contour. Her baby's rhythmic heartbeat and subtle, first movements confirm the reality of her pregnancy.

More than half of surveyed prenatal massage therapists said that their expectant clients begin receiving bodywork in this trimester (Osborne 2009). To be prepared for such women in your practice, you will need to broaden and develop your repertoire for this trimester's characteristic needs.

See Box 4.2 for a summary of maternal developments during this trimester.

Box 4.2

Second Trimester Maternal Developments and Safe Positioning

Common Maternal Developments
- Pregnancy seems more real
- Increased weight
- Back, pelvic, hip, and leg pain may develop
- Round and broad ligament pain
- Stretch marks and other skin and hair changes
- Varicose and/or spider veins
- Constipation and/or heartburn

Safe Positioning
- Supine, with pillow under right hip, up to 22 weeks
- After 22 weeks, switch to semireclining rather than extended supine position
- Sidelying
- Seated

● MATERNAL AND FETAL DEVELOPMENT

Although the expectant second trimester woman may relish her fertile development, she may also begin to feel additional structural stresses. By now, her hormonally softened joints prompt postural adjustments to increased weight, and she experiences a definite shift in her center of gravity. Her baby will grow in this trimester to between 11 and 14 inches, weighing about 1½ lb. Increased to melon size, her uterus reaches her umbilicus. With this growth, her abdominal and lumbar musculature may become fatigued.

Chronic shortening begins to develop in the spinal extensor muscles and the entire posterior myofascial sheath. This superficial back line or articulated myofascial chain extends from the plantar surface of the foot, along the paravertebral musculature, to the skull. It is one of the main "anatomy trains" described by author and Rolfer, Thomas Myers (2009). Prenatal posture changes can influence balance and functioning anywhere on this line. As normal balance diminishes among the abdominal, iliopsoas, and paravertebral muscles, maintaining good posture is more difficult, and she may experience some pelvic and back pain.

Relaxin has mostly accomplished its softening job, allowing gradual adaptation to this trimester's increase in fetal size. With this growth, women often feel the need to compensate for the anterior shift in their center of balance by broadening their standing base. To protect, nurture, and prevent falling, most create a wider stance, by rotating the femur more laterally in the acetabulum. This also creates more area in the pelvis for growth, but muscles and ligaments around the hip joints may begin to strain. She also may feel compressed in these joints, and in her knees and feet, depending on her weight gain.

The uterus not only grows in the second trimester, but it also lifts higher and more into the abdominal cavity (Fig. 4.4). This change usually allows more room for the urinary bladder to fill, bringing some relief from the first trimester's frequent urination. Unfortunately, this growth also may produce intermittent, sharp pain in her lower abdomen, groin, and perhaps down one leg as the uterine round ligaments stretch. Some women describe this as feeling like a rubber band snapping in their groin. It most often occurs with sudden movements of standing from sitting, uncrossing the legs, or when driving. Referred pain in the lumbar and gluteal musculature from the uterine broad ligaments is also common (see Fig. 1.8).

> **REMINDER:** *The second trimester is often a robust 3 months for the pregnant woman. Enhance her enjoyment of this trimester with guidance and techniques that support her postural integrity.*

She also may begin to hyperventilate and suffer heartburn in this trimester. Progesterone's continuing relaxation of smooth muscle loosens the pelvic floor sphincter muscles. With increased uterine weight also stressing them, some

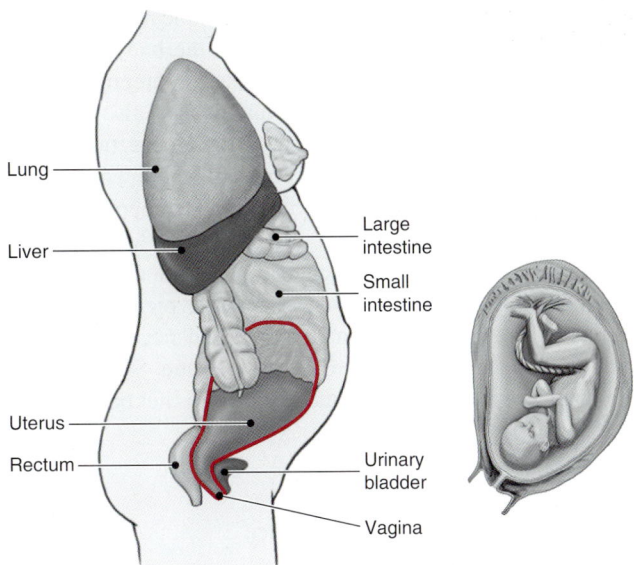

FIGURE 4.4 Fifth month of pregnancy. The middle trimester is a developmental period when fetal organs and structures enlarge and mature, hair grows, and senses, especially touch and hearing, become functional. The uterus begins to push abdominal organs superiorly, posteriorly, and laterally as it enlarges to umbilical level, contributing to gastrointestinal and musculoskeletal discomforts, particularly in the pelvis, hips, and back.

women have urinary stress incontinent episodes. As her uterus and breasts grow, she may discover that her skin feels taut, itchy, and stretched to the point that prominent reddish lines may appear on her abdomen, breasts, buttocks, or thighs, where the connective tissue and the skin have torn.

In addition to stretchmarks, she also may notice many other estrogen-related effects. Some women have increased skin oiliness, acne, and/or hair loss or texture changes, whereas most enjoy smooth, clear, radiant skin and hair. All mucous membranes, including those in the sinuses and vagina, produce more fluid, making sinus congestion and the need for a small pantiliner common (that's often why she will keep her underwear on for her massage sessions). A thin brown line from the pubic bone up to the umbilicus (**linea nigra**) will darken on her now protruding abdomen. Her areola, nipples, and vulva will become even bluish black, depending on her skin pigmentation. A "mask of pregnancy," (**chloasma**) with dark splotches over her forehead, nose, and cheeks, may appear (See Fig. 1.5). She may develop spider veins and/or varicose veins in her legs or rectum (**hemorrhoids**), or at least constipation or strained bowel movements.

Often, the emotional highlight of the second trimester is feeling first movements and hearing the baby's heartbeat. Barely perceptible butterfly-like fluttering in her abdomen will have gradually developed into distinctive rolling, prodding, sliding, and rhythmic movements by weeks 20 to 26. With the aid of a specialized stethoscope or other instruments, her healthcare provider will help her hear the brisk, strong heartbeat of her baby.

Joyous greetings and ongoing communications between the woman and her baby, and between the baby and other family members and friends, will make the pregnancy both more real and personal. But this reality may also generate changes in roles and relationships with the spouse, family, and friends, and cause financial concerns and health worries.

Some women delight in the full, rounded appearance of their breasts, hips, and belly during pregnancy. Many women discover a new sensitivity to their bodies and relish their heightened sexual responsiveness, more typical in this trimester. Others may feel unattractive, and negativity about physical appearance may surface at this time. She may also endure rejection by her husband or partner as her body rounds during pregnancy (Simkin et al. 2010).

● CONSIDERATIONS AND GUIDELINES FOR PRACTITIONERS

As in the first trimester, be alert to signs and symptoms of developing complications of pregnancy. Although most miscarriages occur in the first 13 weeks, later miscarriages and nonviable early births can happen in the second trimester. First-time mothers are more likely to develop pregnancy-induced hypertension, perhaps as early as the twentieth week (Simkin et al. 2010). Increased urination in the second trimester, when less frequent urination is the norm, can indicate gestational diabetes. Note symptoms of other complications and refer these clients to their healthcare providers. (See pregnancy complications, in Chapters 2 and 7.)

Interview clients thoroughly before beginning session work. Remember to update yourself with her developments and most recent checkups at each subsequent appointment. (See Chapter 8 for forms and pointers on both.) If her doctor has no concerns about her pregnancy's progress, then be assured of the pregnancy's normalcy. Of course, you and she should communicate with her midwife or physician if any signs of complications have occurred in the meantime. Observe all of the precautions, guidelines, and contraindications detailed in Chapter 2.

After the first trimester, light abdominal effleurage and rocking is usually soothing and always safe. Of course you won't massage the abdomen if specifically contraindicated by the woman's healthcare provider. If the risk of miscarriage or premature birth is high, you may be more comfortable skipping even light abdominal massage, although this is only a liability precaution. Even though strain to the abdominal and iliopsoas muscles and sluggishness in the colon are common, observe strict contraindications to massage therapy techniques requiring deep pressure into the abdomen. Other modalities, such as pelvic tilting, abdominal strengthening, and reflexive techniques applied on the feet or hands may promote safe relief in these areas.

Because blood clots may develop, avoid all techniques detailed in Chapter 2 that can potentially dislodge clots and cause embolisms. The closer to the pelvic bowl a clot forms, the more serious the consequences, so exercise special caution in the femoral triangle and in the inguinal region. It is safest to assume that all pregnant women have asymptomatic blood clots. Especially if varicose veins are visible, deeper veins may be similarly weakened and harboring blood clots.

Positioning

Adjustments for increased uterine size are a primary concern in this trimester. By this time, the uterus has outgrown the protective borders of the pelvic bowl, and the ASIS will no longer prevent increased intrauterine pressure when in prone position. The sidelying position is the safest position for massaging a pregnant woman's back and pelvis. With the client positioned securely on her side, the practitioner may then safely apply the deep pressure that may be necessary for relieving the posterior structures with little fear of increasing intrauterine pressure (see Chapter 2 for discussion of these topics).

As for supine position, you must now position to prevent supine hypotensive syndrome (see Chapter 2) with bolstering and/or semireclining positioning. Of course, when there are twins or triplets, you will have to make these same modifications earlier in her pregnancy. (Follow the instructions in Chapters 3 and 7 for creating secure, comfortable, and safe positions.)

Selecting Effective Techniques

Structural stresses on the weight-bearing joints and the myofascial structures of the back and hips intensify during the second trimester. Begin and complete each session with guidance in structural balance using visualizations and kinesthetic cues. Emphasize bodywork that is effective for relieving tension and muscle strain, fibrosis, myofascial pain, muscle cramping, and joint dysfunction in the spine, and in the pelvic and pectoral girdles. Include techniques and visualizations that enhance deep abdominal breathing. Carefully apply techniques at the hips and pelvic area that assist blood flow from the legs and reduce pelvic blood and fluid congestion (Fig. 4.5). Encourage her to frequently elevate her legs when sitting or lying to alleviate pooling of blood and ease the pain from edema or varicose veins.

Certain lubricants are helpful in relieving itchy, stretched skin, and they may be effective in minimizing stretch marks (Leduc 1993). One study documented a 22% decrease in the

What Would You Do?

After receiving results of diagnostic testing, your client decides to terminate the gestation of her fetus with a hereditary or congenital defect. What strategies will help you to stay present, nonjudgmental, and supportive of your client despite your own personal beliefs, feelings, and values?

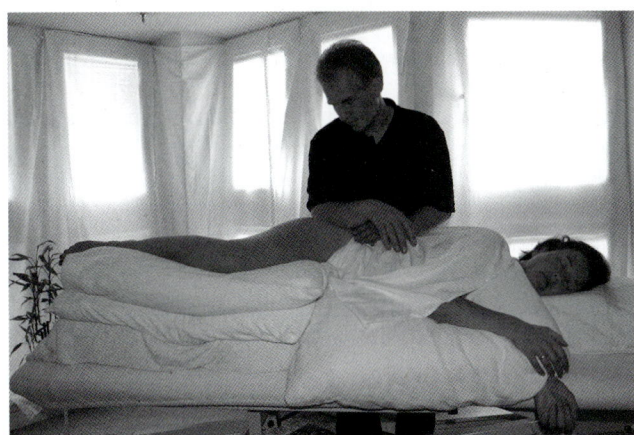

FIGURE 4.5 Second trimester prenatal massage sessions. Weeks 15 to 27. Weight gain and a shift in center of gravity begin to affect the pelvic girdle and hip structures during the second trimester. Clients enjoy deep work in the gluteals and around the hip joint.

likelihood of developing stretch marks when women massaged themselves with a cream including gotu kola extract (*Centella asiatica*), alpha tocopherol (a form of vitamin E), and collagen-elastin hydrolysates (enzymes) (Mallol et al. 1991). In addition to your use, beginning in months three or four, the woman may massage and friction these products, or cocoa butter, into her abdomen, hips, and thighs with a cloth twice daily to also activate skin circulation.

Fatigue contributes to another common pregnancy discomfort: calf cramps. Both the gastrocnemius-soleus complex and/or the peroneals may spasm, especially during the night, causing almost 50% of expectant women to awake in great pain. These cramps may begin in the second trimester, but more often occur in the third trimester (Gibbs et al. 2008). Passive stretching during cramping is effective and may help to prevent spasms when used daily. Also teach women and their partners to gently effleurage her legs and feet daily. Assisted-resisted exercise, kneading, and drainage techniques also assist in removal of waste products produced by cramping and reduce the likelihood of recurrence. (See online resources for specific techniques.) Remember to avoid compressing deeply into the medial surface of the calf, and remind her partner when teaching him. Maintain her foot in a neutral or dorsiflexed position when massaging her feet to prevent possibly inducing a cramp.

Most women thoroughly appreciate Swedish and joint mobilization techniques that ease aching, tired feet. Zone therapy on the feet may help to alleviate many common second trimester complaints: constipation, heartburn, headaches, hemorrhoids, and musculoskeletal pains. Remember to avoid bone-to-bone reflexive pressure at precautionary points detailed in Chapter 2.

Movement modalities also help to alleviate musculoskeletal aches and pains. Use table work modalities such as range of motion (ROM), rhythmic passive movements, and gentle stretching. See the technique manual later in this chapter for many specific techniques to address many of these second trimester needs. Encourage and teach her, if appropriate, to do the most essential of maternity exercises: pelvic tilting, abdominal strengthening, and pelvic floor strengthening (Noble 1995; Calais-Germain 2003). Help her to find other self-exploration modalities and daily exercise that can also increase her comfort as her baby grows: modified prenatal yoga classes, belly dancing, **Aston-Patterning** and walking, swimming and other aerobic conditioning. (See online resources at http://thePoint.lww.com/Osborne-Pregnancy2e.)

Various movements that you regularly include in your sessions can be problematic due to nausea, ligamental laxity, and symphysis pubis dysfunction (Fig. 4.6). Remember that relaxin-soften ligaments are more vulnerable to overstretching, and keep all movements well within normal joint ranges of motion, even if a woman's range exceeds the norm.

● SUMMARY OF RECOMMENDED BODYWORK

Pregnant women in weeks 14 to 26 will derive the most benefit from similar techniques in the bulleted list for the first trimester. In addition, use the following therapeutic activities:

- Cross-fiber friction, deep tissue, structural balancing, passive movements and mobilizations, and trigger point, techniques

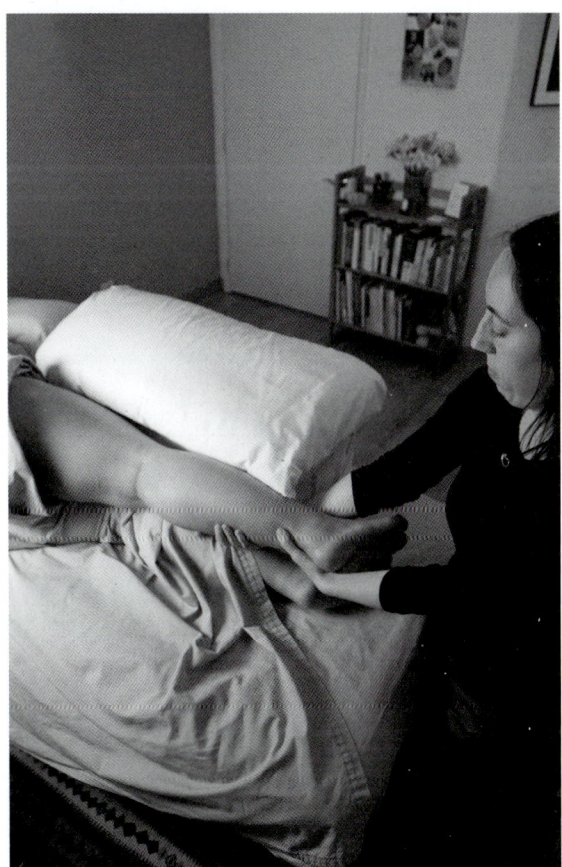

FIGURE 4.6 Movements to avoid during symphysis pubis pain. Avoid leg traction, unilateral pressure on the pelvis, and large-amplitude movements involving the hip joints when a client experiences sharp, midanterior pelvic pain.

to reduce strain to the upper and lumbar spine, especially the sacroiliac, lumbosacral, scapulothoracic, rib cage, and hip joints, the superficial back fascial line, and the erector spinae, intrinsic spinal extensors and rotators, hip rotators, trapezius, rhomboidei, levator scapulae, supraspinatus, scalenes, suboccipitals, pectoralis major and minor muscles
- Myofascial and postural alignment activities to relieve pain from strain to the uterine ligaments
- Swedish, stretching, and appropriate myofascial work to assist in preventing and/or relieving developing varicose veins, cramps, and fluid buildup in her feet and legs

These general guidelines and foci will help you identify techniques you already know that may be adaptable for your second trimester clients. You will find numerous specific techniques detailed in this chapter's technique manual that follows. (See sequential second trimester session sample online.)

Third Trimester (Weeks 27 to 40+)

Most musculoskeletal and physiological discomforts of pregnancy occur during these final weeks of pregnancy, motivating many women to seek massage therapy. In preparation for studying this section on working with third trimester clients, review Chapter 1 for descriptions of these changes and prenatal massage therapy's potential to help with them

See Box 4.3 for a summary of maternal developments during this trimester.

> **Box 4.3**
>
> ### Third Trimester Maternal Developments and Safe Positioning
>
> **Common Maternal Developments**
> - Eagerness and anxiety
> - Further weight gain
> - Increased back, pelvic, and hip pain
> - Diastasis recti
> - Symphysis pubis dysfunction
> - Hyperventilation
> - Heartburn, constipation, or hemorrhoids
> - Edema in feet and legs
> - Wrist or hand pain
> - Leg cramps and "restless leg" syndrome
> - Varicose veins
> - Urinary frequency
> - Braxton-Hicks contractions
> - Lightening
>
> **Safe Positioning**
> - Sidelying
> - Semireclining
> - Seated

● MATERNAL AND FETAL DEVELOPMENT

Pregnancy's final months and weeks often are bittersweet for a woman, as she longs to bask in the feeling of her newborn in her arms, yet is reluctant to move ahead to this new life phase. Her anticipation grows as she and the fetus dramatically increase in size. In this trimester, its weight will more than triple to a typical 7½ lb by birth, and it will almost double to 20 inches. All organ systems are developed by the eighth month, with the exception of the lungs.

This dramatic fetal growth increases anterior weight load and often results in typical musculoskeletal strain and discomfort for the mother detailed in Chapter 1. In summary, these changes include

- Sacroiliac and other lumbar joint and myofascial pain of peripartum pelvic pain syndrome
- Strain to all the uterine ligaments causing referred pain in the buttocks and lower back
- Diastis recti that further weakens the already stretched abdominal muscles, adding more strain to the iliopsoas
- Excessive lumbar curvature (lordosis) (Howard et al. 2000)
- Increased usage of the gluteus medius with chronic tension and trigger points developing here as a result
- Hip joint compression, chronic lateral femoral rotation with painful chronic tension in the deep lateral rotators
- Piriformis syndrome with neurological buttock and leg sensations, including pain, burning, and/or numbness
- Lateral femoral cutaneous nerve compression creating numbness and pain along the anterolateral thigh (Herman 2004)

Relaxin will continue to prepare her pelvis to accommodate the emerging infant. This may mean less pain for those with fibromyalgia and tight ligaments, but more pelvic instability for all. In these last weeks, some women develop dysfunction of the symphysis pubis. They find walking, climbing stairs, rolling over on a therapy table, standing from a seated position, and getting in and out of a car will cause sharp anterior midpelvic pain (Howard 2000).

She will likely experience some normal edema or fluid retention in her feet and legs that may result in varicose veins, carpal or tarsal tunnel syndrome, or posturally induced thoracic outlet syndrome (Herman 2004).

Because the fundus will reach the rib cage, the third trimester woman will become increasingly short of breath, and she may have heartburn, hiatal hernia, constipation, and hemorrhoids (Fig. 4.7). With all of these changes, many women have difficulty with some of their normal activities and are uncomfortable sleeping—reasons that they need more massage in this trimester.

Pregnancy's latest weeks may bring her some welcome relief from shortness of breath as her baby prepares for labor by dropping lower into her pelvis, its head "engaged" against

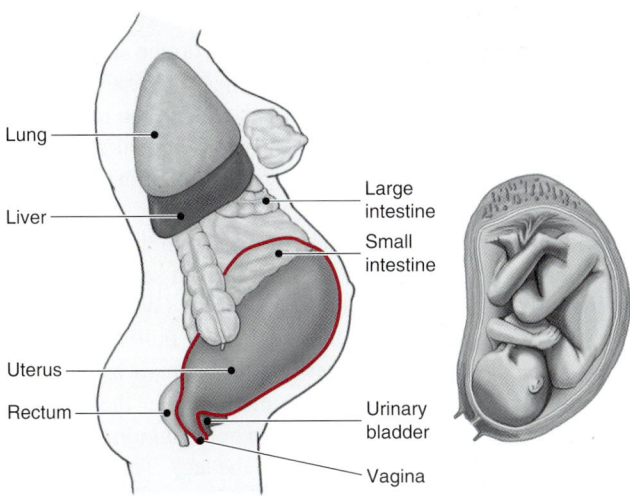

FIGURE 4.7 Ninth month of pregnancy. Now the fetus responds to bright light and familiar sounds, and it chooses a favorite position, usually head down. This is primarily a growth period, and it compresses and displaces all of the maternal pelvic, abdominal, and thoracic organs. Postural muscles must work hard to maintain optimal alignment.

the cervix; however, increased urinary frequency may also result as the baby's head compresses her urinary bladder to less than one third its normal size.

> *REMINDER: Individualizing and emphasizing breath awareness and capability can increase your client's enjoyment of pregnancy and her ability to cope with its challenges.*

As her due date approaches, the estrogen/progesterone balance begins to shift, and the uterus "wakes up" to the bigger baby's weight and movements. The uterus will begin "practice contractions" as the uterine muscle fibers tense irregularly for 15- to 30-second intervals. Although these contractions are usually light, some women find them mildly painful. Changes in activity and position usually will dissipate them. These contractions accomplish only minimal cervical dilatation and effacement, but they do begin to psychologically prepare her for laboring. While called "false labor," most women find these contractions quite real!

Labor begins only if these early contractions dilate the cervix to 2 cm, last 30 seconds or longer, become more rhythmic, and continue regularly each 4 to 20 minutes. Because prematurity is one of the major causes of newborn complications and deaths, the baby may be at significant risk if labor occurs prior to 37 weeks of gestation. Over the last several decades, new procedures, medications, and availability of neonatal care have contributed significantly to improving survival rates for these fragile newborns; unfortunately, acute complications and long-term handicaps occur for fully half of premature babies (Gibbs et al. 2008). (See Chapter 7 for more about preterm labor). Evaluation by her maternal healthcare provider is essential if she suspects that she is in premature labor.

With estrogen levels increasing, labor and birth are imminent, and the expectant woman's emotional state reflects it. Eager, impatient and/or restless, she will begin to "nest." If labor begins prematurely, she may feel unprepared and worried. All of the potential emotional stressors discussed in Chapter 1 often mushroom at this time. While excited, fears for the baby's or her own health may dominate her dreams and thoughts. What she is hearing in childbirth education classes, reading about, and discussing with her friends and family may contribute to her fear, or it can increase her comfort level instead. Labor can be, at least partially, ecstatic, so check the online resources for positive, empowering birth stories and DVDs to recommend. The upcoming birth can bring hidden feelings to the surface and create conscious or unconscious emotional stress (Simkin and Klaus 2004). Most women are at least somewhat awash in joyous anticipation of their baby. Be respectfully sensitive to the depth and range of all the emotions that can emerge when she is under your nurturing hands.

● PRECAUTIONS, CONSIDERATIONS, AND GUIDELINES FOR PRACTITIONERS

Premature labor, or rhythmic tightening and contraction of the uterus prior to 37 weeks of gestation, can result in birth of an underdeveloped infant. Because premature labor may include the common third trimester complaint of low backache, question your clients concerning occurrence of other labor symptoms, such as rhythmic pelvic or thigh pressure, abdominal cramping, or vaginal discharge. If pain persists, regardless of position or activity, this may be an indication of possible premature labor or kidney infection rather than musculoskeletal problems. Typically, referred pain from organs doesn't change with circumstances, whereas musculoskeletal pain will increase or diminish depending on her movements. With any combination of these indicators of premature labor, waiting for communication and written release from the client's healthcare provider is often prudent. Once acquired, your positive presence and therapeutic skills will be comforting and may help prevent premature labor (see Chapter 7 suggestions too) (Field et al. 1999).

The third trimester is when most metabolic complications of pregnancy occur. Continue to collect updated information on her perceptions and prenatal checkup results at each visit. Be especially alert to developing signs of gestational hypertensive disorders such as pitting and/or systemic edema (lymphodynamic). Remember that any edema in areas other than her feet and legs, especially the face and hands, are warning symptoms of possible metabolic imbalances. Wait until consulting with the woman's physician or midwife if systemic edema or any other symptoms of hypertension,

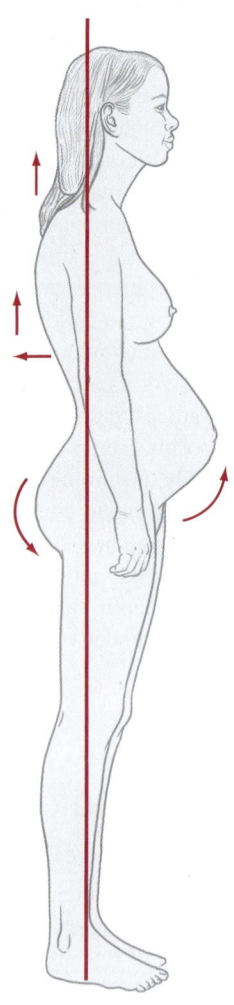

FIGURE 4.8 Optimal prenatal postural alignment. If a pregnant woman's spinal curvatures collapse as drawn here, she may have more pain and movement limitations. Organizing herself toward the vertical polarity shown by moving in the direction of the arrows can help to relieve these discomforts.

preeclampsia or eclampsia, gestational diabetes, premature labor, or placental dysfunction occur. (See complications in Chapters 2 and 7 and bed rest section of Chapter 7.)

Structural stresses on weight-bearing joints during the third trimester usually cause a woman's most intense discomforts. As in the second trimester, erase trigger points, and use deep tissue, cross-fiber friction, passive movements, and other forms of therapeutic bodywork (Howard et al. 2000) in the following areas: posterior spinal structures, rib cage, and posterior pelvis; hip and thigh movers; hip joints; and upper torso, neck, and pectoral girdle. Third trimester women benefit greatly from postural alignment and body-use reeducation for pelvic, ribcage, and cervical alignment (Fig. 4.8). Teach her to regularly correct these postural distortions caused by anterior weight load, and she will suffer less pain, as well as increase her ability to breathe more deeply.

Many women find relief from the weight of the uterus by gently cupping their hands under their abdomen just superior to the pubic bone to hold the baby's weight with their arms. If her partner is willing, teach her partner to do the same for her with a "baby lift." Other women may choose to use supportive undergarments, a prenatal support belt (see online resources), or fabric wrapped in the styles of many traditional cultures to support the abdomen and ease back pain. Supporting the uterus can also reduce venous pressure that contributes to varicose vein development in the legs. Reduce varicose vein discomforts by including modified Swedish leg work in each session, emphasizing raking and light vibrational techniques (Wine 1997).

With as much as nine additional liters of fluid in her body, one of the most common needs of the woman in her third trimester is relief from edema, particularly in the feet and legs. Relieving myofascial restriction in the inguinal area can increase blood and fluid return from the legs. This is accomplished by correct vertical alignment, by performing numerous and frequent pelvic tilts, and by limited, specific myofascial procedures. Positional relief also will be effective, both on and off the therapy table, as will lymphatic drainage and gentle, modified Swedish techniques on the legs. (See Chapter 7 for Points of View discussion on lymphatic drainage during pregnancy.) Acupressure to the medial arch four times daily also may reduce edema in the feet (Stephens 1997).

Tapotement and deep work on the legs, especially the medial surface, and in the inguinal area are increasingly dangerous in the third trimester, when the risk of developing and dislodging thrombi is highest. Continue to avoid reflexive stimulation of uterus-stimulating points on the feet, hands, upper back, and sacrum unless she is past her due date (see Figs. 2.7 and 2.8, and Chapter 7). Remember that women with underlying heart conditions are safer receiving alternatives to Swedish or lymphatic work, such as gentle passive movements and reflexive work, especially in the last trimester.

If calf cramps occur, relieve them as in the second trimester. Remember to prop her so as to avoid her foot dangling down off the supporting pillows or the edge of the table. With increased weight gain, some women develop hip, knee, foot, and **"restless leg"** pain. Approximately 25% of women feel this irritating achiness that gradually intensifies when resting and usually causes an intense need to shake and/or rub the affected leg. Because both leg cramps and "restless leg" are primarily manifestations of physiological imbalances in iron and deficiencies in other minerals, nutrients, salt, water, and hormones (Gibbs et al. 2008), suggest consultation with a nutritionist or her healthcare provider to supplement your Swedish massage therapy and stretching.

Symphysis pubis dysfunction is more common in the third trimester than earlier in the pregnancy, but it can occur sooner with multiple gestations or after several babies. To prevent increasing this intense pelvic pain, avoid techniques that pull on this joint. If a woman has symphysis pubis pain, keep her bent knees together as she rolls over (sometimes a hands and knees rollover is less painful) or minimize position changes on the table. Though uncommon, if nausea occurs, avoid rocking passive movements.

If she experiences hand numbness, pain or weakness, have her hold her posterior hands and forearms together in front of her, then flex her wrists for 1 minute. If pain or numbness results, then it is likely she has carpal tunnel syndrome. This will need medical diagnosis to confirm, but you can begin by first thoroughly draining the arms and hands with Swedish and drainage work. Maximize space in the carpal tunnel with gentle, small-amplitude mobilization and traction. Ice might also be helpful on the wrist.

For whole hand and arm pain, likely to be related to thoracic outlet syndrome, focus on postural realignment activities and relief of chronic tension in the scalene and pectoralis minor muscles (Scheumann 2007). Craniosacral, especially thoracic inlet release, strain and counterstrain, and other passive movements to the rib cage and pectoral girdle are also effective. Locate and extinguish trigger points in the arms and chest as well.

Stretched abdominal skin and muscles will benefit from gentle, rhythmic effleurage to lubricate the skin and ease strain (Fig. 4.9). Usually, the baby will respond to this contact on the walls of its home with distinctive kicks and squirms. Deeper pressure into the abdomen still is contraindicated. See the technique manual later in this chapter for many specific techniques to address many of these third trimester needs.

Positioning

As previously explained in Chapter 3, during weeks 27 to term, position pregnant women on the therapy table only in the sidelying or semireclining positions. Many women labor in the semireclining position. Help her to become accustomed to this position and to learn to achieve maximum relaxation here as preparation for labor. New Zealand midwife Jean Sutton, and Pauline Scott, childbirth educator, argue convincingly against regular and prolonged semireclined sitting in late pregnancy. Their extensive practice-based evidence indicates that this encourages a higher incidence of persistent **occiput posterior** fetal position (see prolonged labor, Chapter 5), often resulting in long, painful labors (Sutton and Scott 1996). Despite this warning, keep in mind that the hour of massage therapy while the client is semireclined will have no negative consequences.

Labor Preparation

In addition to providing relief from common pregnancy discomforts, now is the time to focus therapy on labor preparation. The rationale and instruction in specific techniques to ready women for labor are included in Chapter 5.

Post-Term Concerns

Generally, if a woman gives birth within 2 weeks on either side of her estimated or **expected date of birth (EDB)**, that gestation is considered normal in length. Despite calculations, measurements, testing, and proper prenatal and self-care, 3% to 12% of women's pregnancies go beyond their calculated due dates. The causes of gestation beyond 42 weeks are obscure; however, potential resulting problems include decreased amniotic fluid, fetal fecal contamination of amniotic fluid (meconium), and placental and umbilical cord aging and malfunctioning. The concern with post–due date birth is in large babies (macrosomia) and fetal physiological imbalances, as well as maternal exhaustion, trauma, hemorrhage, fear, and frustration (Gibbs et al. 2008). Discomfort and impatience amplify any anxiety she feels, so more frequent relaxation massage is helpful.

Once a woman is "overdue" (**post-term, prolonged pregnancy, or postdatism**), she may request that you stimulate points on her hand, calf, and foot that have been contraindicated until now. For best results with these acupressure points, teach her their locations, how to work with these points, and encourage thrice daily, 5- to 10-minute self-massage periods (refer back to Figs. 2.7 and 2.8).

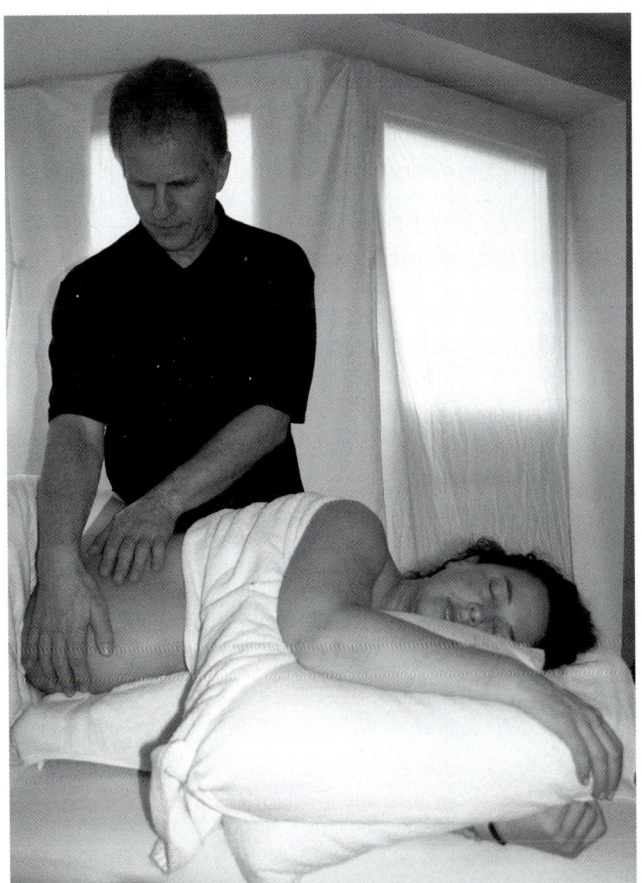

FIGURE 4.9 Third trimester prenatal massage therapy sessions. Weeks 28 to 40 or 42. By the end of pregnancy, many women widen their stance and struggle to maintain vertical alignment, particularly in the lumbar area. In addition to relieving resulting musculoskeletal discomforts, gentle abdominal massage offers soothing contact, communication with the fetus, and lubrication to stretched skin.

Medical management of prolonged pregnancy includes membrane sweeping, and induction via medications that replicate the natural hormones that initiate and stimulate labor. Suggest that she considers and discusses with her maternity healthcare provider nonpharmacological labor initiation techniques (Simkin et al. 2010). Frequently, she benefits from exploring her readiness for motherhood with gentle probes from you such as "Is there any way that I can help you to feel ready for your baby?" "Where in your body do you feel resistant or reluctant to birth?" "What are your fears or concerns?"

● SUMMARY OF RECOMMENDED BODYWORK

In the 27th week through term, pregnant women will benefit from similar therapeutic somatic activities as second trimester women (see bulleted list in previous section). In addition, use:

- Swedish, stretching, and appropriate deep tissue work to assist in preventing and/or relieving pain and increasing flexibility in the thigh adductors
- Relaxation techniques such as visualizations and tense/release or stretch/release progressive relaxation, emphasizing relaxing through intense stimulus and pain, as she will need to do in labor
- Swedish, deep tissue, myofascial, passive movement, and trigger point techniques to reduce leg pain, release chronic tension, and increase flexibility particularly in the adductors, quadriceps, hamstrings, rotators of the hip joint, posterior calf, and the lumbar soft tissues, so that she may more comfortably assume a variety of positions during labor (See labor preparation techniques in chapter 5 technique manual)
- Preparation of the pelvic floor for birth by Kegel exercises and perineal self-massage instruction, as well as appropriate work at the pubic attachments (See online resources for instructional guidelines)
- Instruction to partners in appropriate massage and relaxation techniques that enhance the family's ability to support the laboring woman (see online resources for instructional plans)
- Instruction in infant massage and movement routines to encourage the bonding and well-being of the newborn and its family (see online resources for DVD suggestions) (Schneider 1989)

These general guidelines and foci will help you identify techniques you already know that may be adaptable for your third trimester clients. You will find numerous specific techniques detailed in this chapter's technique manual that follows. (See sequential third trimester session sample online.)

Technique Manual of Prenatal Massage and Bodywork

In this section, you will find detailed instruction in specific prenatal techniques. What follows is not a prescribed sequence or protocol. Instead you have many options to choose from as you prepare for and work with your clients. You can include those most needed by your client, incorporating them into your usual session sequence. If you'd like to use primarily these techniques, you will find a few suggested session layouts in the online resources. You can watch a typical session flow of this work for each trimester in the online video clips. These sequences will help to structure your work until you gain enough experience with pregnant women to more confidently design more individualized sessions.

Each grouping begins with a reminder of the complaints and symptoms these techniques best address. There are many techniques within each group, and each follows this format:

- **Intention** = the intended outcome or purpose of the procedures. Understanding what structures you are affecting and what you are attempting to accomplish forms the foundation for doing any technique in any but the most rote and unimaginative way. Hold this intention in mind as you take the steps indicated, and you'll more likely reach those goals. Understanding these intentions, and their underlying rationale, is also the basis for sharing relevant information that can help to alleviate any fears or concerns that she might have about her experiences.
- **Procedure** = precise instruction in how to accomplish the technique. This is every step you need to execute the technique. Figures in this section include red dots indicating typical trigger points and instructional arrows (white = client movement; solid red = vector of your pressure; dotted red = area to apply technique).
- **Hints** = ways to make the technique easier or more effective or vary it for individual needs. Here's where you'll get pointers on your own body use and ways to adapt the general procedure. When an alternative image or way to create the same effect might be needed for certain situations, you'll find suggestions in this section.
- **Precautions** = adaptations and contraindications for safety. As you apply general precautions and contraindications detailed in Chapter 2, individual techniques sometimes require specific guidance and reminders so that they are not only effective but also perfectly safe.

You will find some recommended lifestyle changes and ancillary ways to help reduce that particular prenatal discomfort in the online resources. Many of these recommendations are not squarely within the scope of practice of most massage therapists; therefore, treat them as ideas for your clients to explore on her own and with her partner and her maternity healthcare provider.

REDUCING EFFECTS OF STRESS AND PROVIDING EMOTIONAL SUPPORT AND NURTURING

Many women find that while pregnancy brings great joy, often they experience the following: stress; anxiety, worries, and fears; difficulty relaxing and sleeping; emotional inconsistency and intensity; problems with family, friends, and coworkers; and stress-related hypertension. This section presents several techniques to address these issues.

Review of Precautions
Observe all safety concerns detailed in Chapter 2, earlier in Chapter 4, and within the procedures that follow.

Technique Suggestions
The following techniques can help to reduce the amount of circulating stress hormones and to promote maternal physical, emotional, and mental integration. They facilitate relaxation; increase kinesthetic awareness; assist her in "grounding" and being more present with the emotional and physical reality of her pregnancy; and create a conducive environment if she chooses to explore her feelings in more depth. Use these techniques to begin sessions or as transitional procedures. Relaxation massage, especially the autonomic sedation series, activates the parasympathetic branch of the autonomic nervous system and may help to lower blood pressure (Longworth 1982).

Diaphragmatic Breathing Reeducation

Intentions

To facilitate relaxation and increased kinesthetic awareness; to reeducate breathing toward complete diaphragmatic activation and maximum lateral and posterior ribcage excursion; to facilitate retraining those who breathe paradoxically to breathe diaphragmatically; to reduce overuse of upper chest and neck muscles that can contribute to headaches, neck and back pain, and thoracic outlet syndrome; to facilitate maximum maternal and fetal oxygenation; to prepare for the breathing demands of labor.

Procedure

This procedure may be performed in any position.

1. Ask the client to place one hand on her lower abdomen and the other on the center of her chest.
2. Instruct her to inhale through her nose and exhale through her mouth gently and deeply without strain (Fig. 4.10).
3. Ask her to visualize the following sequence in her mind's eye:
   (1) See your baby nestled in your uterus, deep within your pelvis. (2) Imagine that your inhaling breath gently touches her or him like a soft, loving hand. (3) As you exhale, see the caressing hand of your breath gently lift from her or him. (4) Watch the movement as you continue to breathe fully in this way for several minutes.

Alternative image (especially useful to increase lateral/costal breathing)

1. Imagine your torso as a folded umbrella with the edge of the umbrella at your lower ribcage.
2. As you inhale, see the umbrella opening.
3. Exhaling, imagine it closed against the center pole.
4. Continue to open and close the umbrella in your imagination as you breathe for another several minutes. (Go online for other breathing guidance alternatives.)

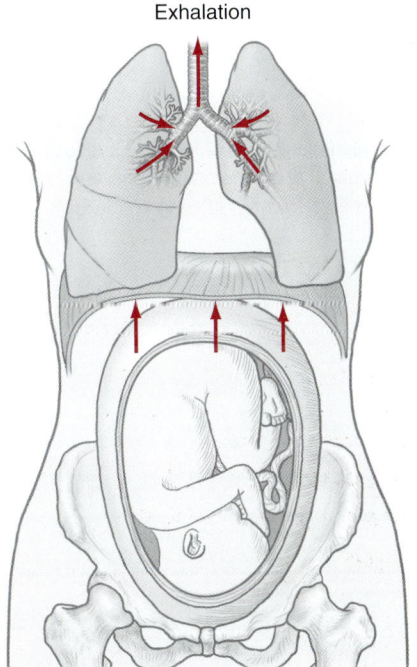
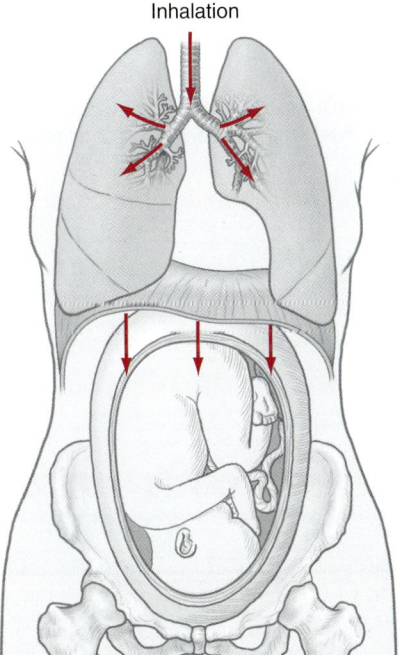

FIGURE 4.10 Diaphragmatic breathing reeducation. In this illustration, red arrows indicate direction of air and diaphragm movement.

Hints

1. Observe any straining, especially any over chest overinflation or activation of the scalenes and other neck muscles with the inhalations. Verbally encourage her to breathe effortlessly, without force.
2. Enhance her awareness by placing your hands on her torso at the specific areas toward which you are guiding her breath.
3. When a client has difficulty with visualizing, switch instead to asking her to place her hands on her abdomen. Ask her to lift her hands away from her spine with her inhale and allow them to sink toward her spine with her exhale.
4. Encourage frequent, daily diaphragmatic breathing and relaxation.

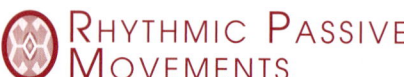 Rhythmic Passive Movements

Intentions

To induce a sedative, calming state; to create gentle joint mobilizations that reduce strain and promote relaxation of the surrounding soft tissue; to evaluate the quality and quantity of joint motion as an indicator of tension and a guide to where to apply deeper work.

Procedures

Best performed with the client in the sidelying position, and may be modified for other positions; described in sidelying.

Spinal Rocking (Fig. 4.11)

1. From a position behind the client's head, but facing toward her feet, extend your hand closest to her feet toward her spine. Gently place either the flat palm or the posterior side of your flexed phalanges directly over the spinous processes of the upper thoracic vertebrae.
2. Shift your weight slowly and gradually into the client's spine, maintaining primarily an anterior and secondarily a caudal direction to your pressure. Release your pressure, but remain in contact with the spinous processes to feel her torso spring back toward your soft hand.
3. After feeling the rebound of the torso back toward you, again press anteriorly, and continue to create a gentle, undulating rocking motion of her spine, ribcage, and pelvis. Keep your pace at that of a relaxed heartbeat.

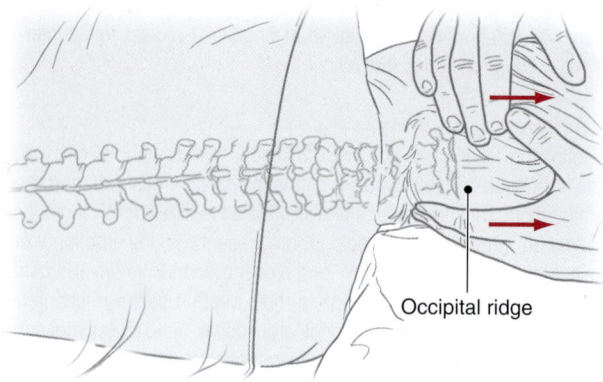

FIGURE 4.12 Rhythmic passive movements: occiput traction and rocking.

4. Rhythmically rock three to five times in that spinal segment, and then move down her spine to the next segment, maintaining your rhythm and contact, to press on the next group of spinous processes.
5. Proceed caudally down the spine with rhythmic, undulating mobilizations to eventually rock the entire spinal column and pelvis.
6. Repeat several times, and/or reverse directions to rock from the sacrum moving up to the seventh cervical vertebra.
7. More specific mobilizations of individual vertebra are possible by focusing the pressure rather that spread over a wider surface. Move vertebra by vertebra up or down the spine, as above.

Occiput Traction and Rocking (Fig. 4.12)

1. Stand at the head of the table, facing her head. Place both hands at her occiput, one hand on the side of her head facing the table and one on the side of her head facing the ceiling. Use your fingers to softly form around the ridge of the occiput. Make room in your hand so that her ears are not compressed.
2. Exert gentle, gradual traction of her occiput away from the cervical vertebrae. Add gentle, slow, microrocking motions to the traction, but do not release the traction as you rock. Maintain for a minimum of 30 seconds.

Transverse Cervical Rocking (Fig. 4.13)

1. Stand at the head of the table and facing the client. Place the middle finger of one hand on the transverse process of the highest reachable vertebra (maybe C2) on the side facing the ceiling. Use the other

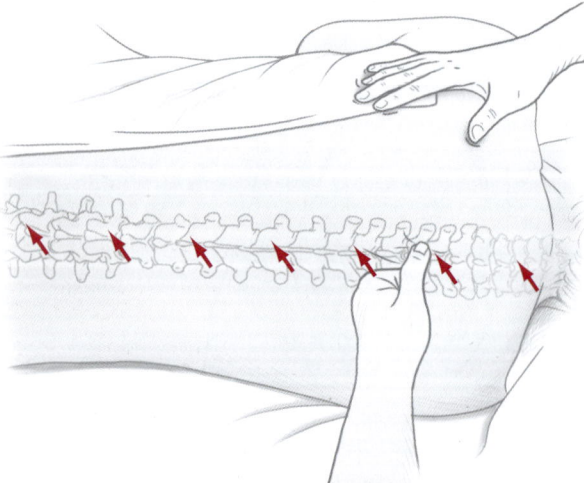

FIGURE 4.11 Rhythmic passive movements: spinal rocking.

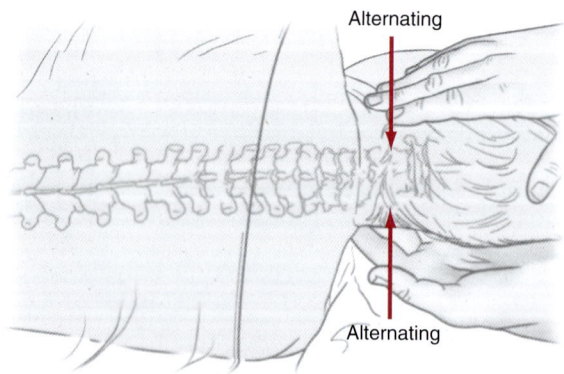

FIGURE 4.13 Rhythmic passive movements: transverse cervical rocking.

hand on the side of the process facing the table of the same vertebra. (Remember that the transverse processes of the cervical vertebrae are roughly in line with the ear, more anterior than many imagine them to be.) Create a slow and fluid transverse rocking motion to C2 by rhythmically alternating pressure on each process for three to five repetitions.
2. Move rhythmically down vertebra by vertebra to mobilize the entire cervical spine one vertebra at a time.
3. Visualize creating more space between each vertebrae and re-establishing fluidity that will help to improve function of the parasympathetic nerves emerging from between the cervical vertebrae.

Pectoral Girdle Mobilizations

1. Stand at the head of the table. Place one hand on the shoulder facing the ceiling, between her neck and the acromioclavicular joint and the other hand over that joint. Press the pectoral girdle toward her feet with gentle caudal- and lateral-directed pressure. Maintain traction of the tissue between her upper back and her neck and add gentle, slow, microrocking motions to the traction, but do not release the traction as you rock. Maintain for a minimum of 30 seconds (Fig. 4.14).
2. Stand behind the client at her upper back and facing her head. Slip the arm closest to her, under hers so that her forearm is resting across your forearm. Gently bend her elbow to tuck it within your own flexed elbow. Place the other hand directly over the scapula or just medial to the scapula (Fig. 4.15).
3. Open the pectoral girdle horizontally with rhythmic, gentle lateral rocking of the scapula and humerus and circular movements of the scapula. Emphasize quality of movement by using only very small-amplitude movements, performed at a slow, relaxed heartbeat pace. Include combinations of all of the movements of the scapula-thoracic junction. Spend a minute or more exploring her movement, stretching tight areas and/or shortening tense muscles to reset tension levels.

Pelvic Girdle Mobilizations (Fig. 4.16)

1. Stand behind the client, facing her pelvis. Place your hand closest to her head gently on her iliac crest and the other hand between her sacrum and her greater trochanter.
2. Distract and hold the ilium from the ribcage by leaning toward the foot of the table and initiating slow, small-amplitude rocking motions. After 30 seconds, slowly release.
3. Using the hand on her buttocks, distract and hold the ilium from the sacrum, then the femur from the acetabulum, by leaning toward her knee and initiating slow, small-amplitude rocking motions. Maintain the traction on soft tissues for a minimum of 30 seconds as you slowly rock, and as you move down the leg with lengthening, rocking movements.
4. If you can perform each of the movements above with ease, then combine them so that you are simultaneously creating space between the ribs and the ilium and between the sacrum and the ilium.

HINTS

Notice the quality and range of motion as you rock. Rigid, resistant areas are places where the soft tissues are most in need of further therapy.

PRECAUTIONS

1. In the sidelying position, maintain her horizontal alignment so that she does not roll forward onto her belly during any of these movements.

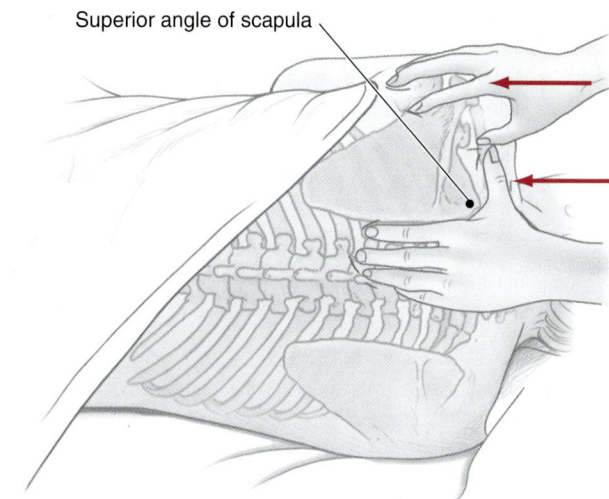

FIGURE 4.14 Pectoral girdle mobilizations: stretching.

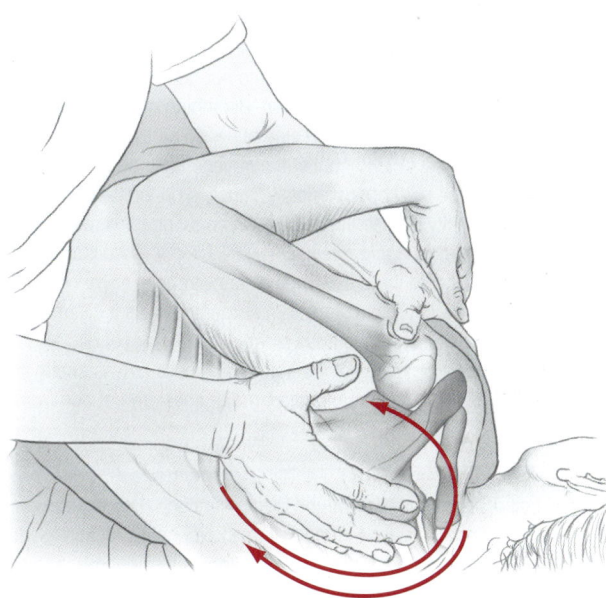

FIGURE 4.15 Pectoral girdle mobilizations: circling.

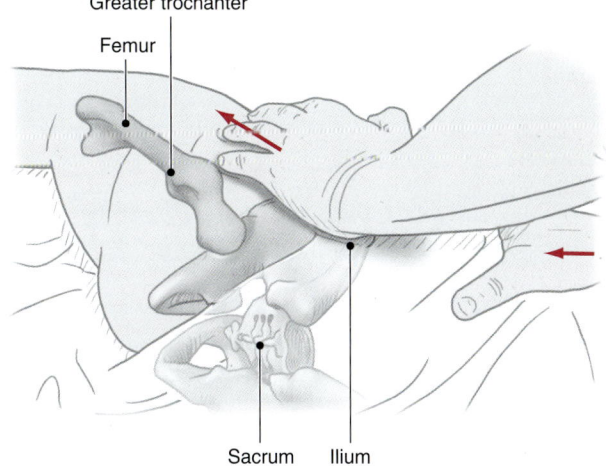

FIGURE 4.16 Pelvic girdle mobilizations.

2. Do not vigorously rock. The most effective movements are those with small-amplitude, slow, relaxed heartbeat frequency and steady rhythm. Avoid extremes of range of motion.
3. If client is nauseated, eliminate these procedures.

Autonomic Sedation Series 3-1-1

Adapted from Longworth (1982).

Intentions

To lower blood pressure by stimulating the paravertebral and sacral plexus parasympathetic nerves; to induce a sedative, calming state; to gather and center the client's energy around her core.

Procedures

Best performed and described in sidelying position.

Paravertebral Raking (Fig. 4.17)

1. Stand behind the client at about her waist level and facing her head. Spread the fingers of your hand closest to her head to create a space between your index and middle fingers. Beginning at the crown of her head, stroke down on each side of her spine sinking to the superficial fascial level, and continue paravertebrally down to her sacrum. Cover the area approximately 2 inches on each side of the spine. Stroke gently and continuously with your fingertips to drag through her skin and fascia, creating a reflexive response through the skin dermatomes into the parasympathetic nervous system.
2. Repeat rhythmically at approximately 1-second intervals for 3 minutes.
3. Pay particular attention to the base of the skull and upper cervicals, where major branches of the parasympathetic nerves emerge between the cervical vertebrae to affect major chest and abdominal organs.

Sacral Friction (Fig. 4.18)

1. Stand just distal of her sacrum and facing her head. Use the same hand as above to perform 1 minute of rhythmic, gentle friction to the sacrum. Use the flat pads of three or four fingers to rub through the skin and fascia, systematically covering the entire sacrum. Take care to avoid bone-on-bone or pointed pressure on the sacrum that could stimulate uterine contractions.
2. Imagine stimulating the plexus of parasympathetic nerves bundled deep to the sacrum that affects the pelvic organs.

Rib Raking (Fig. 4.19)

1. Stand behind the client's upper back, facing her feet. Using the hand furthest from her, spread your fingers into a rake-like formation, and place your hand just distal of her scapula on her lateral ribcage with a finger between each rib.
2. Beginning along the lateral midline, gently stroke lateral to medial following the ribs, continuing all the way to her spine.
3. Reposition and repeat at a frequency of approximately 1-second intervals for 1 minute.
4. If you are able to comfortably reach beneath the ribs on the side against the table, do the same rib raking there for another minute.
5. Imagine as you stroke her sides that you are collecting and solidifying her energy around her spinal core.

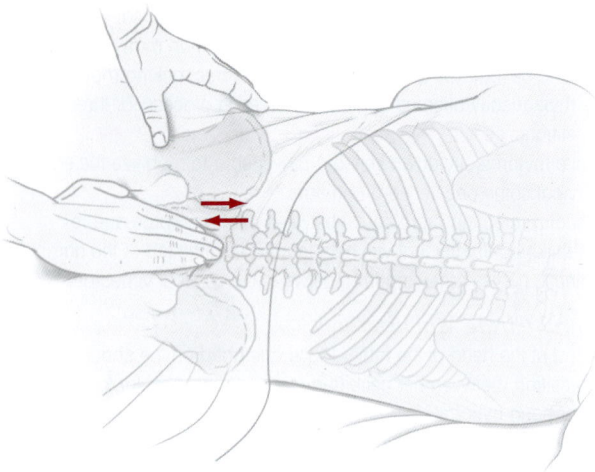

FIGURE 4.18 Autonomic sedation series: sacral friction.

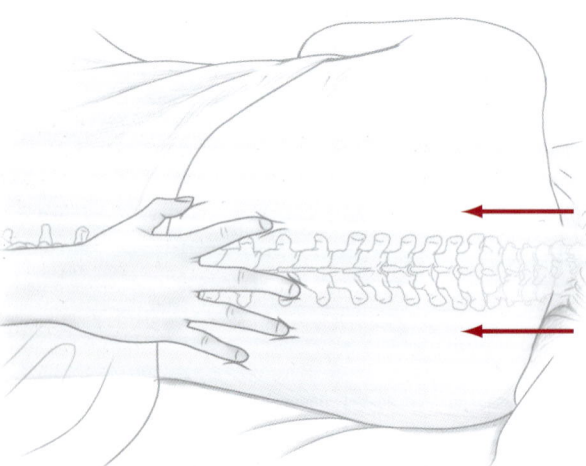

FIGURE 4.17 Autonomic sedation series: paravertebral raking.

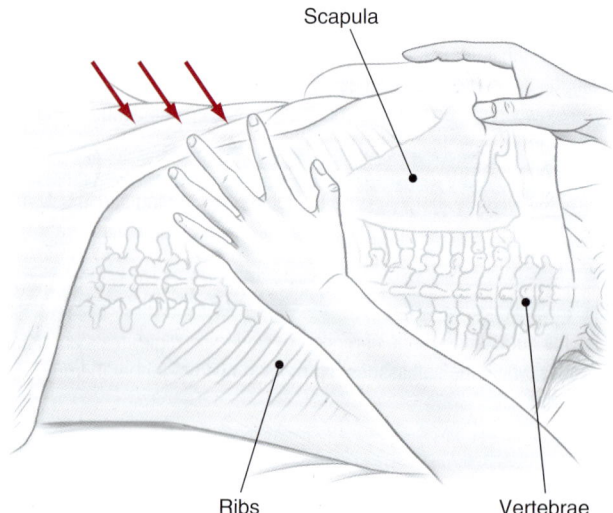

FIGURE 4.19 Autonomic sedation series: rib raking.

Hints

1. This technique is most effective if you perform all three procedures in the sequence described and for the length of time required.
2. If you or your client seems impatient with the repetition and simplicity of this technique, try adding to it a visualization of a peaceful spot or of brushing away her worries and tensions, or have her practice deep abdominal breathing, which will further encourage a deep relaxed state.

Abdominal Massage

Intentions

To facilitate relaxation, especially of the abdominal muscles; to lubricate the abdominal skin, reducing dryness and itchiness; to gently mobilize torso joints; to facilitate connection with the baby; to reduce leg edema.

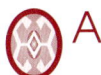 Superficial Abdominal Effleurage

May be performed in all positions, depending on trimester; described for supine or semireclining (Fig. 4.20).

1. From a position beside the abdomen, use your flat, relaxed palms to apply oil with superficial effleurage strokes, circling around her abdomen. Complete a circle with one hand as the other makes a half circle.
2. Going no deeper than when spreading oil, make superficial thumb or finger fanning motions, moving medially from her sides toward her umbilicus.
3. Use your flat fingers in small superficial circles around her abdomen, concentrating in the lower abdominal region.
4. Create long, superficial strokes with your fingers. Stroke from just superior of the inguinal ligament and pubis moving toward the umbilicus.

Other Techniques

Choose strokes and procedures from your own repertoire that promote relaxation, integration, grounding, and emotional support. These may include the following: gentle, full-body Swedish and Esalen-style massage; craniosacral therapy, focusing on stillpoint, occipital cranial base, transverse diaphragm releases, traction, and leverage release of L5–S1; polarity therapy; or jin shin jytsu.

Easing Leg and Hip Discomforts

Second and third trimester women often experience extensive hip and leg pain and discomfort. Some of these affect the entire leg, such as varicose veins, "restless legs," and edema. Most women have swollen calves and feet by midpregnancy. Sometimes, this results in numbness and pain in the first three toes. Calf cramps, knee pain, and hip joint achiness are more common, though. In the second trimester, she might have inner, anterior upper thigh pain, and third trimester women can develop numbness and pain on the anterolateral thigh.

Review of Precautions

Pitting edema, systemic edema, swelling of the face and hands, and first and early second trimester edema are all warning signs of gestational hypertensive disorders. Proceed with any work with caution and with the prenatal healthcare provider's written release. Reduce depth of leg work to protect vulnerable varicose and spider veins. Do not perform cross-fiber friction, deep tissue, Shiatsu, acupressure, and other deep or ischemic pressure in the areas of greatest possible clot formation in the medial leg, femoral, and inguinal regions. Avoid brisk or intense rocking and tapotement techniques on the legs. Do not use any circulatory effect leg massage with women on bed rest.

Do not plantarflex the foot, to avoid prompting cramps in the gastrocnemius-soleus complex. Carefully monitor passive movements performed on the legs and hips of women experiencing symphysis pubis dysfunction so that stabbing, midline pelvic pain is not worsened by traction or shifting of the joint. Omit Swedish and drainage techniques, which can create and increased load on the heart in the third trimester for clients with underlying heart disease. Observe all safety concerns detailed in Chapter 2, earlier in Chapter 4, and within the procedures that follow.

Technique Suggestions

Pregnant women with dependent, lymphostatic edema benefit greatly from Swedish and lymphatic drainage techniques that reduce fluid accumulation in the legs and from techniques that help to relieve pelvic

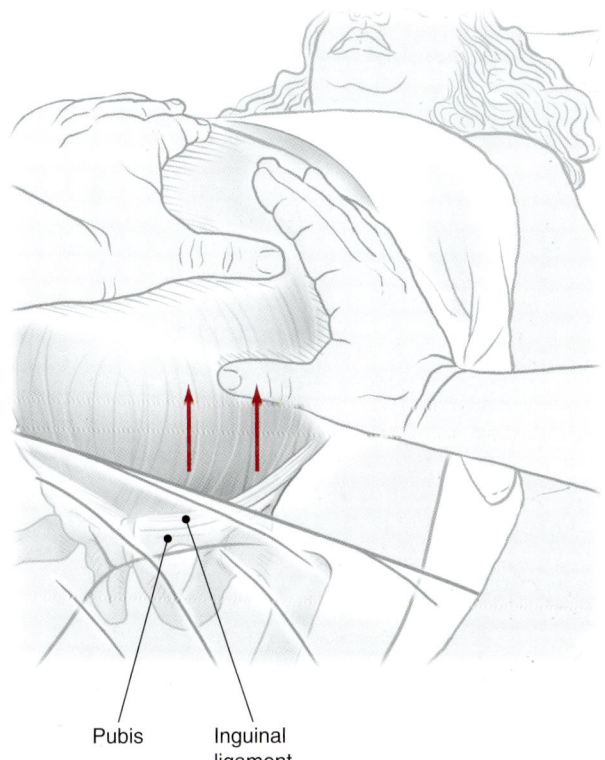

FIGURE 4.20 Superficial abdominal effleurage.

circulatory congestion and obstruction. Deep tissue, passive movements, structural/movement reeducation activities, and other therapeutic techniques help to alleviate pain in the joints and soft tissues of the hips, knees, and feet.

STRUCTURAL BALANCING

This technique is to be performed with the client clothed and standing.

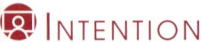 INTENTION

To promote vertical head, spine, and pelvic alignment; to reduce most musculoskeletal and physiological discomforts; to locate areas needing release of tension and those needing muscular toning; to reach more optimal structural balance.

Occipital Lift (Fig. 4.21)

1. Verbally guide the standing client to imagine the area immediately behind her ears lifting upward as it shifts more posterior.
2. After she imagines the movement, place your hand around her occiput. Lightly pull posteriorly and lift toward the ceiling to let your hand guide this movement as she does it.
3. Alternate image: Have her imagine that a string attached to crown of her head pulls skyward, lifting the crown of her head with it and allowing the cervical spine, rib cage, and pelvis to follow.

Rib Cage Alignment (Fig. 4.22)

1. Stand behind your standing client. Ask her to imagine that a string attached from the opposite wall is pulling her sternum slightly forward.
2. After three imaginary movements, ask her to initiate this movement. As she does, use soft hands on the lateral, lower edge of her rib cage to draw her lower ribcage more posterior. Lift her upper ribcage slightly forward as you rotate your thumbs anteriorly.

Pelvic and Lumbar Alignment (Fig. 4.23)

1. Verbally guide your standing client to imagine that an attached string lifts her pubic bone skyward. Have her imagine another attached to her tailbone, extending down toward the earth.
2. After three imaginary movements, ask her to initiate this movement. Guide her pelvis by gently pressing her sacrum to tuck her pelvis under without engaging her buttock muscles.

HINTS

1. Due to proprioceptive habituation, many women will feel as though they are falling forward with these realignments. Where possible, use a full-length mirror so that she may verify that she is indeed more vertical.
2. Encourage her to realign her structure throughout her day and whenever she feels pain, strain, or fatigue.
3. For other approaches to prenatal postural guidance, consult Noble (1995).
4. Note that in Fig. 4.21-23 the red arrows denote both client and therapist's movements.

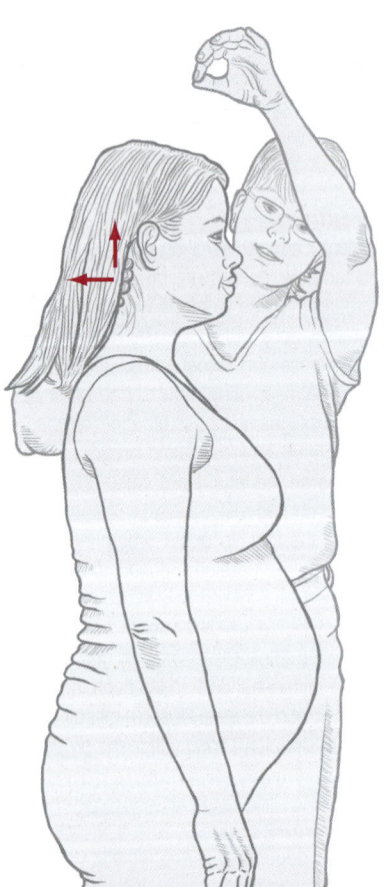

FIGURE 4.21 Structural balancing: occipital lift.

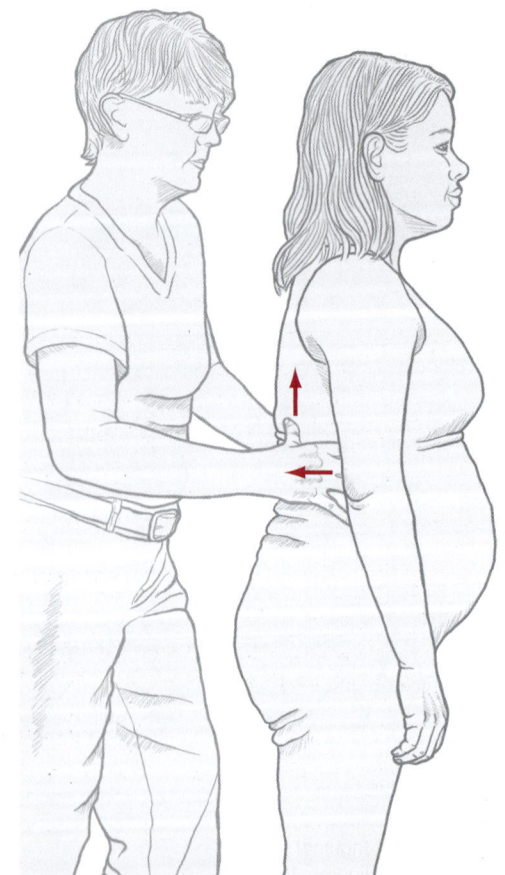

FIGURE 4.22 Structural balancing: ribcage alignment.

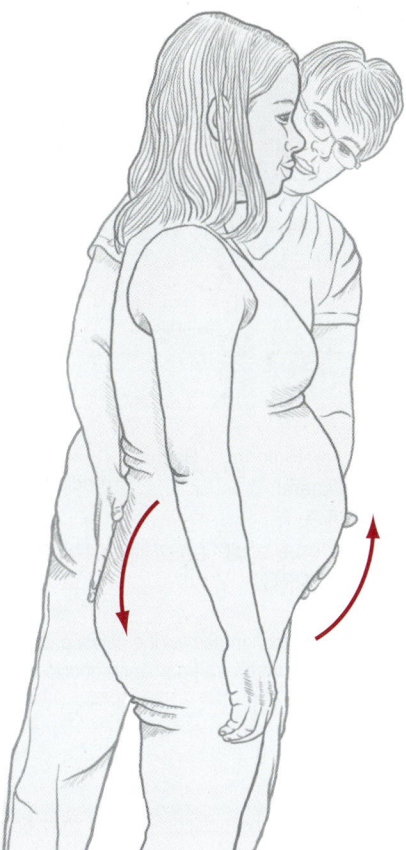

FIGURE 4.23 Structural balancing: pelvic and lumbar alignment.

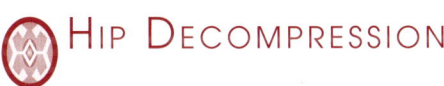 Hip Decompression

Intention

To alleviate compression and chronic external rotation of the femur; to reduce hip joint and surrounding myofascial tissue pain, especially the femoral rotators and flexors and the iliotibial tract; to reduce sciatic nerve compression; and to assist in fluid drainage from the legs.

Procedure

Traction and Rocking
May be performed with the client in all table positions; described for sidelying.

1. Stand behind the client at the client's pelvis level and align your body with the angle of the client's femur as supported by the bolsters.
2. Lightly place your hand closest to her head on the ASIS to fix the pelvis and to stabilize her position (Fig. 4.24).
3. Place the palm of the other hand superior to the greater trochanter and distract the femur from the acetabulum by leaning your weight toward her knee.
4. Hold this stretch for 30 seconds to 1 minute. Initiate small-amplitude rocking motions, if desired and if she is not nauseated.

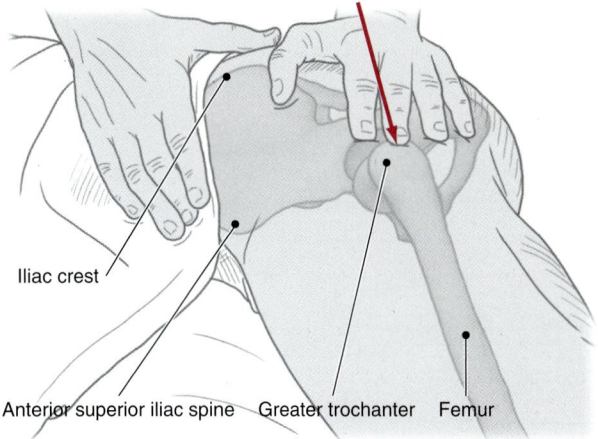

FIGURE 4.24 Hip decompression: traction and rocking.

Precautions

1. Allow the hand on the ASIS to rest passively so that you make the movement by gently leaning rather than forcefully pulling the ASIS. Do not flex your fingers into the pelvic bowl.
2. Maintain the horizontal alignment of the client so that she does not roll forward onto her belly.
3. Maintain a soft hand to avoid painful pressure on the supratrochanteric bursa.

Alternative Procedure: Internal Rotation and Rocking

Described for supine or semireclining positions

1. Stand facing the client's feet. Use the hand nearest her head to gently stabilize the pelvis at the ASIS. Place the other hand several inches below the hip joint to midway to the knee.
2. Traction the femur from the acetabulum with the distal hand. Maintain this traction and initiate small-amplitude rocking motions directed toward her foot. Continue for up to 30 seconds.

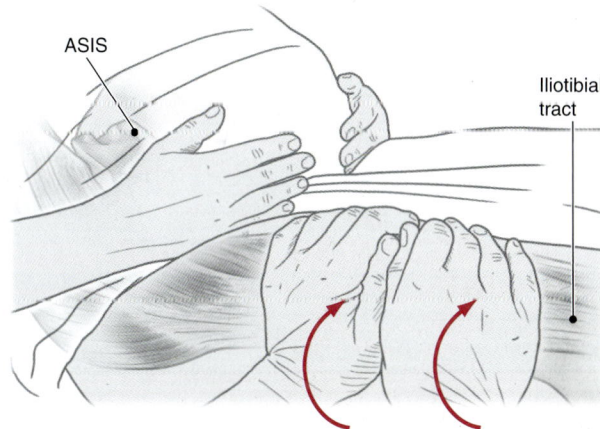

FIGURE 4.25 Hip decompression: alternative internal rotation and rocking.

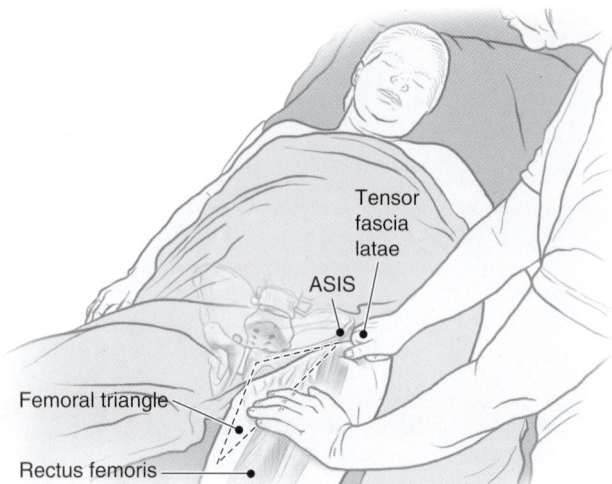

FIGURE 4.26 Hip decompression: deep tissue sculpting of anterior hip.

3. Reposition yourself to face directly toward the table at her knee level. Use the heels of both hands just superior of the knee and posterior of the iliotibial band to internally rotate the femur in the acetabulum and stretch the posterior ligaments of the hip joint. Hold in this position and gently rock for 30 to 60 seconds (Fig. 4.25).

Deep Tissue Sculpting Anterior Hip
Adapted from Osborne (2002) (Fig. 4.26).

1. Stand at the client's pelvis, facing toward her feet, and use the fist or proximal forearm of either arm. Compress slowly and deeply into the attachment of the rectus femoris and sartorius sinking to a level of tissue resistance and creating no pain. Wait a minimum of 30 seconds for tissue relaxation. Work without oil, and glide on the skin only if the muscle fibers elongate to create motion of your working arm.
2. Release your pressure gradually, and reposition your fist or forearm to similarly sculpt the tensor fascia latae by compressing just lateral to the ASIS, and aiming down toward the table. Work without oil, and glide on the skin only if the muscle fibers elongate to create motion of your working arm.

PRECAUTIONS

Be especially careful to be lateral of the femoral triangle, on the lateral side of the rectus femoris and sartorius. Use soft fingers and hands and avoid poking deeply into clot endangerment sites there and on the medial, adductor area of the thigh.

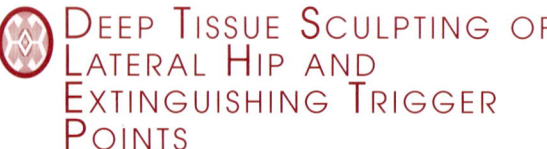

DEEP TISSUE SCULPTING OF LATERAL HIP AND EXTINGUISHING TRIGGER POINTS

Adapted from Osborne (2002) (Fig. 4.27).

INTENTION AND IMAGERY

To relax chronic tension in the gluteals and other femoral rotators, to reduce pain in the hip and posterior pelvic joints, to locate and eliminate

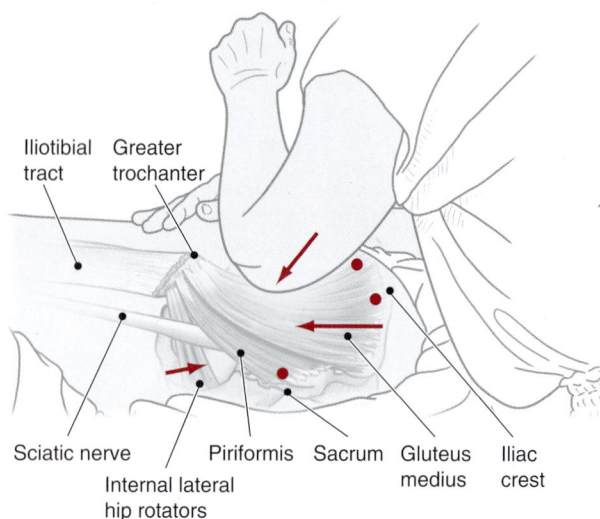

FIGURE 4.27 Deep tissue sculpting of lateral hip and extinguishing trigger points.

trigger points, to assist in realignment of the pelvis and the hip joints, to reduce pain referred from the broad ligaments, and to reduce compression of the sciatic nerve.

PROCEDURES

Best performed in the sidelying position, though may be performed in prone position, but only in the first trimester; all described for sidelying position.

Gluteus Medius/Gluteus Minimus

1. Stand posterior to the client's pelvis, facing toward her feet, and use your proximal forearm or the fist of the arm closest to her. Slowly compress into the gluteus medius sinking to a level of tissue resistance and creating no pain. Begin at its attachment inferior to the iliac crest and hold for a minimum of 30 seconds waiting for tissue relaxation that might move you toward the insertion. Follow any myofascial release that takes you deeper into the gluteus minimus or along the gluteus medius fibers. Release your pressure as slowly and gradually as you applied it. Continue performing a series of compressions for 30 seconds each until reaching the insertion in the iliotibial band. Use no oil and limit any movement on the skin to elongation of fibers beneath.
2. Reposition yourself to slowly work into the gluteus maximus sinking in gradually. Begin at its attachment on the sacrum and posterior iliac spine and continue with slow, melting compressions until reaching the hip joint. If no spider veins, reposition distal of the hip joint, and proceed similarly down the iliotibial tract.
3. Using the knuckles, forearm, or elbow, slowly compress into the channel between the ischial tuberosity and the greater trochanter to relax the bellies of the deep lateral rotators. Maintain pressure for 30 seconds or until the tissue releases, then carefully sculpt their attachments around the greater trochanter.

Trigger Points
Adapted from Howard et al. (2000).

1. As you sculpt, be alert to any points eliciting a jump response from the client or referred pain. Extinguish these myofascial trigger points

with a moderate pressure on the point until any pain initially discovered diminishes, and the client reports no pain remaining. Continue compressing for an additional 7 to 20 seconds. (See technique for ribcage trigger points for more details and methods for finding and extinguishing trigger points.)
2. If possible, stretch the trigger area for 30 to 60 seconds or perform localized strokes over the area.
3. Many trigger points in these muscles and the iliotibial tract refer to the hip joint, thighs, pelvis, and sacrum. (Typical trigger points are indicated by dots on diagrams). Also palpate quadratus lumborum and leg muscles for tender points referring to the hip and lateral pelvis.

PRECAUTIONS

1. The sciatic nerve is embedded beneath the gluteus maximus, within the lateral rotators, and may be sensitive to deep compressions. Change position, direction, or depth of pressure if the client experiences an electrical, burning, numbing, or painful sensation down the posterior of her leg.
2. Avoid creating pain from excessive pressure into the supratrochanteric bursa.
3. When extinguishing trigger points, adjust your pressure so that she experiences only a slight painful sensation. Take care to not defensively activate her sympathetic nervous system.
4. Do not perform these techniques on areas where there are spider veins. Use mobilizations instead.
5. Maintain the horizontal alignment of the client on the table so that she does not roll onto her belly.

FIGURE 8 HIP MOBILIZATION

INTENTION

To alleviate compression and restricted movement of the femur, to reduce pain from the hip joint and surrounding myofascial tissues.

PROCEDURES

This technique may be performed in sidelying, supine, and semireclining positions; described for sidelying (Fig. 4.28).

1. Stand in front of the client at her knee level. With relaxed hands, pick up the top leg and adjust the supports to allow free movement of the ceiling side leg and hip.
2. Slide one hand and forearm beneath her thigh to support gently at the distal thigh and knee. Use the other hand to support her calf. Avoid torque on her knee and creation of pressure points on her medial leg.
3. Subtly traction the hip, then slowly and meditatively move the hip through small-amplitude combinations of its varied motions. Imagine the movements occurring in thick honey so that the pacing is extremely slow.
4. As shown by the red line in Fig. 4.28A, create a figure 8–like pattern of movement, with the center of the 8 being the hip joint. Vary the shape of the 8, making the movement more like an infinity sign.

PRECAUTIONS

1. Avoid squeezing into the medial leg.

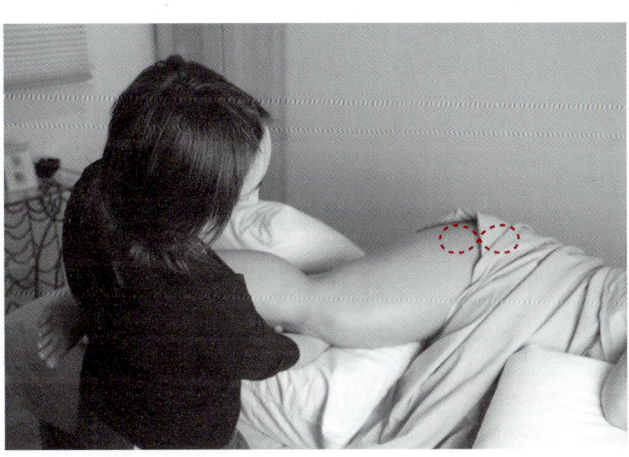

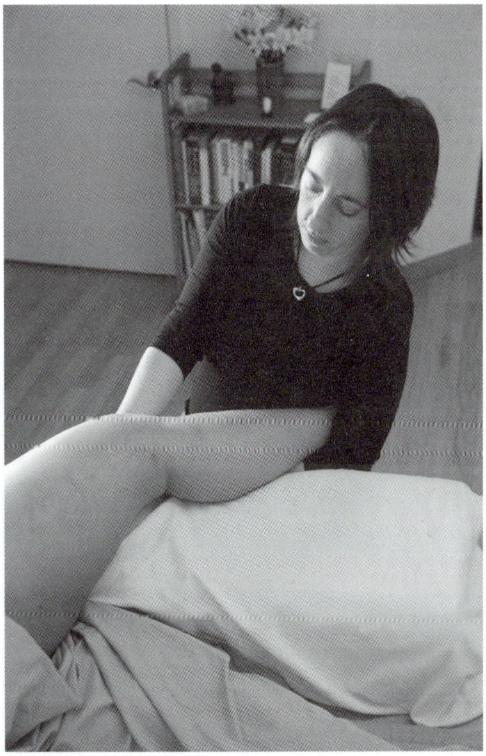

FIGURE 4.28 Figure 8 hip mobilization.

2. Do not move the torso with these movements; instead, isolate movement of the hip joint itself. Avoid hyperextension of joints.
3. Do not perform these movements if client is experiencing symphysis pubis dysfunction or has other pelvic instability.

Swedish and Lymphatic Drainage of Legs

Intentions

To promote movement of lymph, interstitial fluid, and venous blood return from the legs; to promote relaxation of the leg muscles and reduction of fatigue, cramping, and soft tissue pain; and to reduce tarsal tunnel and "restless" leg symptoms.

Procedures

May be performed in all positions.

1. Use strokes from your repertoire of Swedish techniques, such as effleurage, petrissage, kneading, fanning, raking, and chucking.
2. Modify rolling and wringing techniques so that they are very gentle, or eliminate entirely. Do not use tapotement or other vigorous movements.
3. Drainage techniques, both from the Swedish system and other lymph drainage methods, are particularly useful on the legs. For multiple tissue effects, work superficially and then increase pressure so that strokes gradually penetrate beyond the skin and into deeper muscles. Drain proximal areas first. Proceed further distally, but be sure to direct all strokes toward the heart (Fig. 4.29).
4. Modify these strokes when working in the sidelying position, and work on both the leg on the table and the supported leg, maintaining superficial pressure on the medial side of either leg.
5. Emphasize reducing edema with lighter strokes and relieving tension and cramping in the peroneals and gastrocnemius-soleus complex with deeper ones.
6. Raking, very subtle vibration, and acupressure to the medial arch can also help reduce ankle and foot edema.

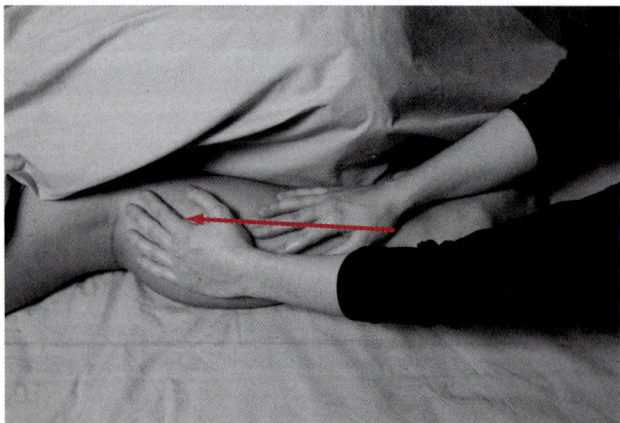

FIGURE 4.29 Swedish and lymph drainage for legs.

Hint

Take care to not push the client's leg so that she feels that she needs to prevent her leg from slipping off of the supports. Often, using one hand for your strokes and the other to create a countertraction to the leg helps to stabilize her on the table and also to avoid compressing the already compressed hip and knee joints.

Precautions

Modify as specified above, particularly on the medial leg, for varicose veins, spider veins, clot endangerment sites, cramping, hypertension and heart disease.

Other Techniques

Choose strokes and procedures from your own repertoire that have circulatory effect; that relieve downward pressure on veins and lymphatic structures in the pelvis and legs; that promote optimal alignment in the pelvis, hips, knees, and ankles; and that reduce myofascial pain. These may include the following: structural integration; craniosacral therapy, especially v-spread at pain sites; polarity therapy; Asian bodywork therapies; trigger point therapy to hips and legs; strain/counterstrain to pelvic points; zone therapy to feet or hands, especially the calcaneus and other tarsal bones and the space between the first and the second metatarsals (avoid pressure at all contraindicated points described in Chapter 2). Also, see the relaxation section of this chapter for superficial abdominal effleurage. Emphasize gentle, superficial strokes from just superior to the inguinal ligament toward the umbilicus. Performed prior to Swedish leg work, this will be helpful to decrease leg edema.

Addressing Pelvic and Lower Back Pain

Second and third trimester women often experience extensive lower back pain, including the following:
- Backache or shooting pain, spasms, cramping, particularly in the lumbar area and sacrum, and achiness over the sacroiliac joint
- Buttock pain
- Stabbing midline pubic bone pain when stair climbing, rolling over, or standing on one leg
- One-sided groin pain that may extend down anterior thigh (round ligament strain)
- Sciatica or sciatic-like pain and other neurological sensations

Review of Precautions

Low back pain can be a symptom of early labor or miscarriage, especially if unrelieved by a positional change. Kidney infections often create back pain as well. Evaluate carefully for other symptoms of complications, and refer to her prenatal healthcare provider for diagnosis. Observe all safety concerns detailed in Chapter 2, earlier in Chapter 4, and within the procedures that follow.

Technique Suggestions

Effectively addressing the "pregnant pelvis" involves techniques that increase range and quality of movement and that relieve strain in the following joints: the lumbar intervertebral and facet joints, the lumbosacral joints, the sacroiliac joints, and the symphysis pubis. Relieve muscle tension, myofascial strains, and trigger points in the following muscles: erector spinae, quadratus lumborum, rotators, multifidi, piriformis, and gluteals. Correct postural imbalances and reeducate movement patterns when possible.

PELVIC TILT REEDUCATION

INTENTIONS

To reeducate the client in efficient iliopsoas activation for proper lumbar and pelvic alignment with the legs, to tone the iliopsoas, to reduce pain referred from the sacrouterine ligament and around the lumbosacral joint, to reduce strain and pain in the lumbar spine and sacrum, to promote femoral circulatory flow by encouraging proper support of the uterus in the pelvic bowl.

PROCEDURES

Performed on the therapy table, in supine, sidelying, or semireclining position. This is a client-activated exercise that you can also teach before or after a session, in lying, sitting, and/or standing positions. Remember that after 22 weeks of pregnancy, women should not lie supine for extended periods.

1. Ask the client to imagine a long monkey tail attached to her tailbone and pulled between her legs, with the end at chest level where she can grasp it.
2. Verbally guide her to imagine pulling her tail to stretch it over her head, then releasing it back to the beginning position at chest height. Ask her to imagine this movement two more times, coordinating the imagined movements with her breath; while inhaling the tail is in front of her chest, and exhaling she pulls it over her head.
3. Standing at her lower back, place the palm of your hand closest to her feet over her sacrum. Spread your fingers gently across her gluteal muscles; lift your fingers away from the gluteal cleft to avoid inappropriate contact here. Place your other hand over her ilium so that your fingertips rest gently on her lateral abdomen just superior of her inguinal ligament. Pay attention to which muscle groups she is using as you now instruct her to continue imagining pulling her monkey tail and allowing the resulting pelvic movement (direction indicated by the white arrow on Fig. 4.30). Encourage her to coordinate the imagery and the pelvic tilting with her breathing as above.
4. Ask her to continue gently tilting and releasing the pelvis for up to 1 to 2 minutes as you refine her muscle usage with each repetition.
5. Encourage her to repeat pelvic tilting periodically throughout her day, in lying, standing, and seated positions to help reduce pelvic congestion and lower back strain.

HINTS

1. Expect some clients to have tiny tilts occur, even when initially only visualizing this movement.
2. She should be contracting primarily the iliopsoas muscles to make this movement, with a slight activation of the lower rectus abdominus fibers. You should feel this underneath your fingertips. If you feel her gluteal muscles tightening under your other hand, she may be using these or other extrinsic muscles, such as the hamstrings, the rectus femoris, or the upper abdominals. This type of large-amplitude pelvic movement creates a pelvic thrust rather than a pelvic tilt, and it doesn't train and tone the iliopsoas. Request that she inhibits use of any extrinsic muscles. She may have to make her tilts smaller or limit herself to simply imagining this movement for several practice times before the psoas can activate in isolation.
3. For other approaches to appropriate pelvic alignment and pelvic tilting, consult Noble (1995), Calais-Germain (2003), and Franklin (2003).

LUMBOSACRAL STRETCH OR PASSIVE PELVIC TILT

INTENTION

To facilitate the client's ability to correctly maintain pelvic/spinal alignment, to reduce hip and lumbosacral pain by stretching these joints, to

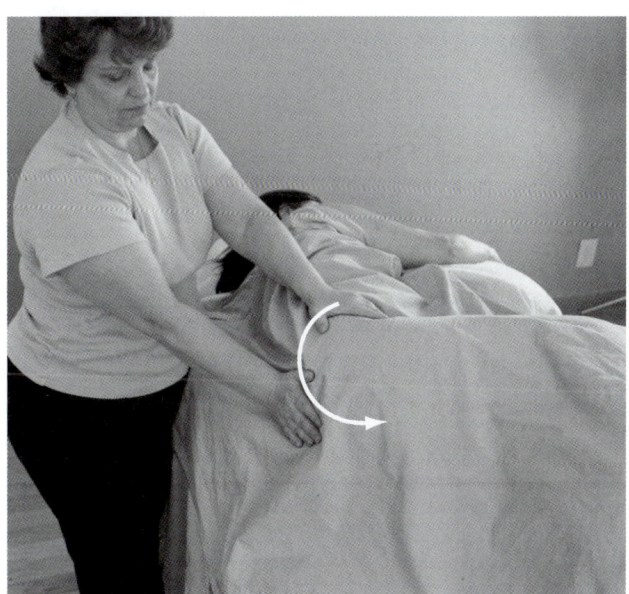

FIGURE 4.30 Pelvic tilt reeducation.

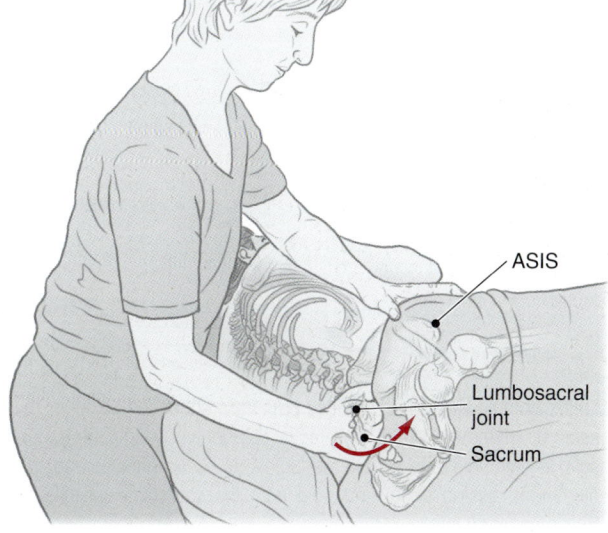

FIGURE 4.31 Lumbosacral stretch or passive pelvic tilt.

reduce sacrouterine ligament referred pain in the sacrum and lower back, to reduce lumbar pain from the intervertebral joints and surrounding myofascial tissues.

PROCEDURE

Best performed in the sidelying position and described for sidelying.

1. Stand behind the client's lower back. Cover her sacrum with your softly fisted hand or the palm of your hand nearest her feet. Place your other hand on her ASIS.
2. Apply firm, anteriorly directed pressure to the sacrum that turns her coccyx, as though tucking a tail. Allow your hand on her ASIS to remain relaxed throughout. Stretch the lumbosacral joint as you rotate her pelvis.
3. Hold this stretch for 30 seconds to 1 minute. Add rhythmic, small-amplitude rocking of the pelvis while holding the tilt, if desired.

HINTS

1. This passive pelvic tilt can lead naturally into instruction in active pelvic tilting as detailed in the procedure above.
2. If common tender points between the first/second and second/third sacral spines are present, use your whole hand to apply anterior directed pressure to the apex of the sacrum and hold for 90 seconds.
3. Teach partners to perform this simple, effective comfort measure so that they may assist in daily relief of hip and low back pain, and for "back labor." (See Chapter 5 for details.)

PRECAUTIONS

1. Avoid pointed, bone-on-bone pressure to the contraction stimulating points that coincide with the sacral sulcuses by applying generalized pressure with a broad tool such as the posterior flat of your fingers or the palm of your hand. (See Chapter 2 for detailed explanation and illustration.)
2. Allow your hand on the ASIS to rest passively so that the movement of her pelvis occurs by gently tucking her sacrum and coccyx rather than forcefully pulling the ASIS or flexing your fingers into the pelvic bowl.
3. Lift your fingers away from the gluteal cleft to avoid inappropriate contact here.
4. Take care to not strain your wrist as this technique requires considerable pressure to be effective. Keep your wrist joint aligned in all planes.

DEEP TISSUE SCULPTING AND TRIGGER POINT THERAPY TO PARAVERTEBRALS

Adapted from Osborne (2002) (Fig. 4.32).

INTENTIONS

To relax chronic tension and reduce pain from shortened posterior myofascial structures, primarily the erector spinae group and lumbodorsal fascia; to eliminate pain from trigger points; to assist in pelvic and spinal realignment, easing strain and pain from the sacroiliac, lumbosacral, and intervertebral joints.

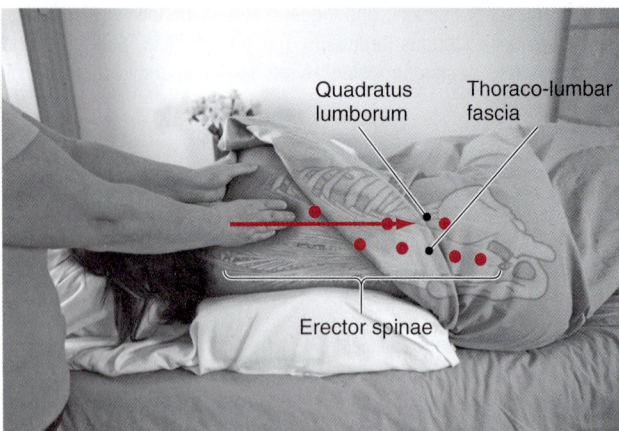

FIGURE 4.32 Deep tissue sculpting and trigger point therapy to paravertebrals.

PROCEDURE

Best performed in the sidelying position; may be performed in the prone, but only in the first trimester; described for sidelying.

1. From the head of the table, begin in an identified area of tension or near the C7 area. Using no oil on your fist, knuckles or fingertips, compress into the paravertebral myofascial structures. Sink to a level of tissue resistance, but create a sensation no more intense than pleasure, on the borderline of pain.
2. Continue to the base of the sacrum, changing which part of your hand or arm you use as tools as the muscles narrow above and over the sacrum.
3. Use fingertips, knuckles, elbows, and/or thumbs to release each side of the back, or you may work both sides simultaneously.
4. If common tender points between first/second and second/third sacral spines are present, apply pressure with a broad portion of your hand to apex of sacrum and hold for 90 seconds.
5. Extinguish any trigger points located during sculpting, especially in longissimus thoracis (T8–T10), in iliocostalis lumborum (L1), multifidus (S1), and quadratus lumborum (dots on Fig. 1.6). Modify your pressure on an identified trigger point until the pain is no more intense than pleasure on the borderline of pain. Request feedback from her about changes in pain intensity. Once her pain dissipates, continue to compress for 7 to 20 seconds.

HINTS

1. Perform all sculpting before applying oil. Do not force an unbroken stroke if the tissue is not elongating. A series of compressions is equally as effective. Remember to hold stationary for a minimum of 30 seconds or until myofascial release occurs. A combination of strokes and compressions will more likely be the release pattern.
2. Change your position to alongside the table and change tools as needed to avoid excessive leaning over the table or discomfort in your hands.
3. As an alternative to sustained pressure on a trigger point, move her to a position that eliminates the pain, and hold her there for 90 seconds. Slowly return her to her original position.

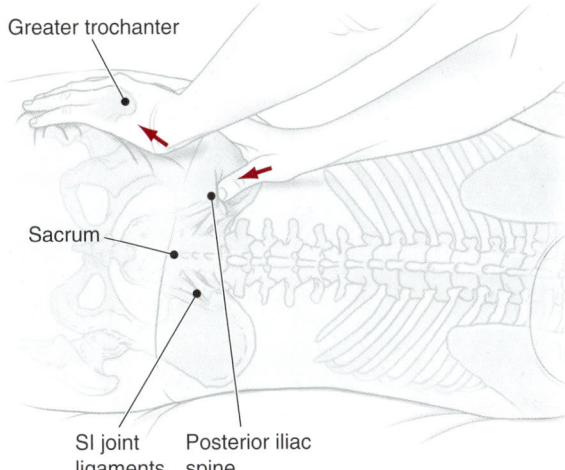

FIGURE 4.33 SI joint releases: rhythmic deep tissue (lateral vector).

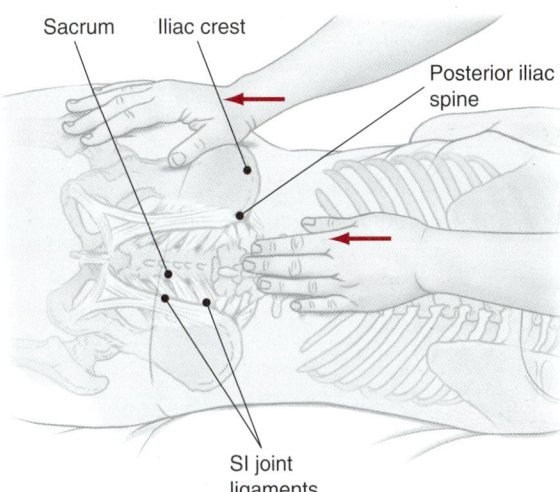

FIGURE 4.34 SI joint releases: rhythmic deep tissue (inferior vector).

Precautions

1. Work in either the muscle bellies or along the lateral border of the erector spinae group. Do not stroke directly over spinous processes.
2. In the lumbar area, be sure to direct pressure more toward the sacrum than anteriorly to avoid excessive lordosis.
3. If lumbar lordosis is extreme, do not use the prone position, even in first trimester.

Sacroiliac Joint (SI) Releases

Intention

To create ligament and myofascial relaxation in and around the SI joint, to reduce SI joint compression and rotation, to assist in pelvic and lumbar repositioning that reduces lumbar strain and pain.

Procedure

Best performed in the sidelying position or okay in prone, but only in the first trimester; described for sidelying; use no oil.

Rhythmic Deep Tissue (lateral vector) (Fig. 4.33)

1. Stand at lumbar level facing the client's feet. Use fingertips or thumb of the hand closest to her head to compress toward the SI joint of the higher hip. Sink just medial to the posterior iliac spine into the SI joint ligaments. Compress to a level of tissue resistance, but create a sensation no more intense than pleasure, on the borderline of pain.
2. Simultaneously place the palm of the other hand between the sacrum and the greater trochanter. Initiate gentle traction toward the knee accompanied by subtle rocking that shifts the ilium away from the sacrum. Maintain this blend of pressure, traction, and rocking for a minimum of 30 seconds for myofascial release.

Rhythmic Deep Tissue (vertical vector) (Fig. 4.34)

1. Change hand position to compress into the client's sacroiliac joint ligaments with the hand closest to her feet.
2. Place the palm of your other hand immediately superior of the lateral iliac crest.
3. Initiate gentle traction toward the feet accompanied by subtle rocking that shifts the ilium longitudinally in relationship to the sacrum. Maintain this blend of pressure, traction, and rocking for a minimum of 30 seconds.

SI Joint Approximation (Fig. 4.35)

1. Stand in front of client facing her top knee. Gently cup that knee and lean into it pressing her femur directly into the acetabulum to slowly approximate the hip joint. Lean further to also press the ilium closer to the sacrum to approximate that joint as well. Add a subtle, slow rocking movement if desired.
2. If you can reach with your opposite hand to the posterior iliac spine, you can monitor this movement and avoid her feeling you might push her off the table. Avoid twisting her lumbar spine.

SI Joint Distraction (Fig. 4.36)

1. Continue from the front of the table. Place one hand and forearm under her thigh, creating no focused pressure points on the medial leg. Lean away from the table to distract the hip joint. Lean further to distract the ilium from the sacrum as well. Add a subtle, slow rocking movement if desired.
2. If you can reach with your opposite hand to the posterior iliac spine, you can monitor this movement. Avoid twisting her lumbar spine.
3. If she prefers approximation or distraction, perform only her preference, and teach her to do this type of relief measure at home.

Hints

1. Use very small-amplitude and a slow, steady rhythm in the rocking motions.
2. On rhythmic deep tissue procedures, do not allow the rocking to jar the thumb or fingertips into the joint area. Maintain a steady, melting compression, while you rock, going deeper only as the myofascial structures relax.
3. Create variations and address other combinations of the SI joint ligaments, the sacrospinous and the sacrotuberous ligaments by relocating the rocking hand or the sculpting hand.

94 Pre- and Perinatal Massage Therapy

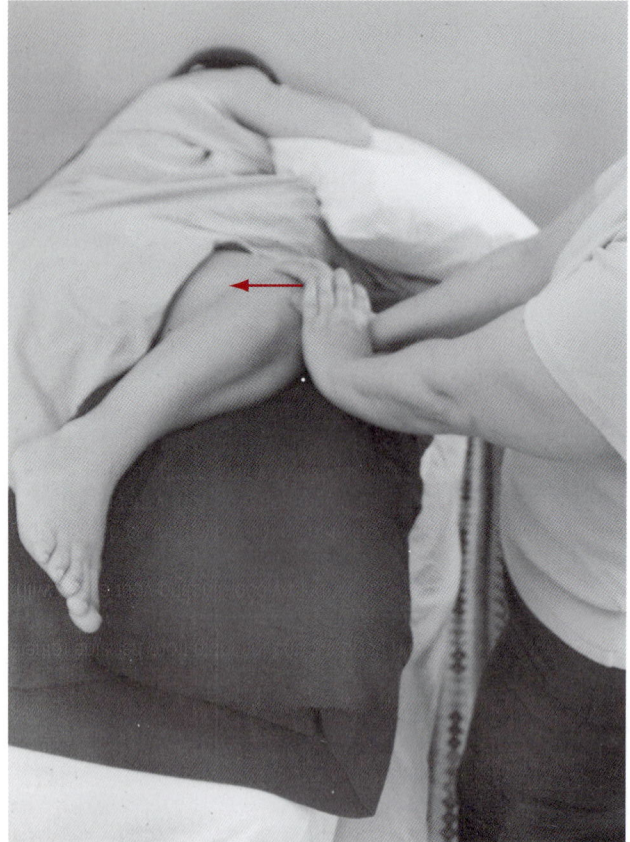

FIGURE 4.35 SI joint releases: approximation.

PRECAUTIONS

1. In the sidelying position, maintain the horizontal alignment of the client so that she does not roll forward onto her belly.
2. If the client experiences any pain, numbness, or tingling down the posterior leg or in the trochanteric bursa, reposition or reduce pressure.

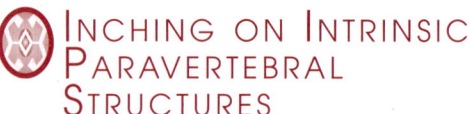 INCHING ON INTRINSIC PARAVERTEBRAL STRUCTURES

INTENTIONS

To relax and reduce pain from the spinal ligaments and paravertebral musculature, especially the more intrinsic intertransverse, interspinalis, semispinalis, multifidi, and rotators; to locate and extinguish trigger points in these muscles; to mobilize the spinal and rib joints.

PROCEDURE

Best performed in the sidelying position, though may be used prone, but only in the first trimester; described for sidelying (Fig. 4.37).

1. Stand at pelvic level, facing the client's head. Spread oil to her back. Place the middle and index fingers of your outside hand near the lumbosacral junction. Sink deeply into the laminar groove of the spine.

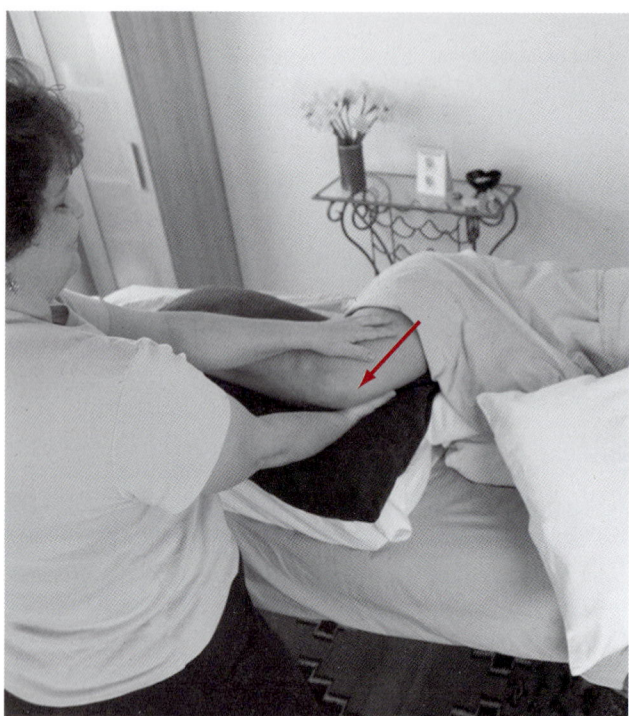

FIGURE 4.36 SI joint releases: distraction.

2. Maintaining your depth, rock your weight further into the spine and simultaneously flex and extend your distal phalangeal joints rhythmically. Slide up the groove parallel to the vertebral spinous processes pressing into the spinal rotators and vertebral ligaments. Work from the lumbosacral junction to the seventh cervical vertebra.
3. Repeat on the other side of the spine.

HINTS

1. Extinguish trigger points as you locate them, or after completing the inching.
2. Perform this procedure alternatively by using the thumb.

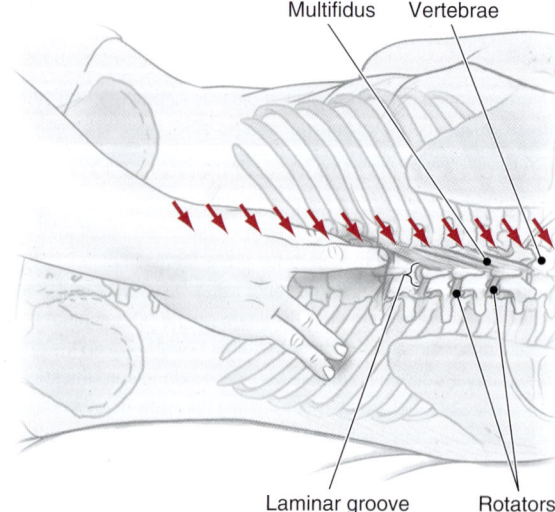

FIGURE 4.37 Inching on intrinsic paravertebral structures.

3. You can create inching variations by directing your pressure more medially or more anteriorly; also, by beginning at C7 and working caudally.

PRECAUTIONS

1. Inch immediately lateral to the spinous processes, but do not press directly on the spinous processes.
2. Maintain the alignment of the client so that she does not roll onto her belly.

Lumbar Lengthening

Adapted from Maupin (2004).

INTENTIONS

To reduce lumbar pain by realigning the pelvis and spine and by reducing strain to the sacrouterine ligament, to reeducate client movement, to improve iliopsoas strength through eccentric contraction.

PROCEDURE

Must be performed in supine position with no pillows or bolsters on the table (Fig. 4.38).

1. Stand at pelvic level facing client's head on the side of the table so that your dominant hand is closest to the table. Direct her to draw each leg up so that the soles of her feet are resting on the table about 12 inches apart. Ask her to rest her knees together as well, if preferred.
2. Instruct her to turn her tail under and lift first her pelvis, then her lumbar and, if possible, her thoracic spine from the table in a bridging movement. Direct her verbally to set her torso back onto the table starting at her upper ribcage. Guide her to slowly drop one vertebra at a time toward the table so that her pelvis comes down last as her spine lengthens as indicated by white arrows on Fig. 4.38.
3. Once the client has learned this movement, have her lift again. Place the palm of your dominant hand as high as possible with your middle and index fingers each lateral to the spinous processes and raised perpendicular to the table top. Let your forearm rest on the table. Place your other hand lightly on her upper chest.
4. Direct her verbally to set her torso back as above. Hook your fingers deeply into the fascia and draw them down as shown with the dotted red line. Elongate through her thoracic, lumbar, and sacral areas as she slowly lengthens her back, flexing her pelvis on her torso, and finally resuming a resting position on the table. Let your other hand lightly follow down the anterior of her torso at the level where your hand beneath is.
5. Repeat two more times.

HINTS

1. Slide your hand between her back and the table from her side rather than going between her legs.
2. Avoid trapping your hand under her by coordinating your stroke with her movement.
3. The words most likely to get her to do the movement as described are: "Begin at the top of your spine, and drop your vertebrae one at a time to the table. Very slowly continue while leaving your bottom up. Let your waistline come down, and now finally your bottom."

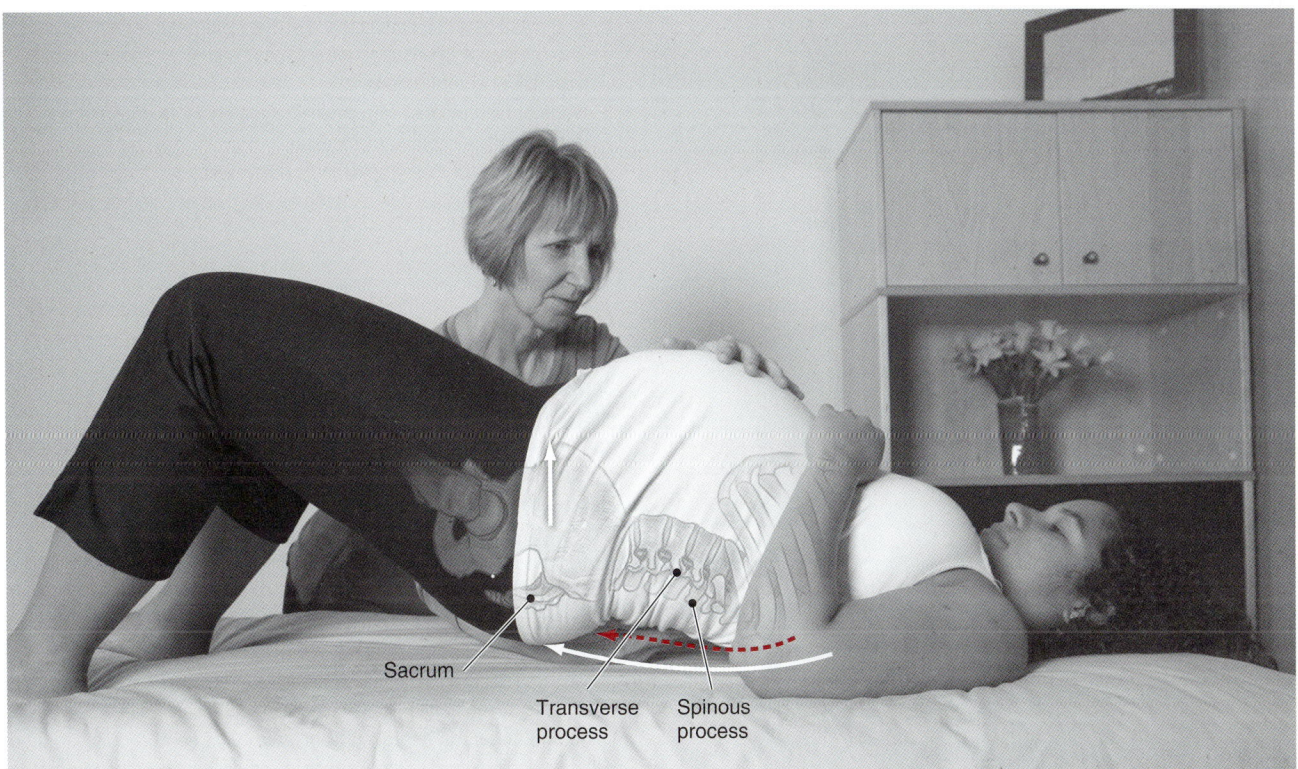

FIGURE 4.38 Lumbar lengthening: (White arrows indicate client's movement, and red dotted arrows indicate therapist's movement on client.)

PRECAUTIONS

1. Do not press into her abdomen.
2. In weeks 14 to 22, remove torso support pillow prior to performing lift. To prevent possible supine hypotensive syndrome, do not exceed 2 to 5 minutes of unsupported supine positioning as you do this technique.
3. Eliminate with high risk/complications.

SYMPHYSIS PUBIS REBALANCING

INTENTIONS

To reduce pain of symphysis pubis dysfunction, to improve motion and/or stability of the joint via resisted action of adductors and abductors.

PROCEDURE

Best performed in supine or semireclining positions.

1. Stand at the client's pelvic level facing her head. Direct her to draw each leg up so that the soles of her feet are resting on the table about 12 inches apart. Ask her to rest her knees together.
2. Hold her knees together as she attempts to part her knees (abduction movement) for 5 seconds and repeat 3-5 times (Fig. 4.39).
3. Release her knees and ask her to part her knees so that one or both of your forearms fits between them. Ask her to attempt to squeeze her knees together (adduction movement) against your forearms for 5 seconds and repeat 3-5 times (Fig. 4.40).

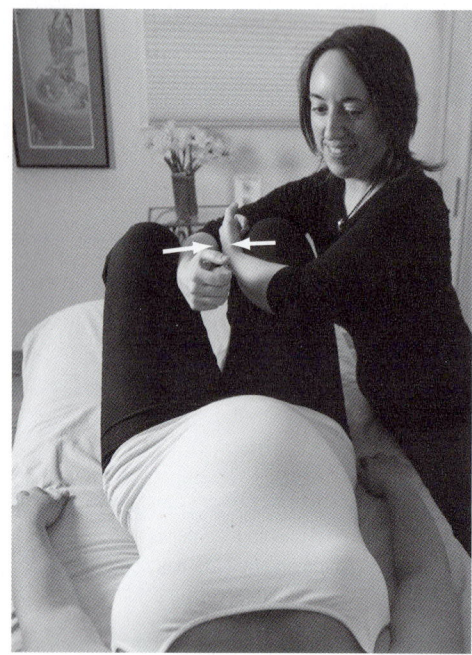

FIGURE 4.40 Symphysis pubis rebalancing: client's adduction movement indicated by white arrows.

PRECAUTIONS

1. In weeks 14 to 22, remove the torso support pillow prior to performing.
2. To prevent possible supine hypotensive syndrome, do not exceed 2 to 5 minutes of unsupported supine positioning. Eliminate with high risk or complications.
3. If one or both of these movements create pain that does not subside immediately, discontinue procedure.
4. If one or both of these movements relieve her pain, teach her to perform the effective one at home on her own or with her partner's help.

OTHER TECHNIQUES

Choose strokes and procedures from your own repertoire that reduce stress on major joints, relieve muscle and ligamentous strain, and retrain appropriate pelvic movement. These may include the following: assisted resisted stretches to the lower torso, pelvic, and thigh muscles; craniosacral therapy, including traction or leverage release of L5–S1, medial compression of ASIS to release SI joints, V-spread to painful sites, and dural tube rocking; strain-counterstrain technique for quadratus lumborum and anterior pelvic points, especially those on the pubic bone; Swedish massage of the lower back and posterior pelvic muscles; zones on the foot for musculoskeletal strain in the back, sacroiliac joint, pubis symphysis, and coccyx (avoiding reproductive organ reflexes), and sacrum; abdominal strengthening exercises; rhythmic passive movements in the spine and pelvis, as described in the relaxation section of this manual; deep tissue sculpting of the lateral hip, as described in the hip and leg section of this manual. Be especially alert to trigger points in the gluteals and piriformis that refer to the SI joint area.

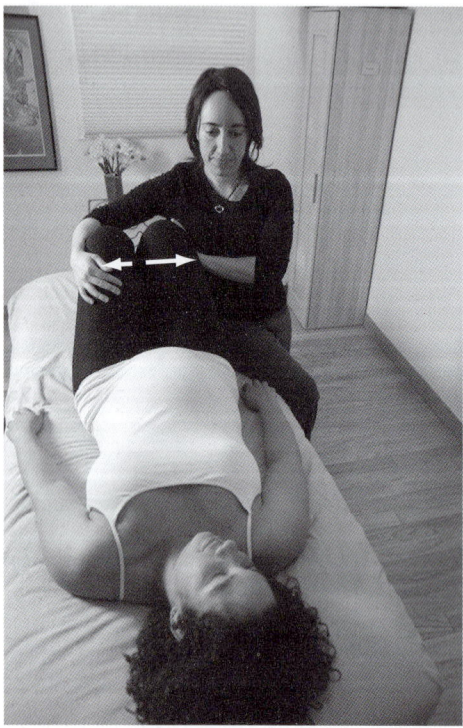

FIGURE 4.39 Symphysis pubis rebalancing: client's abduction movement indicated by white arrows.

Reducing Upper Body Discomforts

Even first trimester women often experience pain and dysfunctions in the neck, upper torso, and pectoral girdle. They may report the following:

- Headaches: either migraine, tension, or sinus in origin
- Neck pain and stiffness
- Tightness and pain between the scapula and across the shoulders
- Rib soreness or pain
- Numbness, tingling, and/or pain down the arm
- Wrist and hand pain

Review of Precautions

Severe headaches, especially with dizziness, nausea, or visual disturbances, can be symptomatic of eclampsia of pregnancy. Severe, persistent midback pain, especially on the right side and shoulder and unaffected by positional changes, also can be referred pain from the liver and/or the kidneys during eclampsia. Edema in the arms and hands can be symptomatic of gestationally induced hypertension. When these symptoms occur, refer the client for immediate evaluation and do not perform massage therapy without a prenatal healthcare provider's written release. Observe all safety concerns detailed in Chapter 2, earlier in Chapter 4, Chapter 7, and within the procedures that follow.

Technique Suggestions

The pregnant woman's upper body is much like that of a nonpregnant client whose tendency is toward a lordotic posture. Many popular massage therapy techniques for neck, upper back, and pectoral girdle tension and pain are effective with expectant women, too. The techniques detailed in this section focus on the most problematic soft tissue areas using deep tissue, cross-fiber, trigger point, and passive movement.

Deep Tissue Sculpting

Adapted from Osborne (2002).

Intentions

To create myofascial release that reduces chronic tension and pain in the trapezius, levator scapula, scalenes, pectoralis major and minor, and other pectoral girdle musculature; to reduce pain by assisting in realignment of the head, cervical, and thoracic spine, and ribcage; to relieve any pressure on the brachial plexus or the ulnar nerve; to reduce pain by locating and extinguishing trigger points.

Procedures

All of these procedures may be performed in any appropriate position; all are described for supine or semireclining.

Upper Trapezius (Fig. 4.41)
1. Stand at the head of the table to use either one or both fists to work either unilaterally or bilaterally.
2. Compress into the upper trapezius beginning near the base of the neck. Sink to a level of tissue resistance, but create intensity no more than pleasure on the borderline of pain.
3. Maintain stationary pressure for a minimum of 30 seconds, and let the speed of myofascial release guide the speed of any movement along or into the muscle. Proceed in a stroke or a series of compressions to the trapezius insertion along the scapula.

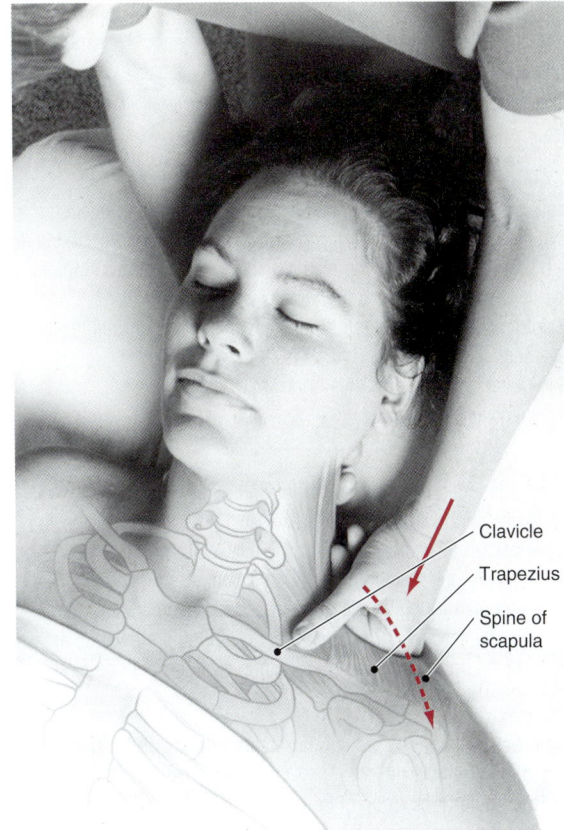

FIGURE 4.41 Deep tissue sculpting: upper trapezius.

4. Extinguish any trigger points uncovered.
5. If performed unilaterally, repeat on other side.

Levator Scapula (Fig. 4.42)
1. From the head end of the table, use knuckles or fingertips to compress into the levator scapula attachment on the superior angle of the scapula.

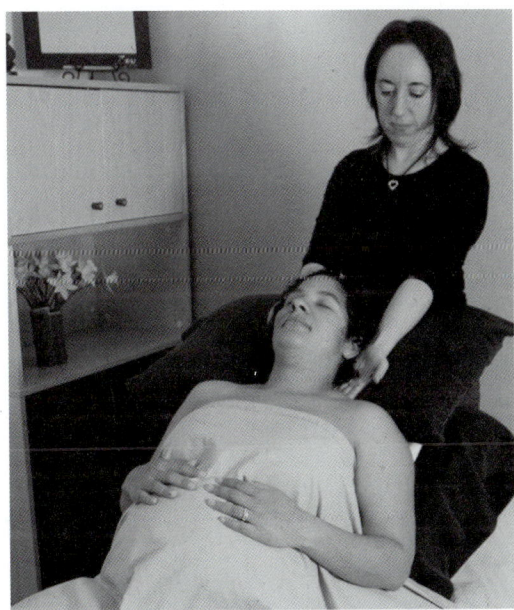

FIGURE 4.42 Deep tissue sculpting: levator scapulae.

2. Maintain pressure for a minimum of 30 seconds or until tissue releases.
3. Extinguish any trigger points uncovered.
4. If performed unilaterally, repeat on other side.

Scalenes
(Fig. 4.43)
1. From the head of the table, use thumb or fingertips to release the scalenes. Apply unilateral compression just posterior to the clavicle at a point just lateral to the sternocleidomastoid origins. Maintain a vector of pressure toward the client's feet.
2. Maintain pressure for a minimum of 30 seconds or until tissue releases.
3. Extinguish any trigger points uncovered.
4. Repeat on other side.

Pectoralis Major (Fig. 4.44)
1. Stand at the client's side facing her opposite shoulder.
2. Using your hand closest to her, sink with your fingertips into the upper pectoralis major fibers (clavicular section) just superior to breast tissue and immediately lateral to her sternum.
3. Progress laterally out to the humeral insertions with either a series of melting, 30-second compressions or a stroke, if the tissue elongates.
4. Move to the opposite side and repeat to work both sides.

Pectoralis Minor (Fig. 4.45)
1. Stand beside the client, facing her head. Slightly abduct her closest arm with her elbow flexed.
2. Use the posterior surface of your inside hand to medially displace her breast so that you may access her axilla without compressing

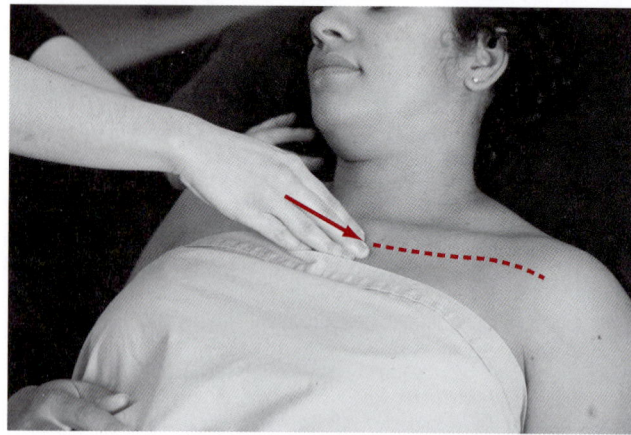

FIGURE 4.44 Deep tissue sculpting: pectoralis major.

into breast tissue. (Alternately, you may ask her to displace her breast.)
3. Use the other hand in her axilla at about the fifth rib level to gently sink into the myofascial tissue just deep to the pectoralis major. Direct the vector of your pressure toward her sternal notch.
4. Shift the nonsculpting hand to the shoulder joint and forward rotate the scapula to sink deeper. Downward rotate the scapula to create stretch of the pectoralis minor against your fingertips.
5. After a minimum of 30 seconds of melting compression, release slightly and redirect your vector of pressure to similarly contact attachments on rib four and then on rib three.
6. Extinguish any trigger points uncovered.
7. Move to the other side of the table and repeat.

PRECAUTIONS
1. Avoid painful and dangerous pressure into the brachial plexus. Redirect vector if numbness or tingling occurs down her arm.

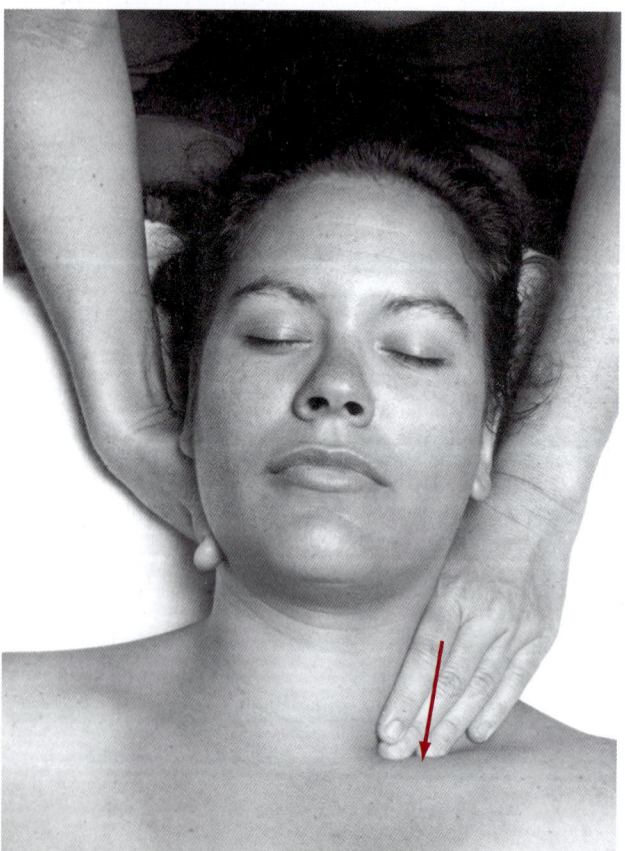

FIGURE 4.43 Deep tissue sculpting: scalenes.

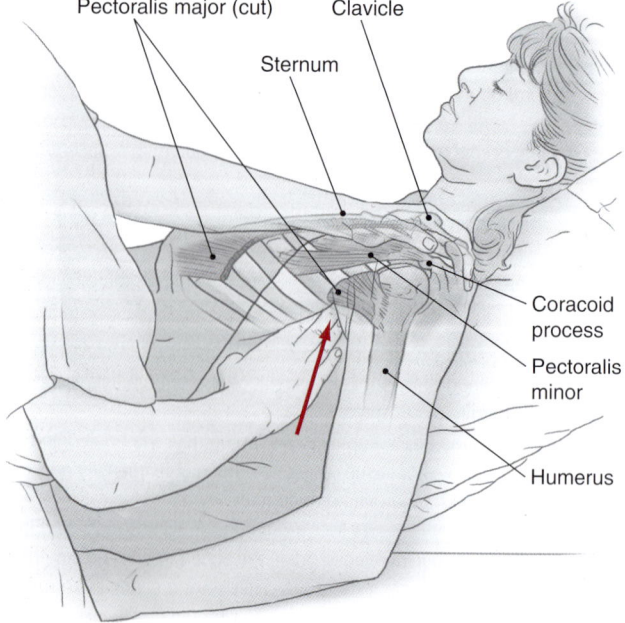

FIGURE 4.45 Deep tissue sculpting: pectoralis minor.

2. Avoid pressure into the "careful triangle" bordered by the sternocleidomastoid, clavicle, and anterior trapezius.
3. Avoid painful pressure on the acromioclavicular joint.
4. Be specific to the superior angle of the scapula when sculpting the levator scapula insertion to avoid the GB 21 point.

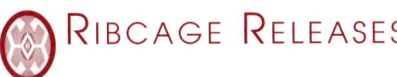 RIBCAGE RELEASES

INTENTIONS

To facilitate ribcage expansion to better accommodate the enlarging uterus; to facilitate deep abdominal breathing by relaxing the diaphragm; to create myofascial release to reduce chronic ribcage tension and pain; to reduce pain from postural imbalances by assisting in ribcage realignment; to reduce pain by locating and extinguishing trigger points, particularly in the external oblique, rectus abdominis, and intercostals.

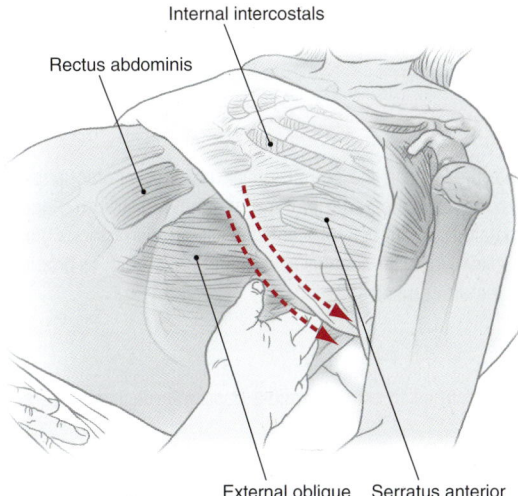

FIGURE 4.47 Ribcage releases: trigger points.

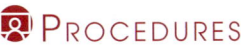 PROCEDURES

Both of these procedures may be performed in all appropriate positions; described for sidelying and semireclining as illustrated.

Distal Ribcage Sculpting (Fig. 4.46)
1. Stand beside your sidelying client at her waist level and facing toward her head.
2. Using the flat of your fingertips of your inside hand, reach between her abdomen and breast to contact the distal border of the ribcage at xiphoid level on the ceiling side of her ribcage.
3. Lean away from the client to gently sink into the myofascia on the ribcage. Remain on the distal costal cartilage, and avoid slipping inferior of it.
4. Wait a minimum of 30 seconds for myofascial release that allows movement along the distal border or deeper into the tissue.
5. Continue until you feel the floating eleventh rib.

Trigger Points (Fig. 4.47)
1. Stand beside your client to either work on her opposite ribcage or on the same side.
2. Spread a very light application of oil, and sink superficially with your fingertips and create a sawing motion into the external oblique, the rectus and serratus anterior ribcage attachments, and then into the intercostals between ribs 6 through 10. Work between only two ribs with each pass.
3. As you make repeated passes in these tissues, seek any areas eliciting a jump response from the client, or any posterior or anterior rib pain. These trigger points are most prevalent in areas of soft tissue dysfunction and spasm.
4. Moderate your pressure on the point until the pain is no more intense than pleasure on the borderline of pain.
5. Request client feedback of changes in pain intensity. Once her pain has dissipated, continue to compress for 7 to 20 seconds.
6. If possible, stretch the trigger area for 30 to 60 seconds, or perform localized thumb fanning-type strokes over the point.

HINT

Encourage additional relief by directing her to more lateral (costal) breathing during these procedures. (See breathing technique in the relaxation section of this chapter.)

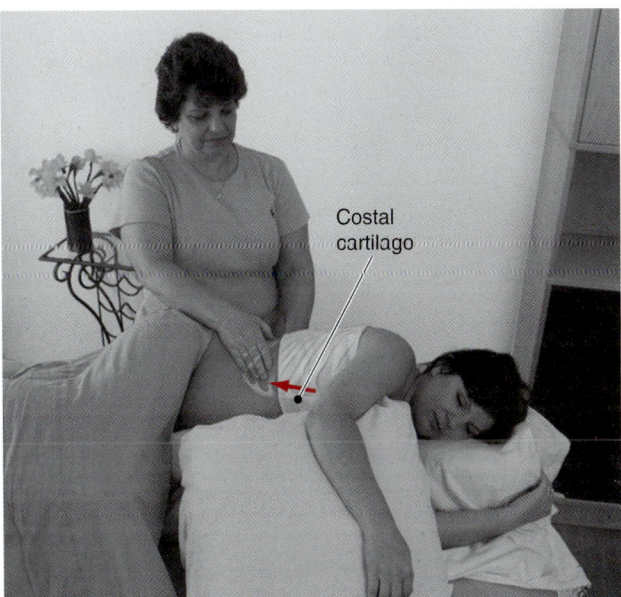

FIGURE 4.46 Ribcage releases: distal ribcage sculpting.

PRECAUTIONS
1. Do not curl your fingertips under the ribcage, and avoid any pressure into the abdomen.
2. Do not press directly on the xiphoid process.
3. Avoid compressing into breast tissue. Use breast drape or ask client to shift breasts if necessary.

Arm Techniques

Intentions

To relieve pressure in the carpal tunnel; to relax chronic tension in the hand flexors; to reduce pain in the arms and wrists from trigger points; to promote movement of lymph, interstitial fluid, and venous blood return and to relieve vascular sources of arm and hand pain; to promote relaxation of the arm muscles.

Procedures

May be performed in all appropriate positions; described for supine or semireclining.

Swedish and Lymphatic Arm Massage
1. Use strokes from your repertoire of Swedish techniques, such as effleurage, petrissage, kneading, fanning, chucking, rolling, and wringing. Drainage techniques, both from the Swedish system and other lymph drainage methods, are particularly useful on the arms.
2. Work superficially and then increase pressure so that strokes gradually penetrate beyond the skin and into deeper muscles.
3. Drain proximal areas first, including the armpit and associated lymph nodes. Proceed further distally, but be sure to direct all strokes toward the heart.

Passive Wrist Movements (Fig. 4.48)
1. Place one hand one on each side of her wrist facing the palm side down. Using your middle fingers, grasp her hand to gently spread apart the hamate/pisiform and tubercle of the trapezium. This will stretch the flexor retinaculum.
2. Hold space between these two bony borders of the carpal tunnel while mobilizing the carpal and wrist joints with small-amplitude, oscillating motions. Avoid extremes of range of motion.

Cross-fiber Friction
1. Use your thumbs or several fingertips to compress firmly into a section of the transverse carpal ligament or flexor retinaculum. Maintain your pressure at that point so that you do not slide on the skin as you move perpendicular to the ligament with a rapid, friction motion.
2. Continue for 3 to 5 minutes of friction in that section, then move to the next segment and repeat, until you have frictioned across the entire ligament and retinaculum.

Sculpting
1. With the client's forearm in anatomical position against the table, sink with your fist or knuckles into the hand flexor compartment, beginning just proximal to the wrist.
2. Compress slowly and deeply to a level of tissue resistance and wait a minimum of 30 seconds for myofascial release. Continue in a series of compressions to the elbow, or stroke on the skin, but only if the myofascial tissues elongate creating motion of your fist. Do not use oil so that you will not slide quickly on the surface.
3. Extinguish any trigger points uncovered while sculpting.
4. Repeat on the extensors and on the other arm.

Hint

Take care to not push client's arm so far toward the opposite side of the table that she feels crooked or that she might fall off. Often, using one hand for your strokes and the other to create a countertraction to the arm and pectoral girdle helps to stabilize her on the table.

Pectoral Girdle Cross-fiber Friction

Intentions

To reduce chronic tension and pain from adhesions in the neck and pectoral girdle, especially in the levator scapula, supraspinatus, cervical soft tissues, and rhomboids; to encourage realignment of the upper torso and neck; to reduce pain from trigger points in the pectoral girdle and neck (Fig. 4.49).

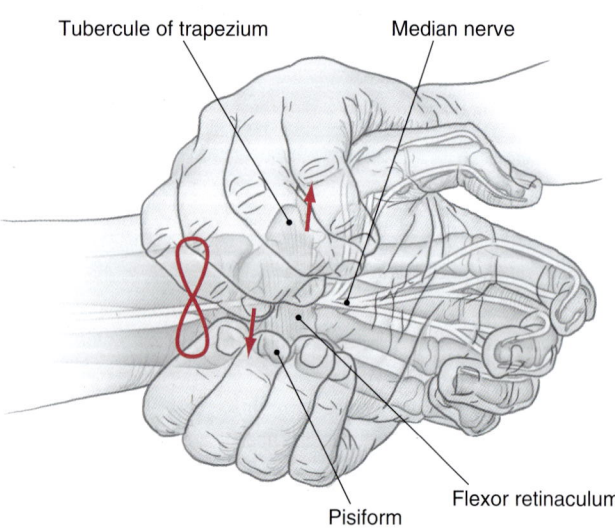

FIGURE 4.48 Passive wrist movements.

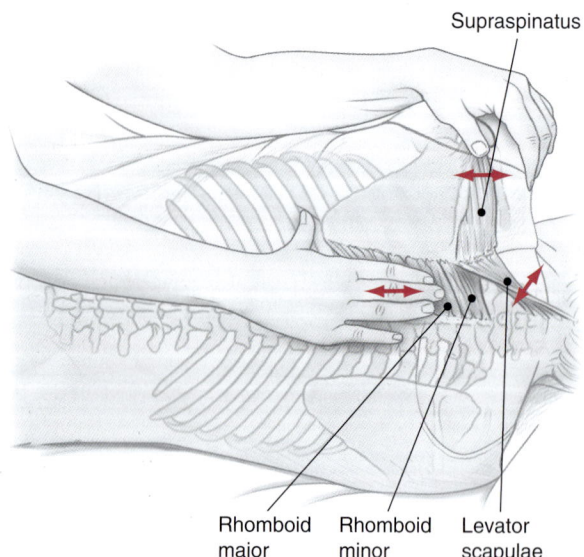

FIGURE 4.49 Pectoral girdle cross-fiber friction.

PROCEDURES

May be performed in any appropriate position; described for sidelying.

1. Stand posterior to the client's torso and facing her head.
2. Use the fingertips or thumbtip of your outside hand to sink to the depth of the desired muscle.
3. Maintain depth of pressure and create a cross-fiber friction to the area by leaning into the client and creating motion from rotation of your torso. Continue, without moving over the skin, for 2 to 5 minutes.
4. Focus on the levator scapula belly and insertion, the supraspinatus near its lateral musculotendinous junction, the insertion of rhomboids, and the posterior cervical extensors.
5. Extinguish any trigger points uncovered during friction.

HINT

Create variations of friction by rocking appropriate joints to rub the affected tissue under your compressing thumb or fingertip.

PRECAUTIONS

Use only broad pressure on the apex of the shoulder and avoid stimulation to the gall bladder 21 point. In the sidelying position, maintain the alignment of the client so that she does not roll forward onto her belly.

OTHER TECHNIQUES

Choose other strokes and procedures from your own repertoire that relieve the strain of anterior weight load, that alleviate musculoskeletal pain and dysfunction in the neck, upper torso, arms, and hands, and that rebalance structural alignment. These may include the following: craniosacral techniques, especially the thoracic inlet and respiratory diaphragm releases, inducing stillpoint, dural tube rocking, and V-spread to painful sites; facial massage, especially to the temporalis, masseter, and frontalis muscles; foot reflexology areas for the shoulder, torso and arms; strain-counterstrain to the anterior and posterior spine, ribs, shoulder joint, and wrist and hand flexors; stretching; structural integration; trigger point therapy to the trapezius, rhomboids, and rotator cuff.

See the previous section on relaxation for details on spinal rocking, occipital traction, transverse rocking, and pectoral girdle movements that would also be helpful with these complaints. The section on the lumbar area explains how to sculpt the paravertebral soft tissues. For the upper body, focus on the thoracic level of the extensors. That section also includes inching for the intrinsic paravertebral muscles.

GASTROINTESTINAL AND URINARY TRACT DISCOMFORTS

Upset stomach, food cravings, and frequency of urination during pregnancy make for many of the jokes and popular stereotypes of expectant women. These discomforts are not a laughing matter for most women.

Complaints and Presenting Symptoms
- "Morning sickness" (nausea and vomiting)
- Heartburn
- Hiatal hernia
- Constipation
- Hemorrhoids
- Bladder and kidney infection
- Urinary incontinence
- Bladder or uterine prolapse

Review of Precautions
- Observe all relevant precautions listed in the first section of this chapter and in the following procedures.
- Do not massage the abdomen in the first trimester or in a pregnancy with increased prematurity or miscarriage risk to lessen possible legal implications in any pregnancy loss. In second and third trimesters, perform all techniques at a maximum depth of the skin level. Avoid pointed pressure into the abdomen, especially at the solar plexus and inguinal regions.
- If nausea and vomiting are severe, proceed with caution and with the prenatal healthcare provider's written release.
- Kidney and bladder infections can become serious prenatal complications. Massage therapy should not replace appropriate medical care. Obtaining the prenatal healthcare provider's written release is recommended after kidney infections.
- Observe all safety concerns detailed in Chapter 2, earlier in Chapter 4, and within the procedures that follow.

Technique Suggestions
Lifestyle adaptations make the most impact on these common pregnancy complaints; however, a few notably effective techniques work reflexively to normalize and balance the involved organs. Acupressure to the Nei Guan (PC-6) point, as shown in figure 7.4, can help relieve nausea. (Belluomini et al. 1994). Deep pressure to zones on the feet may reduce the discomfort of nausea, heartburn, constipation, hemorrhoids, bladder and kidney infection, and other common prenatal complaints (Lett 2000).

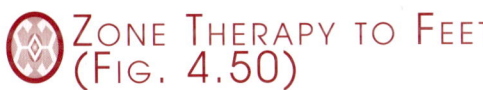

ZONE THERAPY TO FEET (FIG. 4.50)

PROCEDURES

1. Use the side of the thumb and/or a finger to create bone on bone pressure into the foot. Travel with tiny, overlapping movements, compressing the skin and undifferentiated nerves of the foot against the foot bones.
2. Rhythmically inch along or across specific reflex areas or over the entire foot. Press rather than rub to achieve the desired effect. Imagine that your finger or thumb moves like a tiny inchworm.
3. Repeat three times in each zone, specifically addressing the following zones:

- Nausea or hiatal hernia: plantar surface proximal to metatarsal-phalangeal joints
- Constipation: plantar surface of left foot moving across the midline of the foot and toward the heel over the fourth metatarsal
- Hemorrhoids: plantar surface of the foot, on the most distal edge of the calcaneus and along the Achilles tendon from its attachment on the calcaneus to approximately 2 inches proximal (avoid pinching the sciatic nerve)
- Bladder: in the "puffy" area of the medial arch just distal to the calcaneus
- Kidneys: midline of the plantar surface of the foot.

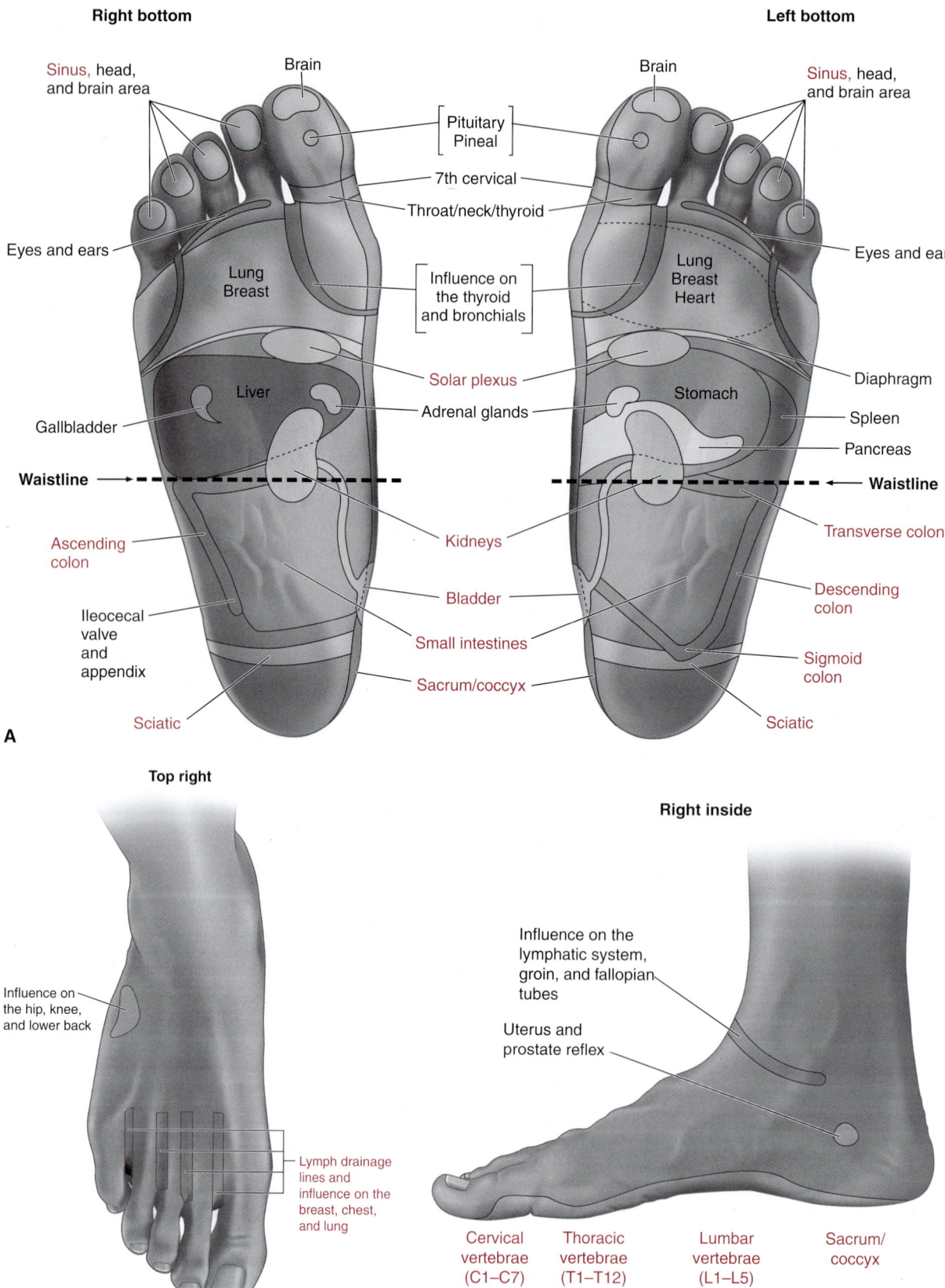

FIGURE 4.50 Foot reflexology (zone therapy). Red labels mark zones most commonly helpful prenatally and postpartum. Adapted from Williams A. *Spa Bodywork: A Guide for Massage Therapists*. Philadelphia: Lippincott Williams & Wilkins, 2007.

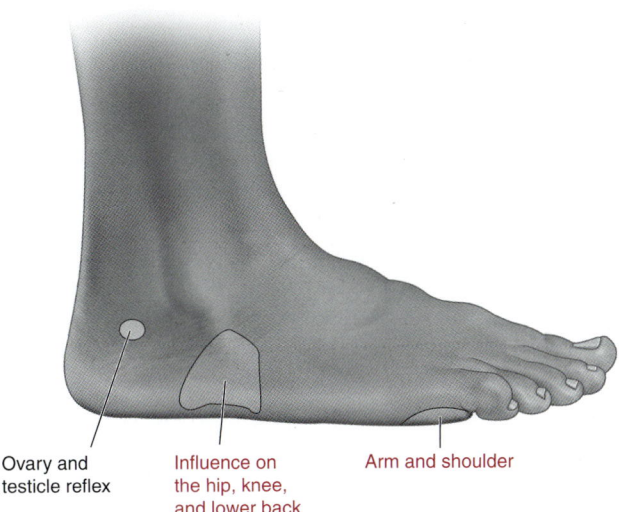

Right outside

Ovary and testicle reflex

Influence on the hip, knee, and lower back

Arm and shoulder

D

FIGURE 4.50 (*Continued*)

PRECAUTIONS

1. Maintain a level of pressure that does not exceed slight pain. If the client perceives high pain levels, move to another area, returning to the painful zone later in the session.
2. Avoid initiating calf cramps by not plantarflexing the foot as you work.
3. Avoid calcaneus reflex zones to ovaries and uterus (see Chapter 2).
4. Exercise caution to avoid overstimulating the endocrine glands.
5. Avoid acupressure points Liver 3, Kidney 3, and Urinary Bladder 60, which may stimulate uterine contractions under certain circumstances (see Chapter 2).
6. Exercise caution with substance abusers, if pregnancy is tenuous, or if first session of reflexology.

◆ OTHER TECHNIQUES

Choose strokes and procedures from your own repertoire that promote gastrointestinal and urinary tract balance. These may include the following: gentle, full-body Swedish and Esalen-style massage; craniosacral therapy; polarity therapy; Asian bodywork techniques; structural balancing (see details in lumbar techniques for details).

CHAPTER SUMMARY

As a baby develops from two cells, growing into maturity, its unique genetic imperatives unfold in generally predictable stages. This chapter has surveyed those fetal developments and the corresponding maternal adaptations normally following along this chronological progression. Now, even if a prenatal client's only input to you about how her pregnancy is going is "fine," you understand the physiological, structural, functional, and emotional states she is likely to be experiencing. You now have guidelines for choosing techniques from your own somatic therapy repertoire that are more likely to facilitate her baby's growth and ease any associated discomforts.

After also viewing the video instructions that elaborate this chapter's technique manual, you can weave additional specific prenatal techniques from a broad range of methodologies into your work. Your sessions can move far beyond just general adaptations of a basic massage. With the specificity, focused intention, and respect for relevant safety concerns of these clinically matured techniques, each of your sessions can reflect your responsiveness to the unique individuals your client and her baby are. Don't forget to review the suggested session outlines available online, but, like a jazz musician improvising on a lyrical theme, let your intuition and creativity infuse your sessions' organic development.

My Story

One of my clients had an unexpected pregnancy a few years after [she turned] 40. This woman was a physical therapist, and, though she had helped many people deal with chronic pain, she had never experienced it herself. As she moved into her second trimester, she began waking up at night with fiery, electric pain in both arms and hands. Her obstetrician diagnosed pregnancy-related carpal tunnel syndrome. Informing this very active woman that her last ultrasound had revealed a potentially dangerous condition called placenta previa, he put her on bed rest.

When she came to see me, she was quite upset about how things were unfolding and was concerned that the carpal tunnel syndrome would last beyond pregnancy. We began our session with circulatory work in the hands and arms, and she was relieved to find that her pain diminished dramatically. We both agreed that the pain was more likely due to fluid in the arms than a structural discrepancy. In subsequent sessions, when I was traveling to her house, we spent some time instructing her husband in the art of Swedish arm massage so that he would be able to offer her some relief during the time in between sessions. Her carpal tunnel syndrome discontinued when she finished breastfeeding.

—*Liz Ellis, Chicago, IL*

Test Yourself

For answers, visit the website at http://thePoint.LWW.com/Osborne-Pregnancy2e!

1. What hormone is the primary cause of many pregnancy discomforts, such as nausea, constipation, and varicose veins?

2. What are the most common first trimester discomforts?

3. List several typical third trimester functional changes in gait.

4. What typical changes might you observe in clients' skin and hair as their pregnancy progresses?

5. What second trimester experiences usually bring women delight and a heightened sense of the reality of their pregnancy?

6. If a prenatal complication were to occur, such as gestationally induced hypertension or gestational diabetes, in which trimester is this most likely to occur?

7. Strain to which uterine ligaments is more likely to occur in which trimesters?

8. What communications with your client should be a standard part of every session throughout her pregnancy?

9. When you need to massage clients' backs, what position on a massage therapy table is usually comfortable and safest in every trimester?

10. Despite the strain to and importance of the iliopsoas in maintaining optimal postural integrity, why is direct massage of this muscle not recommended?

11. What is a unique factor that contributes to the development of carpal tunnel syndrome in pregnant women that usually doesn't occur with nonpregnant sufferers of this type of hand and arm pain?

REFERENCES

Belluomini J, Litt R, Lee K, et al. Acupressure for nausea and vomiting of pregnancy: a randomized, blinded study. Obstet Gynecol 1994;84:245.

Calais-Germain B. The Female Pelvis: Anatomy and Exercises. Seattle: Eastland Press, 2003.

Field T, Hernandez-Reif M, Hart S, et al. Pregnant women benefit from massage therapy. J Psychosom Obstet Gynecol 1999;20(1):31–38.

Franklin E. Pelvic Power: Mind/Body Exercises for Strength, Flexibility, Posture and Balance. Heightstown, NJ: Elysian Editions Princeton Book Co., 2003.

Gibbs R, Karlan B, Haney A, et al., eds. Danforth's Obstetrics and Gynecology. 10th Ed. Philadelphia: Lippincott Williams & Wilkins, 2008.

Herman H. Pregnancy and Postpartum: Clinical Highlights. San Diego: The Prometheus Group. Seminar notes, August, 2004.

Howard F, Perry C, Carter J, et al. Pelvic Pain: Diagnosis and Management. Philadelphia: Lippincott Williams & Wilkins, 2000.

Leduc M. Stretch marks: striae gravidarum. In: Encyclopedia of Childbearing: Critical Perspectives. Barbara Roth Katzman, ed. Phoenix: The Oryx Press, 1993:385.

Lett A. Reflex Zone Therapy for Health Professionals. London: Churchill Livingstone, 2000.

Longworth JC. Psychophysical effects of slow stroke back massage in normotensive females. Adv Nurs Sci 1982;4:44–61.

Mallol J, Belda MA, Costa D, et al. Prophylaxis of *Striae gravidarum* with a topical formulation. A double blind trial. Int J Cosmet Sci 1991;13(1):51–57.

Maupin E. A Dynamic Relation to Gravity, vol 2. San Diego: Dawn Eve Press, 2004.

Mayo Clinic. Pregnancy and Exercise: Baby Let's Move! Available at http://www.mayoclinic.com/health/pregnancy-and-exercise/pr00096. Accessed May 23, 2010.

Myers TW. Anatomy Trains: Myofascial Meridians for Manual and Movement Therapists. 2nd Ed. London: Harcourt, 2009.

Noble E. Essential Exercises for the Childbearing Year. 4th Ed. Harwich: New Life Images, 1995:39–50.

Osborne C. Pre- and Perinatal Massage Therapy: Survey of Massage Therapists, 2009. Available at www.bodytherapyassociates.com. Accessed June, 2010.

Osborne C. Deep Tissue Sculpting. San Diego: Body Therapy Associates, 2002.

Profet M. Protecting Your Baby-to-Be. New York: Addison-Wesley, 1995.

Scheumann D. The Balanced Body: A Guide to Deep Tissue and Neuromuscular Therapy. 3rd Ed. Baltimore: Lippincott Williams & Wilkins, 2007.

Schneider MV. Infant Massage: A Handbook for Loving Parents. New York: Bantam Books, 1989.

Simkin P, Klaus P. When Survivors Give Birth. Seattle: Classic Day Publishing, 2004.

Simkin P, Whalley J, Keppler A. Pregnancy, Childbirth and the Newborn. Fourth Edition Minnetonka: Meadowbrook Press, 2010.

Stager L. Nurturing Massage for Pregnancy. Baltimore: Lippincott, Williams and Wilkins, 2010.

Stephens S. Body work and childbirth, proven wonders. Int J Childbirth Educ 1997;12(4):20–21.

Stillerman E. Prenatal Massage. St. Louis: Mosby/Elsevier, 2008.

Sutton J, Scott P. Understanding and Teaching Optimal Foetal Positioning. New Zealand: Birth Concepts, 1996.

Wine Z. Massage for varicose veins. Massage Mag 1997;66:133–135.

For additional resources, please visit http://thePoint.LWW.com/Osborne-Pregnancy2e!

Massage Therapy as Labor Support

Learning Objectives

After study of this chapter, you should be able to:

1. Plan therapy sessions for pregnant clients and/or their partners that will help them prepare emotionally and physically for labor.
2. Identify and define the stages of normal labor.
3. Describe the role of a massage therapist in assisting women in labor.
4. Describe typical challenges and accomplishments of the laboring mother and the massage therapist at each stage of labor.
5. List specific massage techniques to support typical physiological aspects of each labor stage.
6. Identify key ethical, physical, and emotional challenges involved in assisting at labors as a massage therapist.

Birthing a baby is perhaps a woman's most profound rite of passage. It can be a journey of self-discovery, steeped in mystery, challenge, and discovery of inner strength. A knowledgeable, prepared massage therapist can accompany a woman, offering her meaningful physical and emotional support. This chapter explores the process of labor and birthing and our potential role in it.

It begins with strategies for labor preparation during sessions. Progressing through labor's stages, you will learn to facilitate and encourage the process. You will find options for working with back labor, medications, at home and in hospitals, and for both vaginal and cesarean births. Birthing generates many emotional and ethical issues that uniquely impact you, your client, and the client–therapist relationship. You will learn to navigate these feelings and find guidance for working alongside other birth professionals in various settings.

There's more general information to know about labor and birth than this chapter can cover. Learn about medical interventions, fetal assessment tests, making birth plans, and other such related topics from mainstream books and internet sources and from obstetrical and midwifery texts. (See online resources at http://thePoint.lww.com/Osborne-Pregnancy2e for a recommended list and other supplements.) Take childbirth education and birth doula classes. Use this chapter for what you won't easily find elsewhere: specifically how a massage therapist can nurture a baby's birth and its mother.

This chapter was coauthored by Linda Hickey, RMT.

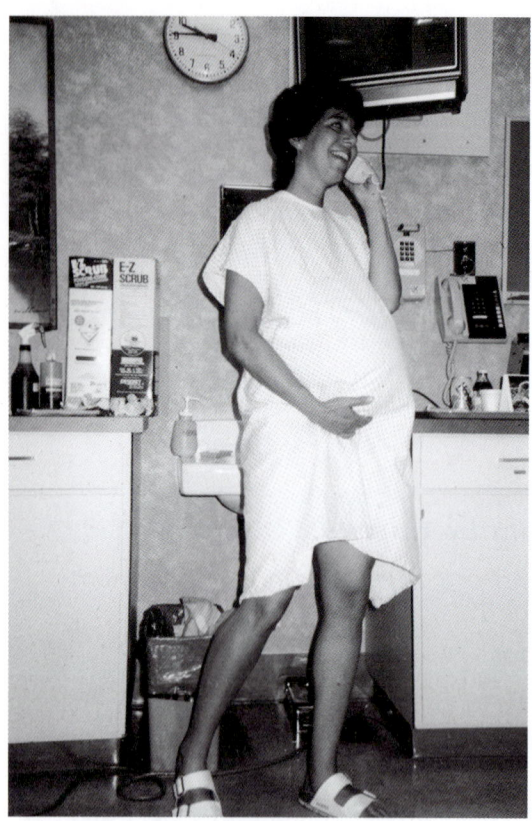
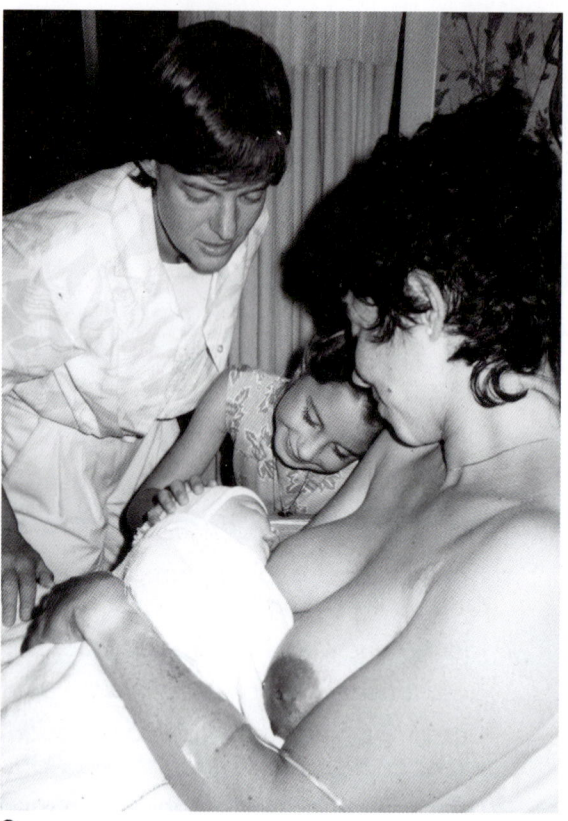
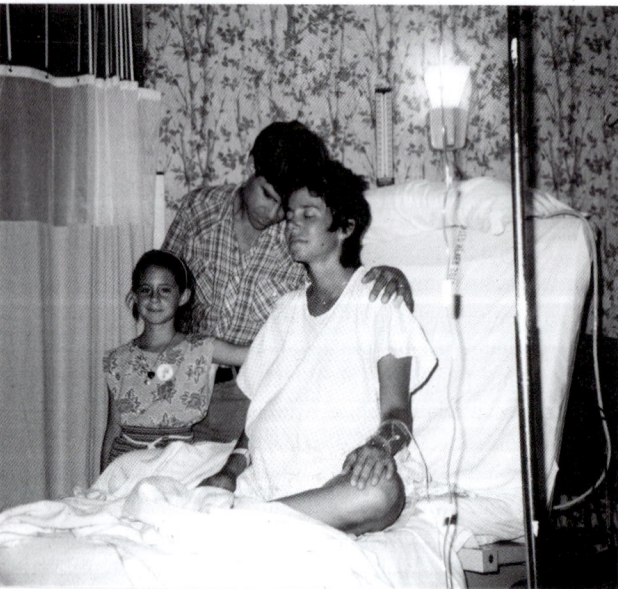

FIGURE 5.1 Labor and birth. Labor normally progresses through **(A)** the early phase of first-stage labor's light contractions; **(B)** more intense, regular contractions of active and transition phases of first stage; and **(C)** second stage of pushing the baby out. The placenta follows in third stage.

Massage Therapy as Preparation for Labor

You can help make labor's stages and phases (Fig. 5.1) more manageable when your sessions include experiences to ready your client's body and mind for labor's challenges.

● RELAXATION AND BREATHING

Women often receive some direction in relaxation and breathing as coping strategies for the pain of labor. These are common topics in books and many childbirth education programs. How much instruction and time is spent rehearsing relaxation and breathing techniques varies among programs from a quick mention of techniques to repeated and continued practice (Simkin and Bolding 2004).

Certainly, the benefits of working with breathing have been recognized over the ages and passed on to women by women, from long, slow, deep relaxing breaths during contractions to the now familiar "Lamaze" huff/huff breathing patterns that are often depicted in media. Most women use breathing strategies as a coping strategy and find them helpful (Sakala and Corry 2009).

With such proven effectiveness, improved breathing and relaxation should be a primary goal of your prenatal work. Even a woman whose labor is the most medically managed, either planned that way or unexpectedly, will need help to calm herself at some point. Your work is not as a childbirth educator teaching labor breathing patterns. Instead, as early as possible in your sessions, observe her normal breathing patterns to help improve each breath. Guide her toward more multidirectional breathing, and suggest that she practices this deeper breathing, particularly in times of pain or tension. Include techniques for any restricted areas, paying particular attention to her ribcage, pectoral girdle, and upper back muscles (see Chapter 4 and online video for specific techniques).

Massage therapy is, by its very nature, a lesson in relaxation. You can also deliberately empower your clients with heightened physical and emotional skills for relaxation. Don't just put your clients to sleep; cultivate a demeanor, touch, and techniques that foster her internal awareness, kinesthetic learning, and ability to let go. Encourage her to create daily relaxation times and to consider prenatal yoga or exercise classes. These can be both enjoyable and helpful in learning to relax, breathe, and otherwise prepare for labor and birthing.

Some well-established childbirth preparation methods offer more thorough and involved relaxation and breathing techniques and practice as part of their curriculum. These programs generally cover many strategies for coping with the childbirth's pain, understanding that the best predictor of how a woman will experience labor pain is her self-confidence in her ability to cope with that pain (Simkin and Bolding 2004). You should develop an understanding of the various approaches to pain management that couples are learning. Although there are many books and Web sites available, actually attending the various childbirth education classes over time is your best orientation (See online box on Childbirth Education, Philosophies and Setting Choice).

> **REMINDER:** *Massage therapy can help women feel more physically and emotionally prepared to labor and give birth with more awe and wonder and less fear.*

IMPROVING FLEXIBILITY

Women need flexibility to labor most efficiently and comfortably. At the very least, she must be able to widely abduct her

What Would You Do?

Having pliable thigh adductor muscles that a woman can relax while experiencing labor's intensity and possible pain often facilitates labor's normal progress. Given the concern about possible thrombi in the medial veins of the leg, how can you safely and effectively work in this area? What types of techniques can you use and what do you need to modify or eliminate from your sessions?

thighs, with her hips and knees deeply flexed. She may find that squatting, kneeling, and being on all fours feel "right" for her. Each of these positions requires further flexibility in her legs and pelvis. To help her have more options for labor positions, include appropriate deep tissue massage, stretches, assisted-resisted exercise, and other passive movements and techniques for these areas. Particularly seek to reduce chronic tension and increase pliability in the thigh adductors, quadriceps group, hamstring group, lateral and medial hip rotators, iliotibial tract, gastrocnemius/soleus and Achilles tendon, and lumbar spine (see Chapter 4 and online resources for specific technique ideas).

PARTNER MASSAGE INSTRUCTION

The last weeks of pregnancy provide an opportunity to enhance partners' connection and support their budding relationship with the baby. Include your client's partner in at one of your individual sessions, or you may want to present a class to your clients and their partners. Teach appropriate techniques, avoiding complicated ones that require advanced anatomical knowledge and extraordinary sensitivity. Long, slow effleurage strokes and kneading to soften tense muscles are good choices. (See online outline of class possibilities.) Demonstrate on both the mom and her partner, and then guide them as they practice. They can continue practicing at home, refining their loving touch and enhancing their family's bonding

The anticipation time of late pregnancy includes different worries for women and their partners. Women's worries may center on the baby, interventions, and the uncertainties involved. The primary worry of their male partners (in this study, only male partners were included) was the severe pain and suffering for their mates, then interventions, the baby, their own powerlessness, and their partners' death (Bainbridge 2000). Certainly, partners will find it meaningful to have specific supportive touch that they can contribute. In addition, an interesting study concluded that the partner's labor massage can positively influence a laboring woman's perception of the quality of her birth experience. Eighty-seven percent of the massaged group in this study reported that partner massage was helpful in providing pain relief and psychological support (Chang et al. 2002).

Techniques to teach partners might include the following from this text:

- Nerve strokes (Chapter 4 technique manual)
- Specific foot reflex zones (Chapter 4 technique manual)
- Abdominal effleurage (Chapter 5 technique manual)
- Pelvic floor relaxation (Chapter 5 technique manual)
- Sacral counterpressure (Chapter 5 technique manual)
- Gluteal double squeeze or double hip squeeze (online technique manual)
- Pelvic press (online technique manual)

● PELVIC FLOOR PREPARATION

The perineal muscles play a dual role in the body. They act as a supportive sling for the pelvic organs and as sphincters for the urethra, vagina, and anus. Many women do not have well-toned pelvic floor muscles before pregnancy. Pregnancy can then add further strain to them, as they adapt to the increasing uterine weight, fetal movement, and the woman's changing posture.

During birth, as the baby's head descends through the vagina and "crowns" or approaches the vaginal outlet, the muscles, connective tissues, and skin of the pelvic floor need to stretch tremendously to facilitate the baby's passage. When tight, restricted by scar tissue or trigger points, or desensitized, a longer, more painful labor may ensue. This is because it appears that the pelvic floor muscles also play an important role in guiding and directing the baby into positioning for birth prior to and during labor (Buckley 2008). A toned and pliable pelvic floor is more likely to remain intact through the birth. It is less likely that postpartum urinary stress incontinence will develop, and postpartum perineal healing may be quicker (Ricci 2009).

Perineal trauma, from a surgical cut (**episiotomy**) or from a spontaneous tear, occurs in more than 65% of vaginal births in the United States. Fear of perineal damage is one of women's top concerns as they approach labor, and you may be able to help reduce this fear. If she is not learning pelvic floor exercises and perineal self-massage from other sources, you may offer to teach her these important preparations. (See online resources at http://thePoint.lww.com/Osborne-Pregnancy2e for further instruction in how to teach both.)

> **REMINDER:** Internal perineal massage is outside of massage therapists' scope of practice. Some jurisdictions also legally limit external work on the pelvic floor and other pelvic structures due to their proximity to the genitals.

Points of View: Perineal Massage

Many studies have sought to validate or invalidate the practice of perineal massage for reducing perineal trauma during birth, with conflicting results (Hastings-Tolsma et al. 2007). Variables such as effectiveness of the teaching of the techniques, timing of performing them, compliance to the practice by the participants, and whether perineal massage was self-performed or done by the partner further complicate getting reliable data.

A summary of the most current literature suggests that performing perineal massage during the last weeks of pregnancy was beneficial in preventing perineal trauma for first-time mothers only (Bodner-Adler et al. 2002). Women who are attempting a vaginal birth after a cesarean section likely would fall into this category, as well. The data are inconclusive for other mothers.

Regardless of the conflicting data, it still may be beneficial for a woman or her to massage her perineal area. Given the intense "ring of fire" sensation as the baby emerges, perineal massage may help women become more familiar with the feel of the perineal tissues stretching and learn to relax. For women with scar tissue from previous perineal trauma, it may help normalize tissue and sensation. Given the importance of postpartum pelvic floor integrity, it may be useful to offer this instruction in the last weeks of pregnancy. Of course, this form of internal vaginal massage is inappropriate for massage therapists to perform on clients.

● IMPROVING AWARENESS AND COMMUNICATION

Some women intend to give birth; others to have their baby delivered. Regardless of on which end of this spectrum of involvement a women falls, she will need good communication skills to succeed. Help her to ascertain the importance of expressing her needs and her desires to her partner, other family and friends, and her healthcare team; to do so, she first needs to be in communication with herself.

Here's how to work this into your sessions. When you ask for feedback, ask a question that requires her to really pay attention. Instead of "how's that feel?" try, "Where do you feel the effects of my pressure?" or "What types of sensations are you experiencing?" As you gently rock her spine, ask her to identify where else she feels the reverberations of your undulating hand. Ask her to bring her breath in as though she could touch where you are working with her inhale. These types of interactions develop her attention to her internal experience and begin training her to express that verbally.

Validate her needs and preferences by asking for them as you work. "Would you prefer to be on your side or semisitting for today's session?" "Silence today, or would you like some soothing music?" "What are the top three places in your body needing to be massaged today?" If you find that she has difficulty with tuning in to herself, you may want to discuss including more of this type of work into your massages.

Other resources to help women "tune in" include prenatal exercise and yoga, childbirth education classes, journaling, and reading realistic, yet affirmative stories of pregnancy and labor. Many women never consider the possibility that labor and birth can be an ecstatic, peak experience in their lives. Encourage them to view DVDs that might expand their familiarity of the varied potential inherent in birthing. (See online resources for suggestions of all of the above.)

Another aspect of communication includes all of the logistics, preferences and decisions, and data related to her labor plans. Know what type of childbirth preparation she has had and where she plans to labor and how. You need to know all the basics of who, what, where, when, and how. Be sure to have verbal and written contact with her regarding all of these details at least 4 weeks before her due date so that you can be prepared. See if she is comfortable to share what her fantasies and hopes are for her baby's birth.

One of the keys to a woman having an empowering birth experience is her feeling of control though successful communication. This is more important to her short- and long-term satisfaction with the birth than whether or not she had an easy or a difficult birth (Simkin 1991, 1992).

Getting Real about Labor Massage Therapy

Before committing to be with a woman in labor, carefully consider of all of the implications. If you reflect on your own motivations, needs, and feelings and on the practicalities of being a reliable professional to laboring women, you will make a good decision about your availability.

● WHAT ARE YOUR MOTIVATIONS?

Much of our understanding of the importance of the role of labor support for women comes from the lifelong work of Penny Simkin and the other founders of the doula movement in North America (Doulas of North America 2009). When writing about the role of the doula, a trained woman caregiver at birth, she provides much information useful to us in our similar role as labor support massage therapists. Thanks to the work of Penny, her colleagues, and the doula movement, it is well understood and accepted through research that women benefit greatly from this type of continuous physical and emotional support. (Hodnett 2007 and see Chapter 1.)

My Story

Perhaps my most gratifying experience with labor massage came with a client whom I didn't even know whether I'd be able to help. After an extremely painful and frightening experience with her firstborn when her epidural medication ran out with no doctor available to refill it, "Margie" was terrified going into this second and last birth. She wanted to manage it as carefully as possible so she had planned an induced hospital birth for her second baby. She was sure she wanted an epidural. I was still in training as a labor massage therapist and offered to be there with her and provide pain relief through massage. In truth, I had only attended women in unmedicated births, and I wasn't sure I could be of any help once that epidural kicked in.

I found that there were actually many ways that my presence helped Margie, but perhaps the most important was reducing the fear factor. She knew that she had someone there at all times who would help her through any pain she might have. And the discomforts were many. The IV had been badly placed and was causing considerable discomfort, interfering with her attempts to rest. We had gone over some advocacy strategies in a previous office visit, and Margie was pleased to find out that she could ask to have it reinserted. She appreciated a hand massage while she waited.

Also, she had been lying on the same side for a few hours. Even through the epidural, she could feel an unpleasant numbness in her bottom leg but was instructed to remain in that position for continuous electronic fetal monitoring. I was able to get her leg circulation going again through massage. When the contractions intensified, she found she could still feel them despite the epidural. Pressure and moist heat on her sacrum and hips helped relieve this pain.

Margie's husband was incredibly responsive to her needs, and we worked together to apply pressure to both sides of her pelvis. I am always grateful when the mother and especially the father invite me into the intimacy of their birth circle. Negotiating that intimacy requires mindfulness of the couple's dynamics and their need for privacy. It can get tense at points, especially when making difficult decisions. The massage therapist needs to know when her absence is more important than her presence.

Margie gave birth to a healthy baby. What stays with me most from this birth is Margie's triumphant smile. She had faced her fear and had come into her own as her child's mother, right before my eyes. It was a profound transformation I felt privileged to have witnessed. I learned that the nurturing behind the touch can be more powerful than the physical relief it provides.

—Karen Salas, Salt Lake City, UT

The cornerstone of supporting a laboring woman is to understand and champion what SHE is looking for in her birthing experience and to bring your expertise to the situation to help her in making that happen. Your scope of practice includes being of service to help the laboring woman feel safe. You can do that through emotional support and physical comfort, and by helping her to communicate her needs and wishes. You must respect her choices and not attempt to direct her medical care. It is critical to examine your own motivation and intentions before embarking on this work. Motivations such as resentment from your own birth experiences, strong beliefs about how birth "should" be, a belief that pharmaceutical interventions are "bad" or "preferable," etc. are more of a personal belief or political position and have no place at another woman's birth.

For example, a therapist may aspire to assist women in birth to, in some small way, respond to the alarming statistical rates of medication and intervention in the birth process. The very nature of our work tends to lead massage therapists to be natural birth supporters. What about the client who, for her own reasons, chooses a hospital birth with pharmaceutical pain relief as soon as it is possible? Ethically, what is your position? Can you objectively and caringly support her? Do you try to change her mind? Taking time to explore and become clear in your intent before pursuing this work protects you, your clients, and our profession from compromised positions and unethical outcomes.

● PRACTICAL AND ETHICAL CONSIDERATIONS

In addition to exploring your intent, you must consider the practicalities of including labor support in your professional practice. The responsibility, as defined by the doula research, is that if we say we are going to be with someone at her birth, then we must be there. Implications in your lifestyle, professional practice, and personal life need to be carefully considered, and personal support needs to be in place so that you can drop what you are doing at any time of the day or night, for however long it takes.

The intimate energy of being with a birthing woman can lead to a deep relationship. In fact, personal connection is necessary for her to feel safe. Open communication about what your and your clients' objectives are in the experience and establishing a system of closure afterwards will protect you both from becoming intertwined in an unhealthy dual relationship. It can be difficult to resume a sense of boundary with labor support clients after the birth. The evidence comes when you find yourself being invited to and sometimes attending not just the original "birth day" but birthday parties in year one and sometimes two!

Here's a little ritual to help put some closure around the birthing relationship and move you back to a more typical therapist–client relationship. After attending a birth, arrange a short visit at the client's home. Bring with you a simple dinner for the family's freezer and a book for their new bedtime story bookshelf. Tuck into the book a letter written for the baby that

My Story

I have practiced as a maternity massage specialist and labor support partner for 10 years of my 15-year practice, attending over 60 births in that time period. In retrospect, I have been called away from my practice nearly all the time. I have missed precious "days off," holidays, and family celebrations. I have declined travel opportunities and arrived at friends' special events only to leave again when that cell phone in my pocket rang!

I chose to include labor support in my practice for a number of personal reasons, all involved with believing it would help make the world a better place. I was not prepared for the whispers of disappointment and other impacts to my friends and family. The other surprise was that I believed my client group would be supportive of my noble endeavors, most being pregnant themselves, but this has not always been so. They wanted their appointment with me in a timely way. With a very full schedule, I was not always able to quickly rebook their missed appointments resulting from my attending a birth. I found it necessary to compromise my rest and recovery time often. And that, in turn, increased the risk that I would resent the labor work over time and not be fully clear and present for my laboring client.

Including labor support in a maternity practice presents many challenges. They are not insurmountable, though, if you can limit the number of births. At this time, I offer labor support in unique situations—home births (I love them), friends, multiples, or VBAC situations—and when my schedule allows, usually three or four times a year.

—Linda Hickey, Calgary, AB

describes the day of his or her birth and a welcome to the world. At this visit, take the time to review details of the day, filling in any gray areas if you can for the parents. Before leaving, book her next appointment at your office to resume her care postpartum. Back in your professional setting, you can pick up where you left off before the birth. Of course, you may still talk about the birth, but it isn't the focus of your interaction.

Certainly, a continued therapeutic relationship is beneficial for the woman as you work with her through postpartum and perhaps further through your practice. The experience of being with her in labor has the potential of making you a more understanding therapist with more insight into her particular body and how it responds to stimuli. Yet the shared experience at birth can lead to a position of dual relationship, beyond massage therapist and client, and you should be alert to the pitfalls of those dualities.

Labor's emotional landscape implies a feeling of vulnerability on the part of the laboring woman. Through your presence and behaviors, you can empower her too. Gently offer her support through information sharing. Repeat instructions and encourage her to look inside to find and communicate her wishes rather than make decisions for her. This is important, even at her most vulnerable moments when she may not initially know what she wants or needs. Your role here also extends to her partner to facilitate, not take over, his or her involvement in the process.

When working with expectant women, particularly in the vulnerability and sensitivity of labor and birth, **transference** dynamics are very common. Transference occurs if a client displaces her thoughts, feelings, or behaviors about a significant other onto you. A woman may then relate to you as though you were someone important from the past, often a parent. Whether the feelings are positive or negative, this dynamic can create other dilemmas that can compromise your care of her. Be aware of this dynamic and do your best not to build or intensify the transference. Don't forget your own vulnerability to countertransference, seeing your client as an important someone from your past or projecting your feelings onto her. You lose objectivity and your connection with HER when this occurs or when you project your own feelings onto her or identify with her (Greene and Goodrich-Dunn 2004).

> **REMINDER:** *Within the extraordinary and intimate process of labor, continue to find ways to maintain professional boundaries with your laboring clients.*

Birthing can appear sexual in its nature. In fact, the same brain centers activated in sexual activity are also energized in birth. Labor may be more efficient if the woman can feel comfortable expressing herself physically. Sounds made, comfort positions, and movements may appear highly sexual during labor and birth. They are signs of the woman connecting with the experience and being "in it." An intellectual understanding of what is going on will help you be comfortable witnessing and sometimes participating and encouraging these behaviors (i.e., holding, rocking, and modeling sound-making to encourage the laboring uterus' work). We must be comfortable in doing these ourselves so we can be fully present and responsive.

For example, it is widely recognized that making low, deep sounds is labor supportive. It helps the jaw and throat to relax, encourages deep breaths, and has a reflexive relaxation effect on the diaphragm, cervix, and abdominal wall (Gaskin 2003). These sounds can be very similar to those of lovemaking. Get as comfortable as you can with them because modeling these sounds for the laboring woman and continuing to sound with her throughout her contractions is the basis of good labor support. It is even more effective when there is an entire chorus going!

All of your draping expertise is often for naught during labor. Some women need to be partially or completely naked in labor to be comfortable while others feel more comfortable and safe in their own or a hospital gown. Many women's inhibitions tend to diminish so any excessive modesty may disappear. This can be unsettling for you, as can her need for contact with you other than your accustomed use of your arms and hands, such as to hold or comfort her.

Because your work must proceed regardless of what is or isn't covered, you need to use other measures to maintain a professional stance. Keep her "covered" by keeping your eyes from being invasive. Use your own clothing barrier and perhaps sheets or pillows between you when you are holding her. Whenever possible, have her partner in close embrace of her rather than you. In your next session after the birth, be sure to reestablish your normal professional draping and physical contact boundaries.

● ROLE OF MASSAGE THERAPY IN LABOR SUPPORT

Like any labor assistant, a massage therapist provides consistent, responsive physical and emotional care throughout a woman's labor. Your refined skill in tactile therapies and pain and stress reduction and as a practiced listener to the nuances of the body-mind is extremely valuable and somewhat unique on most birthing teams. As such, your most direct intentions include the following:

- Supporting the normal progression of labor with physical and emotional support, facilitating relaxation, rhythm, and ritual
- Helping to conserve and regenerate physical and emotional energy
- Facilitating breathing and comfort with massage therapy, stretching, and visualizations
- Assisting in relief of muscle cramping, exhaustion, and pain, especially in the abdomen, lumbar area, legs, and arms (women experiencing less muscular pain tend to have less uterine pain)

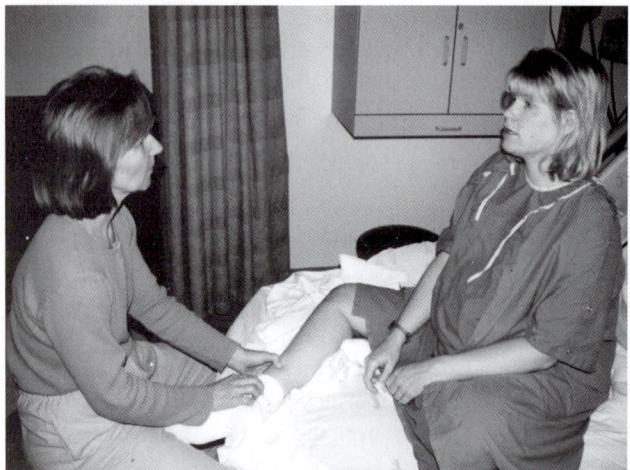

FIGURE 5.2 Massage therapy during labor. Stimulation of feet and leg points to help sustain and energize uterine contractions is an example of the tactile support a massage therapist can offer. Women also appreciate your focused, nonjudgmental listening skills.

- Enhancing the partners' relationship, allowing space and encouragement of the partner's care
- Providing physical and emotional support to the entire birthing "team" (Fig. 5.2)

> **REMINDER:** *Remember your scope of practice centers around nurturing the mother through birthing. A massage therapist does NOT offer medical or nursing advice, assess and determine labor progress, nor make decisions for her laboring client. You also shouldn't assume a partner's or family member's role, unless asked to substitute.*

● COLLABORATING WITH MIDWIVES AND MEDICAL PROFESSIONALS

In North America, it is estimated that over 90% of women will birth in a hospital or medical center under the care of a medical physician or obstetrician or a nurse-midwife (Cassidy 2006). Typically, nurses provide most care in these environments. The nurses will maintain close communications with the doctor or midwife who usually begin to stay with the woman when she is ready to push. Nurses have a primary responsibility in their work to monitor and record the labor progress and well-being of the baby and mother, and to support the mother.

It is in the area of supporting the mother that your role and the nurses' effectively overlap, and you both have expertise to contribute. Many nurses are open to your sharing suggestions to facilitate the mom's comfort and the labor. Perhaps you will have more experience and knowledge of natural birth, that is, birthing without medications and use of technology.

If none of the nursing staff has this perspective, you can be invaluable to a mother who wants a natural birth. Of course, the need to leave your agenda at the door applies not just to preconceived beliefs about medical procedures, but to the personnel as well. The two roles can blend and work well together in most cases. This is especially true when you model respect for their role and you actively support their record-keeping and monitoring responsibilities.

Attending a birth at home or at a free-standing birth center is an opportunity for the labor massage therapist to fully bear witness to the power of natural birth. There you will work alongside midwives and with women who understand, appreciate, and welcome what your presence and your work might contribute as a nonpharmacological form of labor support.

Once the pushing stage has arrived, it is the doctor or midwife who usually directs the laboring woman's actions. Again, your skills will complement their medical expertise and should be focused on the mother's comfort and energy, rather than attempting to supplant her maternity care provider.

● OTHER EMOTIONAL ISSUES

Throughout the course of labor, there likely will be uncertain moments for the laboring mother, her partner, and perhaps even yourself. One predictable time when this may occur is when the attendant announces the dilation after checking her cervix. It is rare that a laboring woman is further along in her dilation than we think! Hearing a less-than-expected number can be a disappointing moment. She (and you) may feel a discouraging sense of failure. Your brain may start to play the "what happens next" game. Instead, take the lead and call for a time-out—a time to regroup.

Encourage your client that she can keep going and that her baby needs her to keep going. Plan a different strategy, have her change positions, and take a positive attitude to get back down to the work of labor. Should the circumstances be that some intervention is necessary or chosen, it is imperative that you do not show any sign of disappointment or judgment of her or her care provider. Adapt, thinking quickly on your feet, and continue to calmly and confidently encourage and support your client through the next minutes and hours of her experience.

Many massage therapists who intent to include labor support in their professional practices take childbirth education classes and read voraciously on the topic. They also pursue doula certification as part of their continuing education. This is an excellent adjunct to your physical work. You have a thorough understanding and experience with the body and how it responds to touch. Doula training can offer you a deeper, broader understanding of the psychological and emotional aspects of birth and provide a network of other birthing professionals for support and information (Doulas of North America 2009). (See online resources for several recommended training programs.)

Preparations for Labor Support

As the due date approaches, clarify everyone's expectations. Cover the details of exchanging phone numbers, getting addresses, and establishing when and how you want to be called. Review their "birth plan," and thoroughly discuss how you see yourself contributing to it. Invite her to share any painful, emotional previous experiences, which may impact the birth. From this, you may also learn how she tends to respond to pain and stress, and what has been helpful to her in the past.

It is good practice to consider yourself "on call" for 2 weeks before and after the baby's predicted due date. It seems to be true that most babies love to be born at night, so it is always a good idea to do a trial drive by the house if you will be meeting your client there and to the hospital or birthing center. Pay attention to technical details, such as ensuring that your mobile phone is charged and on, that you have a plan for calling to cancel scheduled appointments in your office on the labor day, and that, in fact, your bag is packed and ready in your car. (See online resources for a checklist of what you might want to bring.) Ideally, you will have been working with your client throughout her pregnancy and had many occasions for walking through how the actual labor day might go. If not, try to schedule a meeting before the labor to accomplish this important communication.

Your Work in Each Labor Stage

Labor is characterized by three somewhat distinct stages (Fig. 5.3). During the first stage, the contracting uterus thins (**effacement**) and opens (**dilation**) the cervix creating an open passage out of the uterus for the baby. The first stage can be further differentiated into "**early**," "**active**," and "**transition**" phases of cervical dilatation. The **second stage of labor** is the pushing or birthing phase. In the brief **third stage**, the uterus expels the placenta, amniotic sack, and other fluids and tissues. (See glossary and online medical glossary for other labor terminology.)

Your role as a labor support massage therapist will fluctuate as the woman goes through labor's phases and stages. With experience, you will learn to read her body positioning, movements, and birth sounds and to adapt accordingly. Sometimes a continuous, calm and reassuring presence is more useful than any techniques. It is intuition, innate understanding, and experience-based wisdom that will guide you best toward how active your support needs to be.

Laboring women respond with wide variation to touch and massage therapy. Some may prefer to be undisturbed during part or all of their labors. Others cope best when massaged during contractions, and some only appreciate contact between contractions. One woman might require constant cutaneous stimulation to meet her physical and emotional needs. Another may only want certain types of strokes, pressures, or rhythms. A woman might respond best to massage of only specific areas. Often a woman's preferences change greatly over the hours of her labor. Effectiveness of a particular technique might wax or wane.

When a woman has a reasonably normal labor, massage therapy and other forms of nonpharmacological pain relief have proven to be effective. These "natural" coping strategies, including massage, movement, position changes, relaxation, breathing, and emotional support, have few negative side effects (Ricci 2009). Each falls well within a massage therapist's scope of practice.

Most labors are painful, with emotional and physical factors causing that pain. Extreme fear and stress tend to increase physical pain. The uterine muscles pull forcefully on the cervix, stretching ligaments and their fascial attachments, and press the baby through the pelvis and pelvic floor. Massage therapy and other types of labor comfort measures to relieve this pain are based on the **gate theory of pain control**. This concept suggests that local stimulation, such as pressure, stroking, friction, heat, or cold, can fill the brain's sensory receptor sites before pain sensations arrive. This is because painful stimuli travel most slowly of all sensations to the brain. A hypothetical gate in the spinal cord will close the brain to painful sensation so that less pain is felt (Ricci 2009).

Pain management with these stimuli is most effective when you deliver continuous, tactile experiences just prior to and throughout painful contractions. In general, during a contraction, use slow, rhythmic and predictable movements; stationary compressions also are effective. Often the more combinations of sensation, that is, deep pressure during stroking on the erector muscles or deep friction on the sacrum with hot packs, the more effectively the pain gate closes. As your client's labor journey progresses, you will use specific techniques for different needs. Let's go through the typical labor, zeroing in on hands-on strategies with broad recommendations, followed by a labor technique manual at the end of this chapter.

● PRELABOR

At and around 40 weeks of gestation, many elements come together that send signals that it is time for the baby to be born. The full spectrum of physical, chemical, and psychological readiness factors that stimulate birth remains mostly unknown, yet highly speculated upon. What is likely is that a change in the chemical interaction occurring between the placenta and the mother's and baby's brains signals readiness. This interaction initiates shifts in the production of progesterone, estrogen, oxytocin, and **prostaglandins**, the major

114 Pre- and Perinatal Massage Therapy

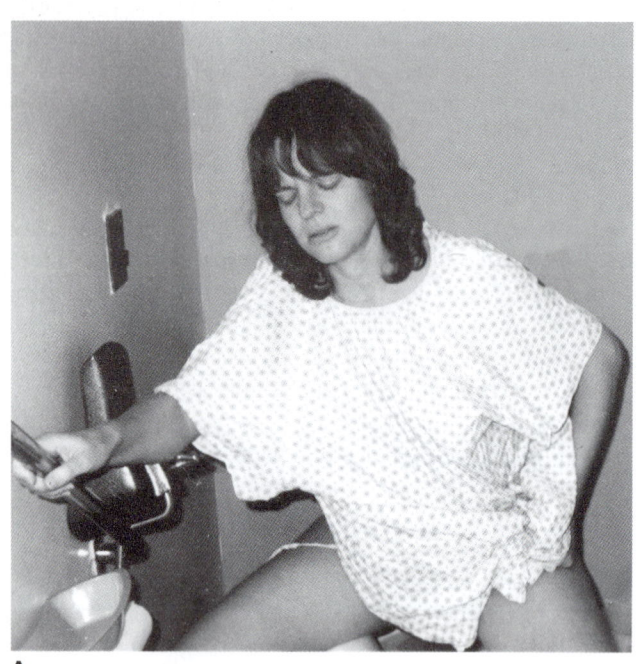

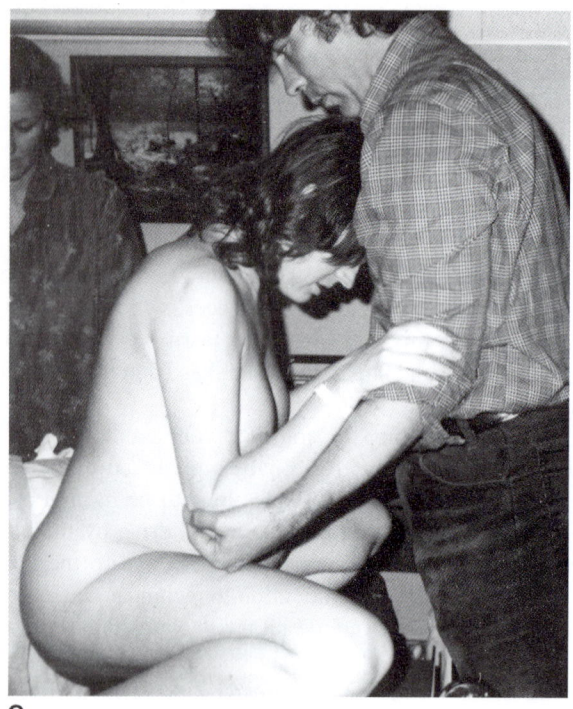

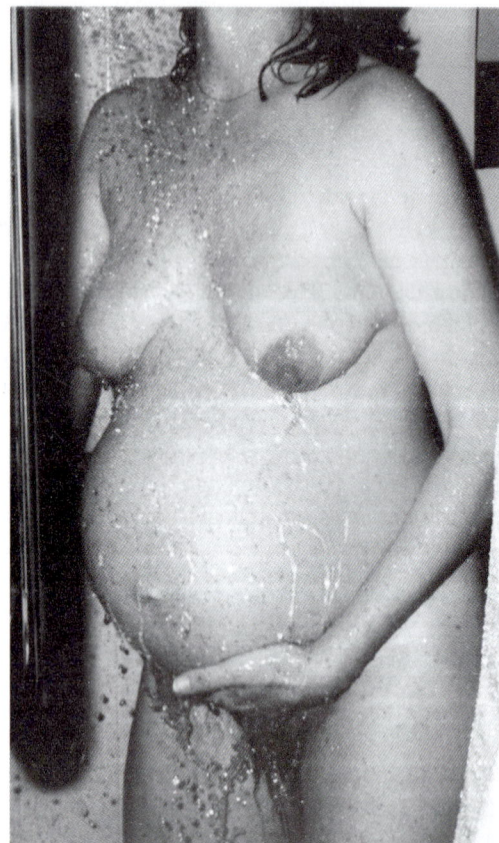

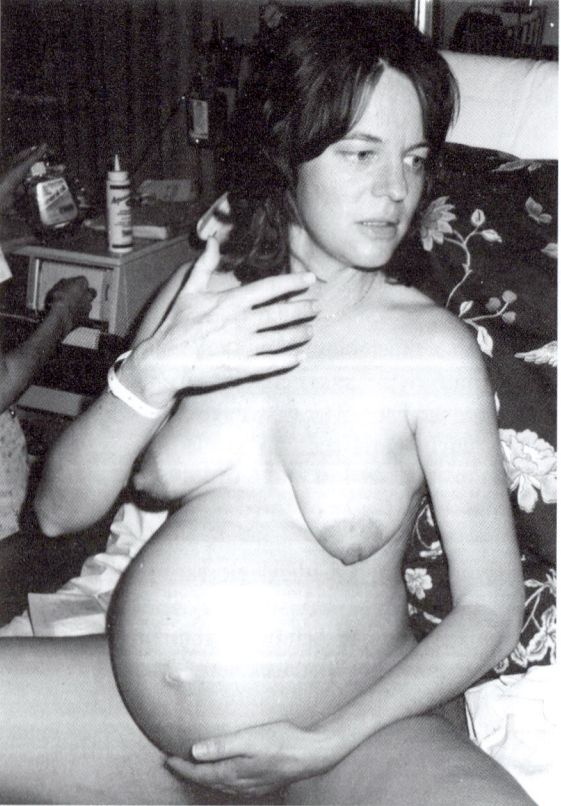

FIGURE 5.3 Stages of labor. Upright positions, water, and a supportive partner help labor to progress from first-stage cervical changes **(A–D)**, to second-stage pushing **(E)**, through to the birth of the baby and then the placenta **(F)**.

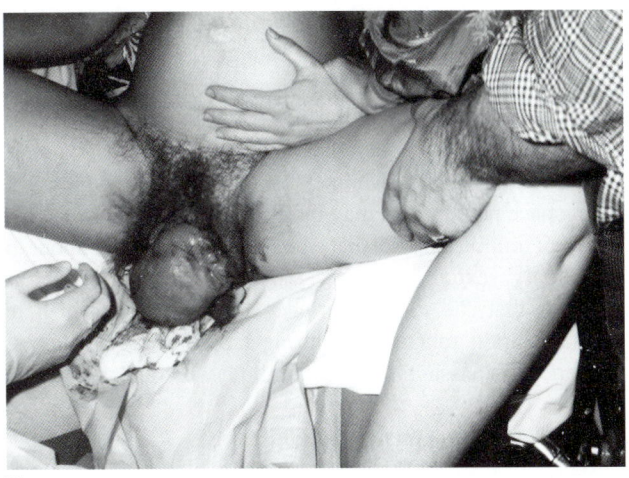
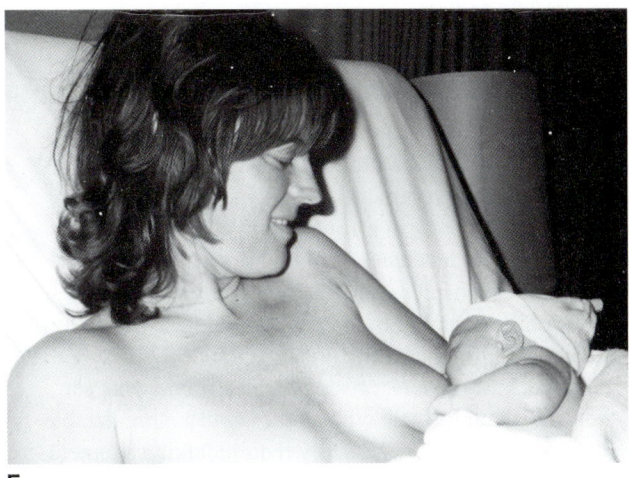

FIGURE 5.3 *(Continued)*

hormones responsible for regulating uterine contractions. (Bainbridge 2000)

This chemical messaging in the mother's body gradually allows the uterus to contract with increasing regularity and strength, moving the baby further down into the pelvis and against the cervix. Under the powerful influence of this circling hormone chain, the cervix grows thinner, or effaces, and also opens or dilates. The **bloody show** or **cervical mucus plug** falling away is evidence of this internal process and a sign of pending labor.

There are other generally accepted signs that predict labor is approaching, including an increase in the number and frequency of practice labor contractions (Braxton-Hicks contractions). Often the baby drops lower into the pelvis, as measured by fundal height (dropping or lightening). This often brings a change in pressure on the pelvic floor and more ease in breathing. Heartburn and other digestive discomforts usually improve too.

The "breaking of waters" or rupture of the amniotic membrane actually occurs before labor has begun in only 10% of cases. More often, the amniotic sac ruptures after labor begins and is well established. Vaginal secretions may increase, another result of shifting hormones preparing for birth, and the mother's breasts may begin to produce **colostrum**, a milk precursor, believed to contain important immune information to protect the newborn. Women often greet this time with a mixture of anticipation (the baby is coming!), relief (I'll be able to see my feet again!), and perhaps a little anxiety about the work that lies ahead.

As labor is imminent, include more specific breath awareness and techniques to improve breathing capacity and rhythm (see section above in labor preparation and in Chapter 4 technique manual). If she has Braxton-Hicks contractions during your session, help her to identify where she tends to tense up and guide her toward relaxing. Remember that until she is actually at her due date and continue the contraindications regarding labor-stimulative points. Maximize her relaxation and help to minimize any discomforts as you have throughout the pregnancy.

● EARLY (LATENT) FIRST-STAGE LABOR: A TIME FOR "DISTRACTION"

When contractions become more rhythmic and occurring without respect to position changes, this signals that the "real" labor has begun. Through these early hours, the uterus gains momentum. Contractions may be subtle and gently erratic as the energy builds. Eventually, they usually will establish a rhythm in which they keep occurring and gradually get longer and closer together (Tornetta 2008).

For the woman and her partner, this time is often one of great excitement and anticipation, "Yes!! This is it!" Early labor usually lasts for more than a few hours, the average being 12 hours for the first-time mother. Ideally, she will be able to go about her regular routine. Hopefully, she will sleep if it occurs at night or can carry on with her daily activities, including resting, eating, and drinking at this latent stage. It is a time for distraction and preparation for the harder work likely to come.

Coping with Pain

Penny Simkin refers to the work of the laboring women, particularly in the first stage, as the three R's: relaxation, rhythm, and, what she calls, ritual, "personally meaningful rhythmic activities repeated with every contraction" (Simkin 2008). These are states the skilled massage therapist is adept in achieving; really, our specialty is using touch rhythmically to promote relaxation. Often women incorporate the rhythm of massage strokes into their coping rituals, developing a pattern of allowing each contraction rather than fighting it. Your involvement in early labor sets the stage for the later, perhaps more challenging, hours of labor.

Techniques for Early Labor

Keep the three R's in mind as you experiment with the effects of:

1. A full-body relaxation or Swedish massage reminding your client about breathing and relaxing all her muscles while her uterus contracts
2. Observing her body in a contraction, addressing areas of tensing with awareness and traditional massage techniques. (See Chapter 4 and later guidelines.)
3. Auditioning a variety of massage techniques: long, slow effleurage during a contraction or static firm pressure at her neck, shoulders, or sacrum. Determine what she feels most comfortable with, and establish a predictable pattern that doesn't necessarily require talking. Remember though that her needs and preferences are likely to change throughout her labor.
4. Deep tissue sculpting of tense muscles to help achieve deep muscle relaxation. (See Chapter 4 and this chapter's technique manual for instructions.)
5. Reminding or teaching the partner some basic massage routines
6. If you are trained in craniosacral work, still point induction and dural tube rocking can help establish an overall relaxed state in her body, helping her to rest and perhaps sleep.

> **REMINDER:** Remember Penny Simkin's three R's: relaxation, rhythm, and ritual, and incorporate each in your massage techniques.

Hormonal Influences on Uterine Contractions

The uterus is composed of interconnected layers of smooth muscle, each in a different orientation for coordinated contractions. The vertical layer pulls the lower uterine portion up and away from the pelvic floor, thinning and opening the cervix. It participates mostly in first-stage labor. Uterine muscle actions are governed hormonally by oxytocin, which gradually increases throughout labor and peaks around the time of birth. The number of oxytocin receptors in the uterus increases at the end of pregnancy, too. Oxytocin is thought to be the prime initiator of the rhythmic uterine contractions of labor, although not the only substance involved (Ricci 2009).

Beta-endorphins are the body's naturally occurring opiates, secreted from the pituitary gland under pain to reduce stressful feelings and induce feelings of pleasure. High levels of beta-endorphins in labor are responsible for the "other consciousness," innate or right-brain orientation that is characteristic of laboring women who are well supported and undisturbed in their labor. Massage therapy may increase the production of endorphins, as well (Ricci 2009).

These changes are known as "the **laboring mind response**." During labor, the brain gradually switches from a logical, rational, left-hemisphere orientation, from which most operate in their daily lives. The intuitive, instinctual, creative right hemisphere becomes more active. As a result, the laboring woman becomes so inner focused that her time and space perceptions may become distorted. This also lowers her inhibitions so that she has less concern about the distinctly sexual positions, movements, expressions, and sounds that she may experience. These changes in hemispheric brain functioning during labor further explain the potency of massage therapy and bodywork as labor support (Jones 1987).

Under right-hemisphere influence, the laboring body is especially responsive to the messages of empathetic, therapeutic touch. The right brain magnifies the many nuances of appropriate touch so that a laboring woman will more strongly receive your tactile communications of nurturance, support, peace, and strength.

While more internally focused, paradoxically, she simultaneously becomes more sensitive to those around her and to her environment. Being more open to mental suggestion in this state, seemingly minor remarks by those around her can negatively influence her. On the other hand, she will positively respond to appropriate encouragement, images, and visualizations. Creative, active imagery, positive statements (affirmations), and prayer are usually dynamically effective during labor (Ricci 2009).

Labor's heightened physical and emotional state can be a rich environment for a woman's personal growth. Meeting labor's challenges and receiving respectful, empathetic care build a good self-image or may repair a poor self-image. Even long, complicated labors are satisfying experiences when a woman feels respected, cared for, and in control of decisions regarding her and her baby's care (Green et al. 1990). There is equal potential for damaging her self-esteem. Every birth has the potential to traumatize or re-traumatize a woman. Labor can also increase her confidence, self-worth, and psychological health. Your nurturing presence during labor is potent in facilitating this type of empowering childbirth experience.

In contrast, the body also produces fight-or-flight hormones **epinephrine** and **norepinephrine** (adrenalin and noradrenalin) in response to the stresses of hunger, fear, cold, and excitement. Together, they stimulate the sympathetic nervous system. In labor, this phenomenon can slow down or stop the contractions by interrupting the synchronized uterine muscle contractions. It can cause the layer of horizontal, circular fibers to contract so that the anxious woman's cervix tightens against vertical muscle contractions intended to open it (Fig. 5.4). Contractions then become more painful but nonproductive and can reduce blood flow to the uterus by as much as 65%. Note that a woman who feels supported and safe can relax into her labor and let the uterus do its powerful work in an efficient pattern (Buckley 2008).

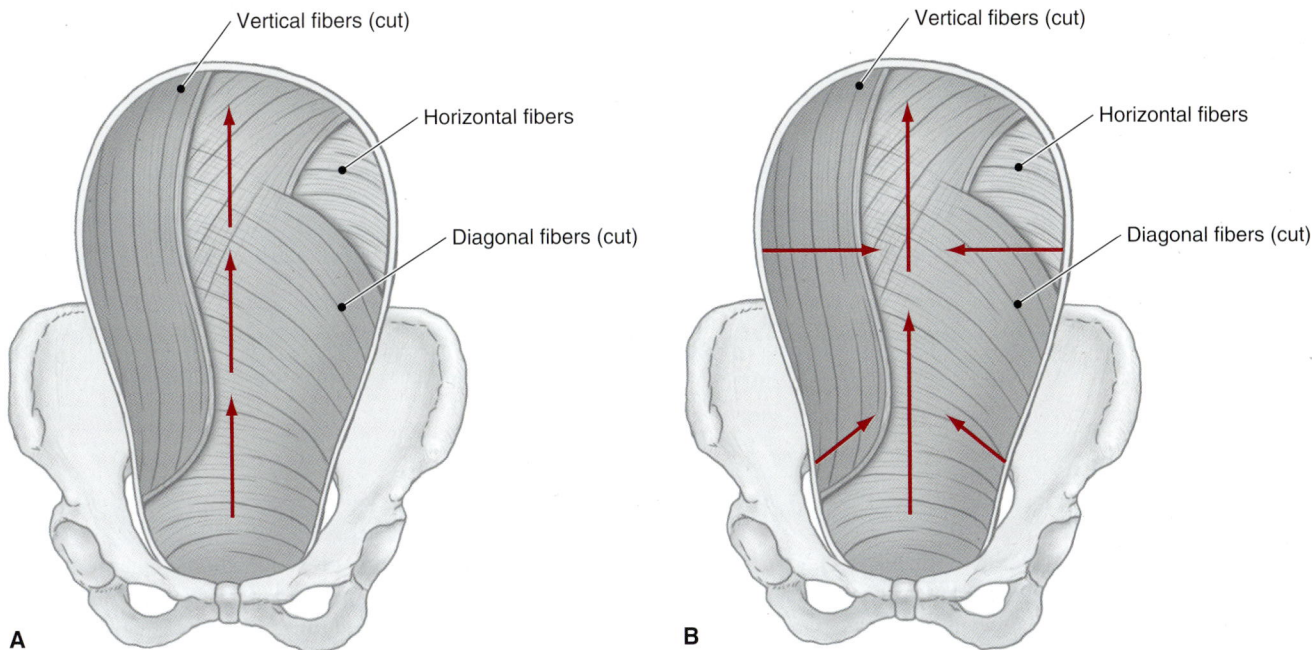

FIGURE 5.4 Effects of stress on progress of first-stage labor. When a woman is relaxed and feeling safe, vertical uterine fibers produce effective cervical dilation and effacement in first-stage labor **(A)**. Under stress, both horizontal and vertical fibers contract, creating a less productive, more painful first-stage labor **(B)**. Arrows indicate direction of contractions.

When early first-stage labor is very slow and painful, your work can be very helpful. First, reduce sympathetic nervous system arousal with relaxing, centering touch employing rhythmic, soothing strokes and holding (see autonomic sedation series 3-1-1 in Chapter 4 and the grounding hold in this chapter's technique manual). Try zone therapy to the entire foot, pressing deeply into the uterus points on the medial calcaneus. Use the labor stimulation points throughout the body. (See Figs. 2.7 and 2.8.) Craniosacral therapy and empathetic encouragement may also help. Try out a variety of gravity-assisted positions, walking, bathing or showering, and rhythmic activities. Unless she requests otherwise, maintain close, supportive physical contact, or have her partner do so.

● ACTIVE FIRST STAGE: A TIME FOR "CONCENTRATION"

Somewhere along the labor journey, the contractions will become closer together and more intense so that the woman will need to stop activity and focus on her breathing and movement. These contractions get her undivided attention. Once the woman's contractions have developed a regular pattern of every 3 to 5 minutes and lasting 60 seconds long, she is considered to be in active labor. The uterus will keep contracting, working at pulling the cervix open and moving the baby's head down against it. What the woman does with her breathing, movement, and positioning supports the uterine action (Tornetta 2008).

This is also the more active part of labor for you. Share with the laboring woman the job of focusing for as long as it takes. There is a common understanding between the medical and holistic care communities that each woman's labor experience is unique and that it takes as long as it takes. Even so, there can be an underlying time pressure to "produce," or interventions to stimulate contractions or operate are urgently suggested. These suggestions can be lifesaving and welcomed, or eclipse the woman's natural labor progress. Help her to stay present with each contraction as the best way to maximize its effectiveness and minimize any real or imagined pressures.

The woman and her caregiver will have discussed when it is she is to call or make her way to the hospital; often, this is during the active first-stage labor. Ideally, you will have begun your support to her to establish strong coping strategies before this transfer takes place. Women need to feel safe and supported to labor effectively and to surrender to the natural process. That may be at home, and she will choose to stay through some or most of her active labor there, transferring to the hospital or birthing center later. Others may feel safest in the hospital throughout labor. If accompanying a woman to a hospital, support her sense of when to go in.

Try to anticipate the next contraction, and have the woman supported and ready for it. You want to have a ritual established, for example, leaning over pillows on the dining room table or the hospital bed with counterpressure on the sacrum while maintaining slow, deep breathing with rhythmic swaying.

My Story

I have had the opportunity to accompany laboring women in many different environments. One memorable time was spent walking throughout a frigid Canadian winter night. I was bundled for the cold; Kathy had her coat wide open and pajamas on underneath! We slowly ambled along the quiet, dark streets, chatting, breathing together arm-in-arm.

At each contraction, with the contractions coming every 4 minutes or so, she would take a deep breath and say, "Here we go." Then she'd wrap her arms around my neck, bend her knees, and we would breathe and sway back and forth for as long as the contraction took, then continue on our way. I remember we shared the night with the deer that had gathered in her wooded neighborhood to snack from the bird feeders there. They were comfortable with our presence, as we were with them. As the sky started to lighten, contractions were closer together and longer, so we made our way home. Kathy woke her partner and then climbed into the tub I was preparing. Dan called the midwives, who soon arrived and determined she was at 8 cm and her baby was near.

—Linda Hickey, Calgary, AB

There may be several such rituals that she chooses from depending on where she is in her home or the hospital room.

Avoid excessive watching when and how long contractions are lasting. Instead, tune in to the contractions' rhythm and the welcomed, inevitable rest between. This can be a challenge if she is laboring in a hospital with fetal monitoring, as the machine announces the contraction and its waning. Especially for partners, you may want to turn down the volume, move the monitors away from the bed, and increase the focus on the woman.

In recent years, women in North America have been able to rent a **birthing pool** that is set up in their homes for home births. With appropriate attention to water temperature, duration of the time spent in the water, and other safety precautions, baths for labor (if not actual birthing) are effective in reducing labor pain (Simkin and Bolding 2004). When the attending midwife determines that labor is well established, submerging chest deep in a warm pool or tub can promote labor progress. It is more appropriate for her partner to be in the tub with her to work at supporting and holding her. Certainly, her neck, shoulders, and head are accessible for your relaxation bodywork.

General Technique Guidelines

Use static or very slow-moving strokes during the contractions, with slow and steady mobilizations matched to her instinctive rocking or swaying movements. If she isn't gently moving through her contractions, "whisper" it to her through your hands. Initiate the movement and guide her in its rhythm. In standing positions, your hands can be on her shoulder and sacrum; in kneeling, on her hips to gently rock her.

Between contractions, use cleansing, faster, and sometimes more energetic strokes to her back, shoulders, neck, and limbs to encourage relaxation. Communicate a steady, sure, calm presence with your hands and movements as well as your words to help set the tone.

Keep an eye on the partner. Engage him in the rituals and physical support of his partner, and safeguard his body mechanics, too. Keep in mind that it is also the partner's birthing experience. Your presence should enable him to be more engaged and to spend more time with his partner, not less. (Use of the masculine pronoun is not intended to exclude females who make up between 1-5% of birth partners.)

Sometimes the laboring woman has chosen to have others at her birth, such as a close friend, a parent, or perhaps siblings. Your attention to their involvement and how your client is responding will guide you in gently moving them closer or farther away. For example, someone may be fearful and bring that fear into the situation, distracting the mother or her partner. Sometimes, it is necessary to be directive and send her off to the kitchen, laundry room, the store, or wherever, giving her a special job to do. Certainly, one of your many hats at a labor is that of a protector. You help to hold the space for the laboring woman, being creative in ensuring that she is surrounded by people who believe in her abilities and can support her in realizing them.

Specific Techniques for Active Labor

Find the appropriate sections in earlier chapters, at the end of this chapter, and online that are usually effective in active labor. These include the following:

- Contraction distraction (Chapter 5)
- Sacral counterpressure in various positions (Chapter 5)
- Labor stimulation points acupressure (Chapter 2)
- Circulation support in between position changes (Chapter 5)
- Cervical and pelvic floor relaxation (Chapter 5)
- Hydrotherapy (Chapter 5)
- Sculpting sacroiliac joints/ligaments (Chapter 4)
- Cramp relief (online)

If dilation is very slow during active labor (**protracted labor**), there may be many causes. From within your scope of practice, use similar approaches as above for a slow early phase. Chapter 7 has suggestions for when cervical progress stops for 2 or 3 hours (**arrested labor or dystocia**) and for other labor complications.

Back Pain in Labor

In most births, babies are positioned head down, facing their mothers' backs, with arms folded at their sides. The sloping, sculpted sides of their mothers' pelvis guide them into this position. This **occipital anterior** (OA) position is considered the ideal position for the mother's ease of birthing (Bainbridge 2000).

Many situations result in other fetal positions, including fetal size, an umbilical cord issue, a uterine anomaly, multiple gestations, and pelvic shape and size. Restrictions in the pelvic soft tissues and positions that the mother assumes in pregnancy's last weeks and during labor also can impact the baby's position. The occiput posterior (OP) position, in which the baby is facing forward with the back of the head against the mother's sacrum, is the most common alternative. An estimated 50% of babies are not in OA position at term (Midwifery Today 2009).

When babies are in an OP position, the woman's labor is usually more painful and/or longer (Tully 2009). She feels the pressure of the baby's head intensely in her back, usually at the sacrum. It is longer because there is a larger dimension of the baby's head in the pelvis, making it harder to move through the pelvic outlet. As a result, babies in an OP position are also more likely to be born by cesarean section or instrumental birth than those in OA.

Most of the time the contracting uterus, aided by a woman's upright position, helps the baby rotate to an OA position by the time of birth. Excess time (several hours daily) spent in a semireclined, lounging position impacts fetal position in the third trimester. For extended periods, many pregnant women are now being advised to sit leaning slightly forward, knees lower than the hip rather than lying back into a soft chair or sofa (Tully 2009).

Obstetricians, midwives, acupuncturists, and chiropractors have effective techniques for turning babies from OP and from breech positions. Refer to these professions when appropriate, remembering that "turning a baby" is outside your scope of practice. In addition, there are self-care practices, midwifery, and doula techniques for helping babies shift their own uterine position. Although they are not massage therapy techniques, understanding their principles sheds light on some massage techniques in this chapter. Some attendants use a long scarf or *rebozo* to lift and jiggle the uterus and baby (Tully 2009). Positional changes that can work include a standing lunge, leaning into the raised hip and pelvis. These help with any uterine or joint ligament imbalances that might be restricting a fetal shift. Others have the mother lie semi-prone or roll over in a sequential pattern to help reposition her baby, using gravity and any fetal inclination to move toward either the left or the right side (Simkin and Ancheta 2011). Gentle, directive abdominal massage can suggest to the baby a more favorable position, and the baby lift can give the baby more room to turn. (See online resources at http://thePoint.lww.com/Osborne-Pregnancy2e and this chapter's technique manual for procedures and precautions.)

In most cases, a baby ideally has rotated into an OA position prior to labor. Even so, back labor can occur, and it

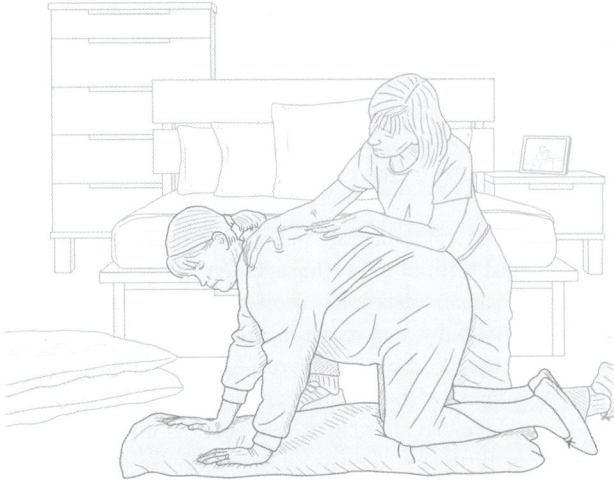

FIGURE 5.5 Coping with back pain. Firm, deep sacral pressure usually provides the most effective relief of "back labor." Many women find hands and knees and similar positions more comfortable too.

necessitates an active approach, for both the mom and you. The hands and knees position often gives most relief. This position, coupled with deep sacral pressure during the contraction, will help her to cope. Use heat and/or ice on the sacrum and try massage tools such as firm tennis balls or an ice-filled bottle for sacral pressure or rolling. (See this chapter's technique manual.)

Try other techniques for back pain in labor, such as the following:

- Sculpting erector spinae and gluteus medius and maximus (Chapter 4)
- Passive and active pelvis tilt with rocking (Chapter 4)
- Sacroiliac joint releases (Chapter 4)
- Gluteal double squeeze or double hip squeeze (online)
- Sacral counterpressure (Chapter 5) (Fig. 5.5)
- Labor TENS (Transcutaneous Electrical Nerve Stimulation) unit (online resources)

Epidurals in Pain Management

While there are various types of pharmacological means of managing labor pain, epidural anesthesia is the most commonly used method during hospital labors. Estimates put epidural use at over two thirds of these labors (Buckley 2009).

What Would You Do?

Your 34-week client is distraught that her baby is in a breech position, rather than head down. A cesarean birth terrifies her, and she asks you to help turn her baby from the breech position. How can you best support her in this difficult situation while staying within your own scope of practice?

An epidural is a pharmaceutical injection into the space around the tough covering, the dura, that protects the spine. It blocks the sensory and motor nerves as they exit from the spine, usually providing effective relief from painful sensation in the lower body. To continuously deliver this medication, a small tube (catheter) remains in place until after the birth.

Widespread epidural use is controversial in some circles as a standard form of labor management. Some studies suggest that it can slow labor, has short- and long-term unknown effects on the baby, can result in further interventions, and, in a small number of births, can result in maternal complications. Awareness of these potential outcomes is often the reason women choose alternative care such as midwifery and/or home or birth center births, where epidural anesthesia is not offered or provided. These concerns also underlie some women's interest in your services as a nonpharmacological form of pain management.

Women generally report high satisfaction with the pain relief an epidural gives. They can be less satisfied with the birth process, however, probably because of the increased other interventions associated with epidurals. With all that said, there are situations in which an epidural can prevent more intervention, in that it can provide a mother a much needed rest and time to regroup in a long or stalled labor, or when she is experiencing overwhelming pain and is actually suffering.

The debate about epidural safety and advisability is spirited. Within your scope of massage therapy practice, what is most relevant is understanding the process and how to best help your client who has an epidural. One primary consideration is that receiving an epidural basically confines the laboring woman to the bed. Before the epidural, she will have an IV inserted for quick administration of any other needed medications. The IV is also for fluids, hopefully to prevent hypotension (Buckley 2009). And because babies can react negatively to the epidural, the use of a continuous fetal monitor is standard care.

Other instruments monitor her blood pressure because up to 50% of all women who receive an epidural have a significant drop in blood pressure. The decreased sensation in her lower half impacts bladder function so catheterization is often necessary, further tethering the mother to the bed. All of these restraints and equipment limit what techniques we can use to continue to encourage and support the labor and the woman. They especially limit her in her use of gravity-assisted positions to speed the labor along.

Your primary role of physical and emotional support for the laboring couple doesn't change in the event your client chooses epidural anesthesia. During the 15 to 60 minutes it can take the anesthesiologist to insert the catheter and establish pain control, you can help her manage contraction pain and reassure her. Your continued presence can help her stay in touch with her baby, her body, and the pressure she still feels as she loses the painful sensations of the contractions. Use abdominal effleurage and guide her to keep physical contact with her baby. She can hold her belly, using words and visualizations of the baby dropping down, cervix opening, and uterus being strong and "hugging" the baby down and out. Try the grounding hold in the technique manual that follows, too.

You need to become acutely aware of your client's position with an epidural. Use the comfortable, supported sidelying position; remember to place a pillow under her belly and to keep her ceiling-side leg high and horizontally supported for comfort and safety (see Chapter 3). More equal distribution of the medication and possible help for the baby's descent occur when she moves every 20 to 30 minutes. Passive ROM to the hip and leg can also encourage downward movement. For such moves, for examinations, and when she is pushing, assist her movement and protect her joints. Ligament laxity is exacerbated, and ligaments are more vulnerable to overstretching when she cannot feel the movement. This is especially true for clients who have had pelvic instability.

You also can assist with fluid circulation with epidurals and when women are laboring in bed for other reasons. The lack of movement and increased fluids via the IV can result in fluids accumulating, in the arms and especially in the legs. Include drainage from those limbs, respecting the medial leg contraindications, of course. Be sure to get permission for the client to change sides. Left sidelying position only is often required, especially if there have been blood pressure changes.

> **REMINDER:** When you massage during labor, continue to observe all contraindications and precautions regarding blood clots in the legs.

You can also use the quiet times that can come with an epidural to work reflexively with her hands and feet. Involve the partner, if he or she is not taking this time to rest, working thoroughly and gently. Remember that your client can perceive the pressure of your touch, but not pain, so err on the side of being too superficial. Especially work the uterus, pelvic, and labor-stimulating points.

Because women generally can feel the pressure or the tightening of the contractions when they have an epidural, some can continue to actively work with their contractions. The goal of the epidural is decreased or eliminated sensation of pain; however, occasionally she may experience "breakthrough" pain or patchy pain relief. In a small area, usually a few inches in diameter, she can still feel the contraction's intensity. Approximately 10% to 15% of women with an epidural will experience only one-sided pain relief (Buckley 2009). When any breakthrough pain occurs, continue to work with that area in the same ways as without an epidural: counterpressure with slow rocking, deep effleurage, and verbal coaching. If the breakthrough area is on the abdomen, move to gentle energy work, such as gently holding the area with your palm.

Continue to involve and support the partner as he or she is available. Often, after the epidural is given, both partners rest and sleep for an hour or so as the labor nurse stays close, monitoring the anesthetic's effects. Take a short break, too, with the mother's awareness and permission to leave to make calls, get some dinner, or regroup. For some, the decision to have an epidural, especially if she had been planning for a natural birth, is emotional and not made lightly. She may need extra emotional support and encouragement. It is an important time to check in with your own expectations, too. When it is your wish for women to birth in a certain way, the request for epidural can be a disappointment. Remember it is not about you!

● TRANSITION PHASE: A TIME FOR "SURRENDER"

Once the cervix is approaching 10 cm, or fully dilated, the contractions' rhythmic nature changes into a more erratic and sometimes aggressive pattern. Contractions become longer, sharper, closer, and tighter, sometimes with no break in between. During this relatively short phase, the uterus is transitioning or reorganizing its contractile pattern for pushing the baby out. All layers of uterine muscle, particularly the diagonal and horizontal fibers, now work simultaneously toward that goal. The rituals and techniques that you have been using for the hours and centimeter dilation up to now may not work. Your client may appear frightened and unsure at this point (Tornetta 2008).

Transition phase is a time of surrender for the laboring woman (Fig. 5.6). Become solid ground for her so she can yield to the intensity. This usually involves firm holding and communicating, perhaps taking a stronger role in directing her breath, keeping eye contact with you, or trying a different position or movement. She might have wildly varying needs that change from moment to moment, including her desire for touch assurance, warmth, and position changes. Nausea and vomiting are common during transition, as is leg and arm trembling.

During this phase, avoid touch that distracts her. Often a firm, still hand on a tense area is the only touch she will find beneficial. She might welcome slow, rhythmic massage or zone therapy on her feet. Backache is common, even with an anterior presentation baby, so concentrate on firm, deep pressure on her sacrum, SI joints, and paravertebral muscles. Rhythmic soft effleurage moving proximal to distal on her inner thighs may help calm her trembling legs.

It is usually a short time until she feels an urge to push, often signaling this with a grunting or guttural noise that creeps into her breath at the contraction's height. At this point, a nurse or doctor will likely do a vaginal check to ensure the full cervical dilation and to give the "ok" to the woman to push with her contractions.

Occasionally, the cervix has not contracted equally around its circumference, leaving a thickened edge known as a **cervical lip**. The concern of pushing without full dilation

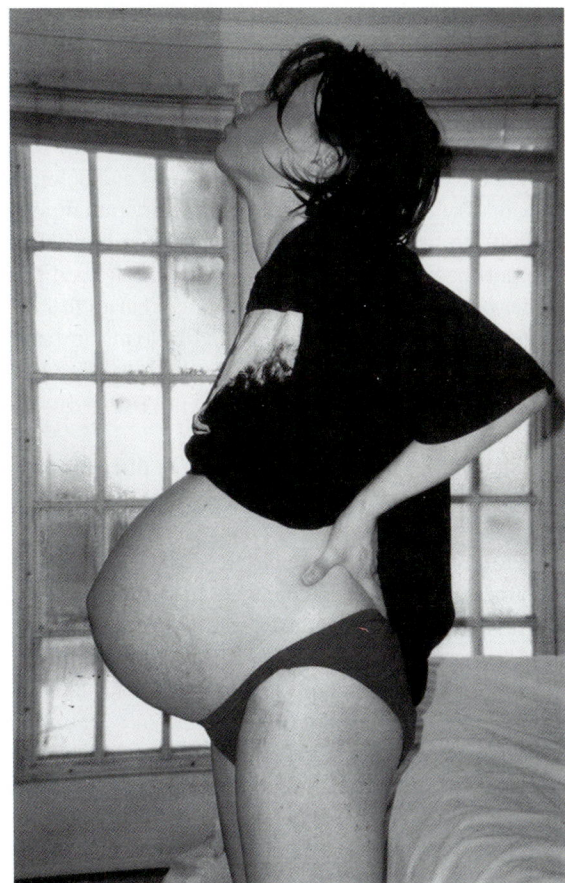

FIGURE 5.6 Surrendering to labor. The transition phase demands internal focus and surrender to the forces of the laboring uterus.

is that swelling or edema will occur at the cervix, preventing the baby's passage. The guidelines of staying upright and changing positions for most of labor are intended to, in part, prevent this from happening. The general antidote is for the woman to change position under the staff person's direction. She may need to pant through a few contractions to avoid her diaphragm assisting the uterus in pushing prematurely. These strategies can allow for time and/or gravity to assist the cervix in completely pulling back over the baby's descending head. As it is very challenging to NOT push when one feels the need to, she will need your extra attention, support, and direction to help her through this difficult situation.

● SECOND STAGE: RESTING, PUSHING, AND THE BIRTH

With cervix opened and the head past, the uterine fibers need 10 to 30 minutes to tighten up around the smaller fetal body. This creates an apparent rest, when the unknowing or impatient can think that labor has stalled. It is best if everyone involved can enjoy the break from intense contractions, regroup for the work ahead, and wait for an urge to push. For most women, that sensation usually becomes as involuntary and uncontrollable as the most urgent bowel movement or vomiting, with all the force of the strongest muscle in the body (Fig. 5.7).

With that urge, your role as labor support massage therapist shifts once again. At this time, you may assist the woman in hearing the doctor or midwife's directions and helping her with them. Try being near her head and ear so that you can talk quietly to her directly. A **birth bar** on a **birthing bed** can support her upright. You might sit up on the bed behind her if her partner is not able to. Encourage her to follow her instincts in breathing, positioning, and relaxing in between contractions. You can continue to use both touch and firm holding to ground her energetically and physically (see technique manual and online video).

Holding one's breath while pushing or directed pushing is often considered problematic in the more natural birthing circles. They instead advocate encouraging the woman to tune into and follow her innate instincts, matching her efforts to her internal messages of when and how to push with the contractions ("laboring down"). Some data indicate that trauma to the perineal tissues is lessened when women follow their instincts in positioning and when and how to push (Sakala 2009).

It may be that the hospital protocols haven't yet made this adjustment and will take a "cheerleading" coaching approach to pushing. They might instruct the woman to take and hold a big breath and push, believing this increases the power behind the contraction and thereby shortening pushing time. Your encouraging words spoken gently near her ear can help offset the higher frantic energy that she may feel and help her focus internally to work with her urges.

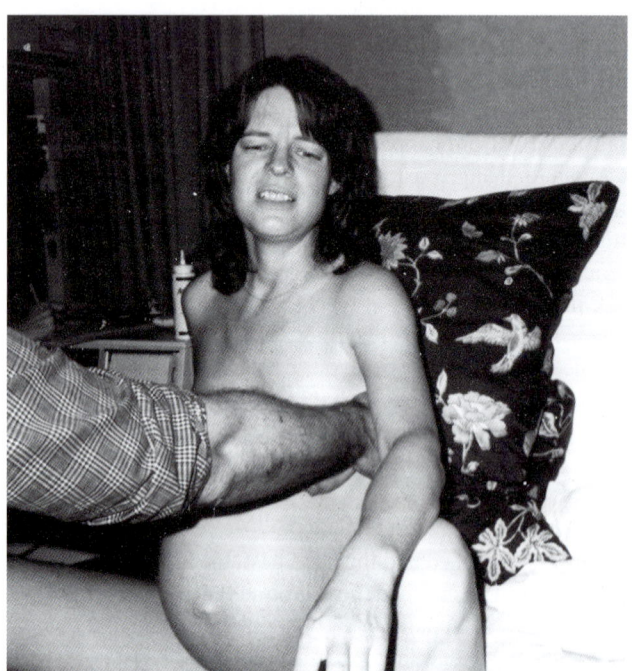

FIGURE 5.7 Pushing. Supported gravity-assisted positions usually widen the pelvic outlet and increase the uterine muscles' efficiency in birthing the baby.

It is also important at this time to stay aware of the woman's positions and any potential compromise to her joints. Caregivers often hold a laboring woman's legs for her in pushing: knees and hips flexed, abducted, and externally rotated, opening the pelvic floor. It is easy for everyone to get caught up in the excitement of the baby's arrival and lose focus on their hands and holding, compromising the woman's vulnerable spine, hip, and knee joints. If you are helping support her legs, protect her joints, and you can also incorporate the acupressure and/or pelvic relaxation techniques in this chapter's technique manual.

Maintaining clear and present focus with the woman and her experience is paramount in this phase of labor. Keep your eyes on her face, ready to make supportive eye contact as needed. When you have established a cooperative working relationship with the labor nurse, doctor, or midwife, you can offer other techniques such as the passive pelvic tilt and rhythmic passive movements (Chapter 4), pelvic press (online resources), or reflexive pelvic floor and adductor relaxation points (Chapter 5) as supportive measures during pushing. The descent of the baby through the vagina to complete birth can take a few minutes or two to four hours of hard work. Most women, their partners, and you will likely be energized by her progress. Nevertheless, help her to rest and regroup between contractions, to push effectively, and to open her body and heart to her baby's birth.

● THIRD STAGE: PLACENTAL SEPARATION AND EXPULSION

As the new mother and her partner usually focus on their baby, discharge of the placenta is often very anticlimatic. For around 30 minutes, the uterus keeps contracting to clamp down on the blood vessels between the uterus and the placenta. The placenta then pulls away from the uterine wall and slides out. The new mother may not be aware of the process as the uterus is now close to empty and with the distraction of the baby in her arms.

In settings, where a clock may be in play, or if she begins hemorrhaging, pitocin may be given to encourage uterine contractions if it wasn't given to augment contractions earlier, and the placenta is manually prompted to expel. The mother may need some help to relax and breathe through this procedure and through the examination and stitching of her perineum, if needed.

Caregivers may also give active and sometimes painful fundal massage to encourage the uterus to keep contracting and expel the placenta. Throughout this time, you will generally be at the sidelines, giving the family time and space to be together. Stay vigilant, ready to step back into your supportive role as needed. Depending on the hospital's family-centered practice and the baby's condition, the perinatal staff may remove the baby for measuring or examination, her partner might stay with the baby for these procedures, and you can rejoin the mother during that time for some soothing massage.

Cesarean Section Births

Currently in North America, approximately one in three women will have their babies surgically, via a cesarean section or c-section birth. Only 5% to 10% of births absolutely indicate a surgical delivery due to an urgent health situation for the mother or baby, yet the US cesarean section birth rate was 31.8 in 2007 and rising. (In Canada—26.5% and in Britain—23.5% even with the higher midwifery care there.) (Buckley 2008) Other situations when a physician might recommend a cesarean birth may include a previous cesarean section, prolonged labor or failure to progress, **breech position** of the baby, changes in fetal heart tone, and in cases of multiple births.

It is this second category of situations that is the subject of much debate and controversy and that is likely the cause of the increasing surgical birth rate (Buckley 2008). There also appears to be a growing trend in North America and other countries of first-time mothers requesting a cesarean birth (Evans and Aronson 2005). Many doctors are against this growing trend, as are proponents of natural birth, citing concern for the potential risks to the baby and mothers. Like many childbearing decisions, this is a decision made between the woman and her doctor. These situations present

> *My Story*
>
> One of the teaching hospitals in my city has a viewing area attached to the surgical suite on the obstetrical floor. On the occasions the labor I was attending ended with a cesarean birth, I have waited in the viewing area and stayed energetically with my client, keeping eye contact with her throughout the procedure. At each of these births, the midwife or doctor has acknowledged my participation in the event for the mother by bringing the baby over to the window to say hello and show me all is well. Smiles of joy were all round, even those behind a mask.
>
> —Linda Hickey, Calgary, AB

an opportunity for you to explore your own beliefs on the subject and practice nonjudgmental, active listening.

● THE OPERATIVE PROCEDURES

In a cesarean section birth, a surgeon makes several incisions through the multiple layers of skin adipose, and connective tissues, then through the uterine wall, with the muscle layer and bladder pulled to the side (Fig. 5.8). The surgeon

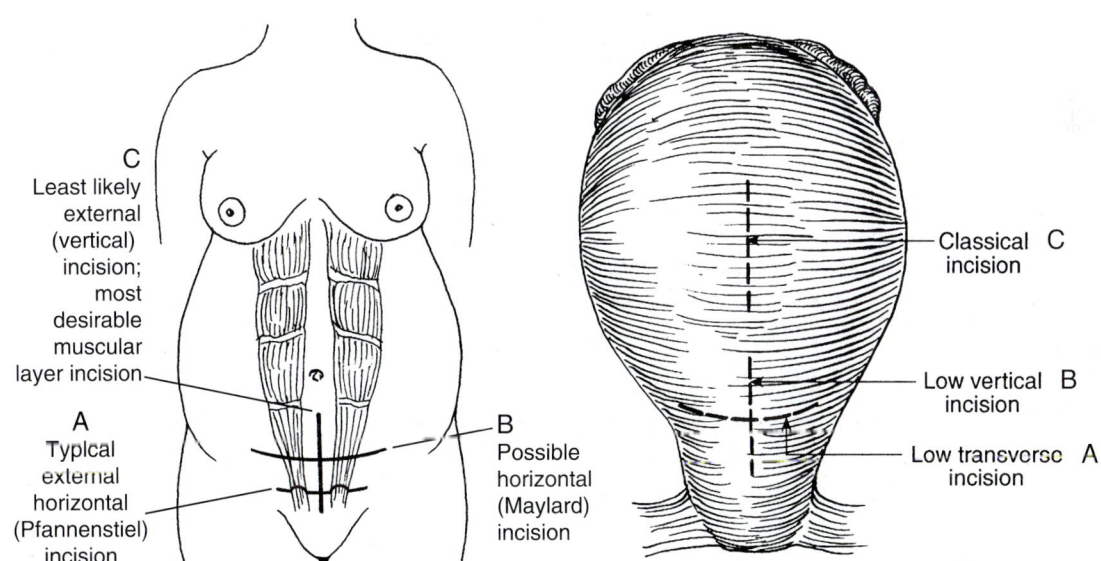

FIGURE 5.8 Cesarean section incisions. Understanding the probable direction of incisions made during surgery can make your postpartum scar work more effective. Note on the left illustration **A** and **B**, the most likely horizontal incision through the skin, and what you will see. **C** is the cut most likely on the internal layers through any unseparated linea alba that you may feel at the midline of the visible scar. Surgical birth continues with retracting the bladder away from the uterus and another horizontal incision on the lower uterine segment line **A** on the illustration on the right. **B** and **C** are the less common uterine incision sites. Finally, the surgeon lifts the baby out through all incisions then repairs all layers. Adapted from Beckmann CR et al. Obstetrics and Gynecology, 5th ed. Philadelphia: Lippincott Williams & Wilkins, 2006.

manually lifts the presenting part and then the entire baby. After the placenta spontaneously detaches or by manual removal, sutures or staples are used to close the incision. Many women report surprise at the sensations of tugging and pulling they feel during these steps.

● HOW YOU CAN HELP

Whether anyone or only the partner is allowed in the sterile operative environment is a matter of hospital policy; the same is true for the recovery room. Should your client request you to come with her and you are allowed, you will dress in surgical scrubs. Cooperate with all medical staff, and expect a great experience. Keep your attention on her, with unwavering eye contact and help her breathing, relaxation, and awareness of what is happening. You may be able to hold a hand, or her shoulder, head or neck, the accessible areas of her body above the draping. As with all births, it is easy for the activity happening at the far end of her body to distract you.

When an immediate concern for the mother or baby's well-being prompts a surgical birth, it will likely happen quickly, maybe leaving you and her family alone in the labor room. If you aren't in with her, stay in contact with the nursing desk and the family. If allowed and requested, resume your support for her and her partner in the recovery room. It could be two hours or longer before she is in her own postpartum room, but you should at least check in with them before leaving. Reconnecting with the mother when you can is essential for her to feel completion with you. Seeing that all is well is important for your own well-being, too.

In situations in which the outcome is an unexpected cesarean birth, women may experience feelings of failure or, in some cases, some symptoms of posttraumatic stress (Buckley 2008). You can be helpful in her positive recovery emotionally. Continued emotional support and comparing stories help to fill in any missing pieces she may need to help her integrate her experience. (See Chapter 7 for guidance with perinatal death and illnesses.)

In both planned and unplanned cesarean births as with vaginal births, bringing your caring, unconditional, nonjudgmental support to bear helps to deal with any negative outcomes. Remember and remind her that your work throughout her pregnancy aids her development of effective labor skills. You prepare her body in physical and kinesthetic ways, nurturing her and sharing information. This will help her to grow trust in her abilities to birth and flexibility to cope with the unexpected as events arise. Your work can help her to feel her safest, and that can decrease the likelihood of a cascade of interventions to the normal progression of her labor.

My Story

I believe that if it wasn't for my pregnancy massage during my labor with my daughter, it wouldn't have gone as smoothly as it did. I was in active labor, but the massage put me in such a relaxed state that I could get some rest and complete my labor without any drugs. My first was a cesarean section, but this time was a "stop and drop" delivery, and vaginally. Just a few good pushes and my daughter was born. I mention my labor massage experience to every woman whom I meet who is expecting.

—Jessica

A Few Final Thoughts about Assisting at Labors

Because labors may last from 2 to 42 hours or more, you must have great endurance. Remember to eat, stay hydrated, and take mini-breaks for stretching and tension relief when possible. Efficient body mechanics help to conserve energy and reduce overuse injuries, especially to your hands, wrist, and back. Reduce back strain from leaning over low, wide hospital beds by adjusting the bed height and having her close to the bedsides when possible. A rolling stool can be very handy, too. When using deep, sustained pressure, as for back labor, align hand, wrist, and shoulder joints. Use elbows, knuckles, knees, and legs whenever possible.

Expect utterly unexpected events and outcomes at any birth. An apprehensive woman can burst into confidence and strength when she gets into labor. Some women describe their birthing experience as empowering, orgasmic, or ecstatic. On the other hand, even the most prepared, healthy, positive woman, who appears to have done everything "right," can have a very difficult, complicated labor that progresses very differently than anticipated. If this occurs, you may feel as though you failed her or even caused some of her difficulties. Frightening events and strange equipment and procedures may disrupt your composure and focus. Your own personal issues regarding birthing or other "emotional baggage" may disturb your ability to be fully present with your client. (See Chapter 7 for labor complications and special needs.)

Develop your regrouping and concentration skills to be more prepared for these moments. Establish support for yourself to "debrief" after each labor so that you may unburden yourself of any negative feelings you may have developed. Record the labor in your client's chart as soon as possible after the birth.

Technique Manual of Labor Massage and Bodywork

As in Chapter 4, this section includes detailed instruction in how to perform selected techniques. This chapter's technique manual focuses on preparing a woman for labor and supporting her during the process. You will find techniques grouped according to the stage in which they are most likely to be useful; however, take those groupings very loosely. Remember that some of these will be helpful throughout labor. Others may seem ineffectual at first, and then in later stages, they may be the only thing that keeps a woman going. All women will not respond favorably to all techniques nor need all of them. Labor massage therapy is truly an adventure of spontaneity, careful observation, and trial/error/success. You will need to modify for client position and for monitoring and other equipment that may be used. Do not interpret the order of these techniques as a sequence or a ranking of priority.

As in Chapter 4, each technique breaks down into the following segments:

- **Intention:** the intended outcome or purpose of the technique
- **Procedure:** precise instructions in how to accomplish the technique
- **Hints:** ways to make it easier or more effective or to vary it for individual needs
- **Precautions:** adaptations and contraindications to remember to safely use the technique

In addition, you will find a section of each technique grouping suggesting auxiliary approaches to addressing the labor stage involved. Table 5.1 summarizes these techniques. See the online resources at http://thePoint.lww.com/Osborne-Pregnancy2e for videos of some of the techniques presented here and for additional labor techniques.

Labor Preparation Techniques

Much of your prenatal work can help ready a woman physically and emotionally to have the maximum options available to her in how she meets labor's ups and downs and maximizes its pleasures. Begin specific labor preparation in the last 6 to 8 weeks before a woman's due date with the techniques below and any others you know that will accomplish the same intentions safely.

Precautions
Remember all of the general contraindications and precautions for prenatal massage therapy covered in detail in Chapter 2 and those discussed earlier in this chapter. Some of the techniques below also have their own specific precautions.

Technique Suggestions
In addition to the breathing, relaxation, communication, education, and other techniques discussed earlier in this chapter, use the following techniques in your prenatal sessions.

Passive Relaxation of the Thigh Adductors

(Fig. 5.9).

Intentions
To induce relaxation and passive stretching of the thigh adductors; to promote ability to squat and abduct the thighs during labor; to prepare emotionally for the exposure and vulnerability inherent in birthing; to assist in resolving issues related to prior births, medical procedures, sexual abuse, or other experiences that may negatively impact the birth.

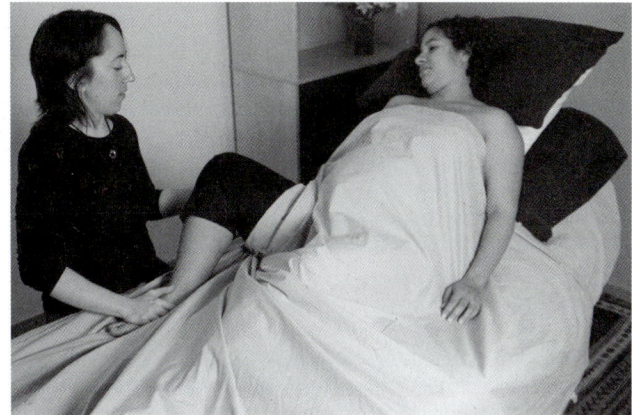

FIGURE 5.9 Passive relaxation of the thigh adductors.

Procedure
Best performed in semireclining position

1. Stand facing the client. Slide the leg bolster out from under her closest leg, and flex that knee to place her foot flat on the table near her other knee. Support this foot with your hand closest to the table to prevent it from sliding, but allow it to evert with the following movements.
2. Place your other hand laterally on her bent knee. Ask her to give over her leg weight to you by relaxing her inner thigh. Receive and distribute the entire weight of her leg into your legs to provide stable support.
3. Induce adductor relaxation by initiating very small amplitude, rhythmic adduction and abduction movements while gradually externally rotating her hip. Initiate movement from your own legs rather than with just your arms.
4. Continue the small rocking movements as you gradually take the knee from her midline to maximum hip ROM, without creating pain.
5. Allow the weight of the leg to further stretch the adductors for 30 seconds to one minute and/or perform assisted-resisted stretches.
6. Return the leg to the midline with similar rocking movements.
7. Relocate the bolster, extend this leg and then repeat on the other leg.

Hints

1. If the client has difficulty releasing her leg to your movements, ask her to imagine your hand as a powerful magnet and her leg

as metal. Have her imagine that the attractive force of the magnet makes it impossible for her to hold the weight of her leg.
2. Whenever the muscles contract to regain control of the movement, reverse the direction of your movement to return to an angle where she was passive. Repeat your rocking movements through the resistant area until she is able to relax again.
3. With expressed client consent, improve acceptance of the exposure inherent in birthing by repeated performance of this technique to her level of comfort following this progression in subsequent sessions: fully clothed and draped, fully clothed, with underwear and draped, without underwear and draped.
4. This technique is also sometimes useful during labor to relax the adductors between contractions.

Precautions

1. Do not perform when she experiences symphysis pubis pain.
2. If pain occurs in SI joints or other pelvic areas, provide pillow support under the lateral thigh to reduce maximum ROM.
3. Avoid overstretching ligaments.

First-Stage Labor Techniques

This effacement/dilatation of the cervix stage is a time for relaxation, pain relief, and comforting. Sometimes, changes in maternal or fetal positioning will help normalize labor, and others will help maintain robust, productive contractions. Choose relaxation techniques from those below, from the Chapter 4 technique manual, and any others in your repertoire that create these effects. You will likely find some of the second-stage techniques further below to be helpful in the first stage too. See online resources for other techniques.

Precautions

Remember all of the general contraindications and precautions covered in detail in Chapter 2 and those discussed earlier in this chapter. Some of the techniques below also have their own specific precautions. As labor progresses, the intensity and intimacy of labor may prompt changes in the ways you relate to your client. Balance her needs and your professional commitment to scope of practice, boundaries, and the transference/countertransference and other emotional and ethical dynamics discussed earlier in this chapter.

Modify techniques for the laboring woman's position. In general, supine and sitting positions may interfere with labor progress and can cause supine hypotension; they are usually to be avoided in labor. In most cases, encourage frequent positional changes (every 20–30 minutes), including the following: gravity-assisted positions (squatting, standing, dangling, and kneeling), all fours (in bed or on floor), semireclining, seated, sidelying, and using birthing equipment, such as birthing beds, chairs, stools, bars, or balls or household furniture (Ricci 2009).

You should always observe the laboring woman's preferences in the use of any bodywork techniques during labor. Remember that she may not want to be touched or disturbed during part or all of her labor.

Technique Suggestions

In addition to the techniques discussed earlier in this chapter, use the following techniques to nurture, reduce pain, and stimulate labor.

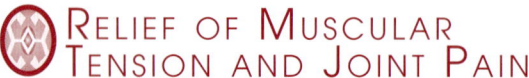

Relief of Muscular Tension and Joint Pain

Intentions

To relax generalized tension and specific muscles tensed in response to pain and to ease strain on pelvic joints as the baby descends and exits the pelvis. The most commonly tensed muscles during labor are as follows: masseter and temporalis; trapezius, levator scapulae, and other upper back muscles; hand and finger flexors; hamstrings and quadriceps; adductor longus, brevis, and magnus; erector spinae, quadratus lumborum, and other lumbar muscles; levator ani, transverse perineal, and other pelvic floor muscles; and gastrocnemius, soleus, and toe flexors. The most strained joints are as follows: the SI, symphysis pubis, lumbosacral, intervertebral, and hip joints.

Procedure

1. Dissipate unproductive tension in these muscles by molding your hand to the area and asking her to focus on relaxing there.
2. During contractions, apply firm, stationary, deep tissue sculpting compressions with knuckles, fist, fingers, or elbow. Cause no pain, and maintain consistency of touch. (See Chapter 4 technique manual for general instructions and principles applicable to any of these areas.)
3. Kneading, effleurage, and other Swedish strokes help to relax chronically tightened muscles and prevent cramping. Perform rhythmic, firm strokes during or between contractions, as she prefers. Between contractions also use passive stretches, assisted-resisted stretches, and/or shortening of tensed muscles to relax these areas by eliciting proprioceptive adjustments in muscle length.
4. Other prenatal techniques that may be effective for muscle tension from Chapter 4's technique manual include the following: inching to intrinsic paravertebrals, rhythmic passive movements, and autonomic sedation series 3-1-1.
5. Other prenatal techniques that may be effective for joint strain from Chapter 4's technique manual include SI joint blended release, knee press and traction, lumbosacral stretch, rhythmic passive movements, hip decompression, figure 8 hip mobilization, and symphysis pubis rebalancing.

Hints

Use visual imagery to enhance the effectiveness of your massage techniques.

Precautions

Avoid clot endangerment sites as blood-clotting factors reach their highest levels during labor to prevent hemorrhaging.

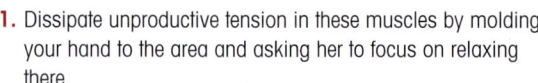

Circulation Support Between Contractions

Intentions

To assist in the circulation of blood and fluid that may have accumulated in ankles, knees or hips, and wrists, elbows, or hands during labor positions and movements; to bring the laboring woman's attention to these areas for conscious relaxation; to bring energy to the limbs in preparation for the next contraction.

Procedures

Legs

1. Use your cupped, soft hands to quickly stroke up from knee to hip 5 to 10 times, covering the circumference of the upper leg. If accessible, vibrate for 30 seconds, with featherlight pressure behind the knee, and then repeat the cupped hand light strokes 5 to 10 times on the lower leg, working your hands around the circumference of the leg again. Gently squeeze around the ankle and the top of the foot. End on the leg with a few upward full leg strokes beginning at the ankle, ending at her hip. Repeat for the other leg.
2. If kneeling, your client may choose to rest between contractions sitting back on her lower legs. Perform quick superficial upward strokes on the lower legs, and do gentle ankle and foot squeezes as she moves forward to hands and knees position readying for the oncoming contraction.

Arms

At any time when your client is holding a bar, has hands clasped, or is leaning forward on bent wrist or forearms, use cupped hands and light touch to quickly stroke from wrist to shoulder. Cover the circumference of her arm with your hands. Grasp and circle her wrist with your palms and strip upward toward her shoulder several times and massage her hands before the next contraction begins to build.

Hints

1. Movements between contractions, depending on her position, that can help circulation include knee high slow marching in place; arms above head or out to sides and shaking; rotating shoulders; walking.
2. Encourage change of position every 20 to 30 minutes, and suggest she attempts to urinate every hour.
3. If sitting on a ball, take care not to destabilize her balance on the ball with your strokes.

Precautions

1. Suggest a change of position to a standing forward leaning position if your client experiences numb or tingling sensations in her legs from the weighted flexion of her knees when kneeling or on hands and knees. Place pillows for space and padding behind or under her knees too.
2. Observe precautions concerning no deep, pointed pressure on the medial aspect of the leg in pregnancy. During labor light, fluid moving strokes are appropriate.
3. When your client has an epidural or is limited in movement, use featherlight drainage techniques as above to lateral, anterior, and posterior aspects of the leg only. Avoid the medial leg entirely due to the increased risk of clots due to inactivity.

Localized Massages

Some women relax best to massage therapy in only one or two areas, particularly their head, hands, or feet.

Intention

To stimulate parasympathetic arousal that increases relaxation.

Procedure

1. Experiment with gentle, soothing facial massage, especially to the scalp, forehead, and jaw. Hair stroking is very nurturing for many. Include her neck and upper shoulders. Gently undulate her cervical spine, and the atlanto-occipital joint. (See Chapter 4 technique manual.)
2. Thoroughly massage both of her hands, especially if she has been clenching them during contractions. Firm, midline palmar pressure simultaneous with friction on the dorsal surface of her hand simulates a traditional labor technique of clenching a comb or other object without generating maternal forearm tension. Simkin theorizes that this technique's effectiveness is due to the abundance of pressure sensors in the palm and the interaction with the gate theory (Simkin 2008).
3. Use Swedish, passive movements, or reflexive work on her feet. Use firm, rhythmic inching pressure to create bone-to-bone contact at the zones reflexive to areas of tension and pain. Concentrate on the pelvis, perineal, and back reflexes. To encourage contractions, press the uterine points on the medial calcaneus. (See illustration of points in Figs. 2.7 and 4.50.)
4. Craniosacral therapy fosters relaxation and balance in all body systems, particularly maintaining physiological equilibrium (homeostasis). Use the biodynamic craniosacral approach (Shea 2008). Or induce still point of the craniosacral fluid rhythms by holding and then releasing the ebbing and flowing fluid with light pressure against the mastoid area of the temporal bones, through holding the legs, or at the sacrum. Follow with release of the occipital cranial base, the thoracic inlet, and the pelvic and respiratory diaphragms. Relieve pelvic pain with sacral compression/decompression techniques. Use the V-spread to focus healing energy at specific painful areas (Upledger and Vredevoogd 1983).

Abdominal Effleurage

Intentions

To facilitate relaxation, especially of the abdominal muscles; to facilitate connection with the baby; to create space for the baby to reposition himself/herself; to facilitate the opening of the cervix.

Procedure

May be performed in all positions, depending on the laboring woman's preference; described for semireclined, as this is a likely position if an epidural is in place

1. From a position beside the abdomen, use the flat, relaxed palms of your hands to apply oil with superficial effleurage strokes circling around her abdomen. Complete a circle with one hand as the other makes a half circle to spread the oil, to make connection with the mother and the baby, and to warm the tissue.
2. If a need of a fetal position change has been decided, go no deeper than the abdominal muscles, making superficial thumb or finger fanning motions. Concentrate on the area to encourage the baby to move to. For example, to encourage a rotation from posterior to anterior, work on the lower segment of the abdomen superior to the pubic bone and on the side opposite the baby's face if already partially turned.
3. Use your flat fingers in small superficial circles around her abdomen, concentrating in the lower abdominal region.

4. Create long, superficial strokes laterally across her abdomen moving in the direction of a desired fetal movement (left to right or right to left).
5. Hold gently at the edge of the baby's back with flat, relaxed hands, and gently rock and undulate the abdomen.
6. When no position change is desirable, reinforce the uterine muscles' action on the cervix with your effleurage strokes on the abdominal muscles. During the first stage, stroke gently from the pubic area upward toward the umbilicus to simulate the lifting force of the longitudinal muscles. Amplify this effect by suggesting that she visualizes each contraction gathering the cervix into the uterine walls to open it. In the second stage, let your strokes flow downward from the ribcage toward the pubic bone while she visualizes the baby moving down.

Hints and Alternatives

1. If a position change is desired, try the above procedures with the mother on all fours or on knees and elbows so that gravity might shift the baby's head slightly out of the pelvic inlet. This will give a bit more space for the baby to rotate in response to the suggestion in your abdominal massage.
2. In one of the above positions, wrap a folded sheet around the mother's abdomen. Stand behind her holding both ends of the sheet. Gently rock her abdomen back and forth as an alternate version of the rocking movement above in step 4 (Tully 2009).
3. Wrap the folded sheet around the mother's hips and rock her pelvis instead.
4. Encourage visualization and conversation between the mother and the baby to suggest the desired effect of the massage.

Precautions

1. Work with the midwife, nurse, or doctor to determine the baby's present position, the optimal preferred position, and to monitor the baby's response.
2. Secure her permission before touching her abdomen.
3. Maintain pressure so that you are not penetrating deeply into the uterus. Be sure to use a flat, soft surface of your hand. Avoid tense fingers that poke or press beneath the ribcage, into the pelvic bowl, or in the inguinal or solar plexus regions.
4. Do not forcibly or aggressively attempt to make a baby move. This is a technique of suggestion and possibilities, not imperatives. There may be a very good reason that a baby is staying in one position, despite the difficulty of that position for the mother.
5. If the client is nauseated, do not perform the rocking. Always avoid vigorous rocking motions.
6. When the belt of an electronic fetal monitor restricts long strokes, shorten your strokes, and emphasize rhythm and the stroke's purpose.

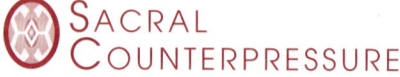

Sacral Counterpressure

(Simkin 2008)

Intentions

To relieve pain in the sacrum and lower back, especially for those who have more extreme "back labor" due to the baby being OP; to stimulate uterine contractions through activating the urinary bladder 31 to 34 points that correspond to the sacral sulcusci. See Figure 5.6.

Procedure

1. From a position behind the client, use your elbow, knee, or knuckle to apply very deep compressions on the sacrum. Protect her lumbar spine by simultaneously directing your pressure inferiorly toward her coccyx, creating a passive pelvic tilt.
2. Search for one or two specific points that, when firmly pressed, afford relief ("sweet spot"). Maintain firm pressure continuously during each contraction. You may wish to support her pelvis with your other hand to keep her pelvis more aligned under your pressure.
3. Relocate further distally or switch to the other side of her sacrum to find a new "sweet spot" when relief begins to diminish because the baby has moved.

Hints

1. Encourage her to try an "all fours" position on her hands or forearms and knees or on a birth ball to facilitate pelvic tilting and rocking of her body forward and then back. These movements, especially in combination with the sacral counterpressure or cold packs, are often effective in reducing or eliminating back labor.
2. If you have sufficient balance and control, you can use other bony body parts such as your heel, knee, or ischium rather than your arms or hands.
3. A knobble, T-bar, large cooking spoon, or hairbrush handle might be a good tool for getting sufficiently deep and pointed pressure.
4. Heat or cold, shower water, or a vibrator applied to the sacrum also may be effective in sending competing stimuli to the brain.

Precautions

1. Do not press the lumbar spine anteriorly with your pressure. Be sure that you or whomever you teach to do this is on the sacrum, not on the lumbar spine.
2. If she has carpal tunnel or other wrist or hand pain, guide her to rest on her forearms or her fisted hand rather than on the palms.
3. Because very deep pressure is necessary to create sufficient counterpressure, use efficient structural alignment as you apply your body weight to avoid injuring yourself.

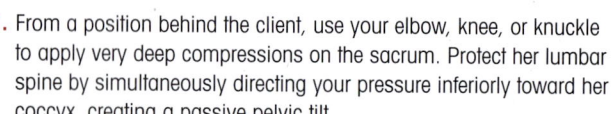

Hydrotherapy

Intentions

To reduce pain sensation by sending competing stimulus to the brain; to relax tense muscles; to comfort and soothe.

Procedure

1. Place a heated device on the lower abdomen, back, or groin to ease pain. There is some evidence that warmth applied just below the ribcage to the fundus of the uterus can stimulate uterine activity (Simkin and Ancheta 2011). Use a hydrocolator pack or other hot pack, a hot water bottle, or a rice- or husk-filled sock heated in a microwave.
2. Place an ice bag, cold wrap, frozen washcloth, or frozen peas or corn on the sacrum or low back to ease pain. Use a can of frozen drink or other object to roll firmly over her lower back.

3. Try other local applications of heat or cold that can soothe and relieve including warm blankets or towels to reduce trembling; warm compresses on the perineal area to help relax the vagina and perineum; cool washcloths for wiping her face, neck, and anywhere it feels good to her.

Precautions

Test the temperature to be sure that you can easily hold any hot or cold object in your hand. Put fabric between the object and the client's skin.

Labor Stimulation Points

Intention

To initiate and strengthen uterine contraction by activating certain Chinese acupuncture points. See Figs. 2.7 and 2.8.

Procedure

1. Press firmly with thumb tip or fingertip bilaterally into each of the points illustrated in Figures 2.7 and 2.8 that were contraindicated prior to her due date. On the foot and leg: liver 3, kidney 3, bladder 60, and spleen 6. On the hand: large intestine 4. On the torso: gall bladder 21, urinary bladder 31 to 34, stomach 36, and urinary bladder 67.
2. Work on each point consecutively in six cycles of 10 seconds of pressure on and 10 seconds off. If not effective, extend your pressure to as long as 1 minute on and 1 minute off.
3. Work bilaterally if possible through all the points, with a 15- to 30-minute rest period between starting again at the feet.

Hints

1. Use a marker or pen to mark each point on your client so that you can teach others to work these points too.
2. These points are their most potent during a labor to stimulate contractions and reduce pain, maintaining the normal progression of the labor. They may help strengthen and increase contractions when a labor has slowed or stalled. They are usually most effective if you are trained in energy work via the meridians.

##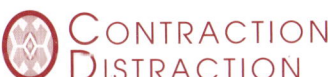

Intentions

To flood the brain with pressure and pleasurable sensations that distract from pain of the cervix stretching, uterine ligament strain, and other anteriorly felt pain; to relax the lower back. See Fig. 5.10.

Procedure

1. Use fingertips, thumbs, knuckles, or elbows to compress firmly and directly perpendicular to the paravertebral muscles at the level of T10-L2. Apply this stationary, deep pressure into the lateral borders of the erector spinae and also at the lumbosacral junction during contractions to compete with uterine sensations.

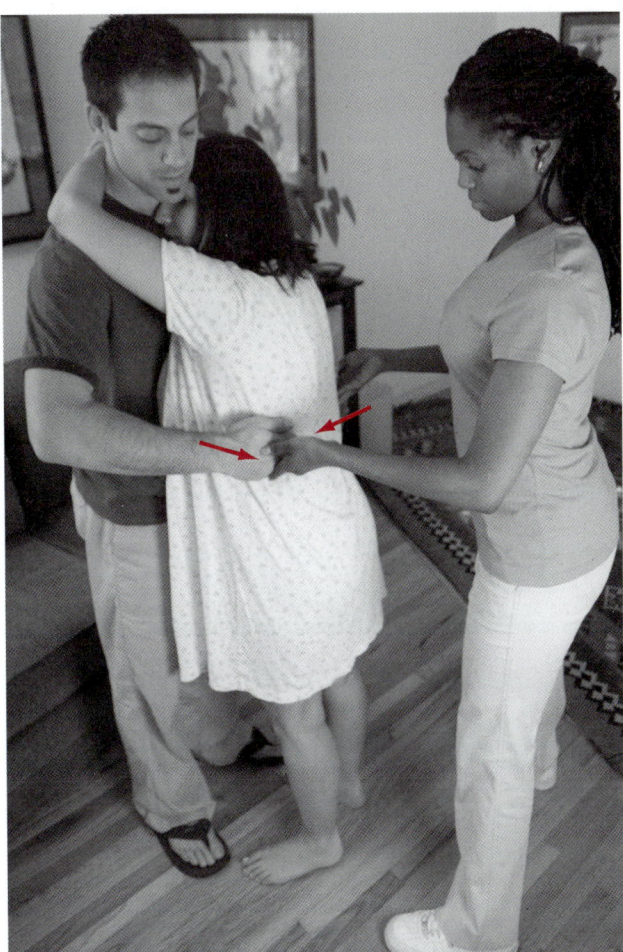

FIGURE 5.10 Contraction distraction.

2. Perform rhythmic effleurage, kneading, thumb fanning, and/or nerve strokes to the area and to the entire sacrum during contractions.
3. Encourage rhythmic pelvic tilting during contractions.
4. Provide more general distraction with gentle abdominal effleurage; long, delicate strokes down the arms or legs; or soft, soothing fanning motions across the brow.
5. Reflexively address pain by stimulating Chinese acupuncture point, bladder 67. During contractions, apply firm pressure bilaterally with a fingernail into the flesh at the lateral, proximal corner of the nails of the fifth toes.

Second-Stage Labor Techniques

Support the effort of pushing by helping with positioning and supporting the mother's body, conserving her energy, promoting relaxation of the pelvic floor and thighs, and maintaining strong uterine contractions. Many of the first-stage techniques continue to be useful now. Some may even become more helpful, particularly in combinations. In addition to these described below, experiment with all first-stage techniques except for the baby lift. Try the Pelvic Press (Simkin 2008), a popular doula technique for widening the pelvic outlet, particularly if the baby is low and no longer moving down (see online resources).

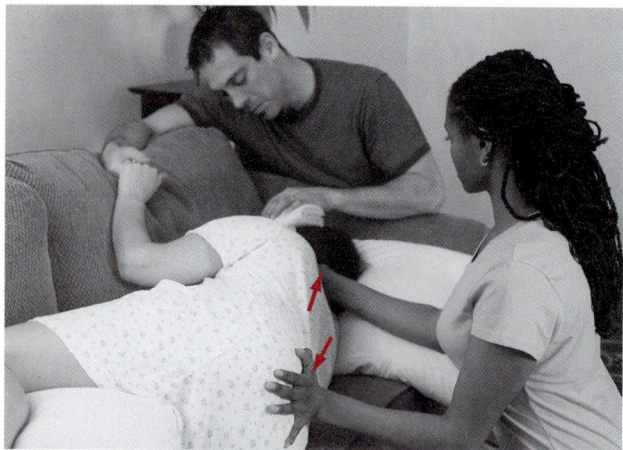

FIGURE 5.11 Grounding hold.

GROUNDING HOLD

Described in the semireclined position, and modify for other labor positions (Fig. 5.11).

INTENTIONS

To gently curve and encourage the spine into flexion for guiding her baby out, counteracting the natural tendency to pull away from the painful sensations of pushing; to relax tense muscles at the occiput and sacrum.

PROCEDURE

1. Position yourself at the bedside at her shoulder height.
2. Slide your top hand under her neck, gently cupping her occiput. Slide your other hand down to hold her sacrum in your palm, the back of your hand against the bed. Your hands stay in this position throughout the push and rest cycle.
3. In the resting minutes between contractions, promote parasympathetic stimulation by circling your sacral hand. With your superior hand, gently knead the cervical muscles and occipital attachments.
4. As the contraction begins, still both hands, and then gently spread them apart and hold, encouraging her head and upper chest into flexion and her sacrum into a pelvic tilt.
5. Hold this lengthening and gentle spinal flexion throughout the contraction and pushing.

HINTS

1. The intent is to guide the subtle movement of the spine—not position and hold her.
2. Use open, soft hands, making your palm the contact area.
3. A subtle rocking between your hands for mobilization may also feel supportive to her.

PRECAUTIONS

Avoid epidural site if she has one, around L3-L4.

CERVICAL AND PELVIC FLOOR RELAXATION

INTENTIONS

To relax the cervix, making it more responsive to dilate and efface; to relax the pelvic floor so that the client will more readily yield to the power of contractions rather than resist them; to relax the pelvic floor through relaxation of the jaw and mouth.

PROCEDURE

1. Encourage open-mouth exhalations to prevent her from clenching her jaws in response to the pain.
2. Validate and support any low-pitched, guttural vocalizations she makes such as groaning, moaning, and repeated sounds. If her vocalizations become high pitched and strident, she may be expressing fear, and she will be tighter in her upper body. Use your own voice to lead her to lower sounds that will calm her, bring her awareness deeper into her belly, relax her throat, and help to keep the masseter and temporalis muscles relaxed.
3. Grasp the three medial toes of both feet simultaneously. Press the three toes firmly together. Hold, or rhythmically release and hold at 2- to 4-second intervals during contractions to create a relaxation of the pelvic floor and/or the adductors.
4. Use imagery and visualizations to assist in opening of the cervix and relaxation of the pelvic floor muscles. For example, ask her to imagine that her cervix is the bud of her favorite flower. As each contraction begins and peaks, encourage her to imagine the bud slowly and easily opening into a large beautiful blossom, adding as much sensorial detail as possible.

HINTS

1. The toe grasp may work by stimulating meridians or medial fascial planes. If you are familiar with these systems, use visualization and energetic intention to supplement your pressure. This technique is more effective when the client's legs are completely supported.
2. Keep the concepts of Sphincter Law, as described by Ina May Gaskin (Gaskin 2003) in mind as you work with these procedures: sphincters function best in an atmosphere of intimacy and privacy; sphincters cannot be opened at will; sphincters can close down when upset, frightened, humiliated, or self-conscious; and relaxation of the mouth and jaw is directly correlated to the ability of the cervix, vagina, and anus to open fully.

CHAPTER SUMMARY

Accompanying a woman through labor and birth as a member of her birthing team is an honor you should consider experiencing. A massage therapist's functions as facilitators of relaxation, mind-body awareness, and physical and emotional nurturance can enhance the woman's experience, her family development, and indirectly the world. Performed by practitioners who are sensitive and attentive by nature, massage therapy lends itself beautifully to the emotional, energetic, and physical support that is necessary for a woman to calmly and confidently labor and birth her baby. Massaging laboring clients is an incredible opportunity for you to fully experience the power of touch.

Table 5.1 Summary of Massage Therapy for Labor

Stage	First — Early (latent) Phase	First — Active Phase	First — Transition Phase	Second: Pushing to Birth	Third: Placental Separation and Expulsion
Centimeters dilated General relaxation techniques	0–3 Visualization and imagery Abdominal breathing Craniosacral techniques Swedish/Esalen massage	4–7 Foot reflexology Face and hand massage Grounding hold Rhythmic passive movements	8–10 "Grounding" Eye contact Reassurance Sounding Autonomic sedation series Craniosacral	NA Swedish/Esalen massage	NA
Techniques for relief of localized painful areas		Pressure and pleasurable techniques to tight areas Hand molding Swedish/Esalen massage to legs and arms Abdominal massage and rocking Open-mouth exhalation with jaw massage and vocalizations Reflexive focus on spinal and pelvic areas of feet Contraction distraction Hydrotherapy "Back labor" techniques Acupressure Bl 67 points Rhythmic movement—passive and active Stretching—passive and active Inching to intrinsic paravertebrals SI joint releases Lumbosacral stretch Hip decompression and figure 8		Focus on adductor tension, arms and legs cramp relief, and fatigue Perineal massage by birth attendant Sounding	
Techniques for stimulating the progress of labor		Uterine foot reflexes Acupressure points Gravity-assisted positions Support positioning changes Rhythmic movement Grounding hold Abdominal massage and rocking Double gluteal squeeze		Toe press Pelvic press Encourage gravity-assisted positions	

Test Yourself

For answers, visit the website at http://thePoint.LWW.com/Osborne-Pregnancy2e!

1. List three main focuses of your work to prepare a woman for labor and birthing.

2. List the three Rs of labor support according to Penny Simkin.

3. Describe three to five functions of a massage therapist attending a client's labor.

4. Describe the differences in uterus contraction patterns in early and active labor.

5. Describe the effects of stress on uterine contractions, particularly in the first stage.

6. Describe three to five strategies and/or techniques that could reduce the severity of laboring women's back pain.

7. Describe the goals of massage therapy in conjunction with epidural use.

8. Describe three possible aspects of the massage therapist's role with a client having a cesarean birth.

REFERENCES

Bainbridge D. Making Babies The Science of Pregnancy. Cambridge: Harvard University Press, 2000.

Bodner-Adler B, Bodner K, Mayerhofer, K. Perineal massage during pregnancy in primiparous women. Int J Gynecol Obstet 2002.

Buckley S. Gentle Birth, Gentle Mothering: A Doctor's Guide to Natural Childbirth and Gentle Early Parenting Choices. Berkeley: Celestial Arts, 2008.

Buckley S. Epidurals: risks and concerns for mother and baby. Available at www.sarahjbuckley.com. Accessed June 29, 2009.

Cassidy T. Birth: The Surprising History of How We Are Born. New York: Grove Press, 2006.

Chang M, Wang S, Chen C. Effects of massage on pain and anxiety during labour: a randomized controlled trial in Taiwan. J Adv Nurs. 2002 Apr;38 (1):68–73.

Doulas of North America (DONA). Available at www.dona.org. Accessed July 5, 2009.

Evans J, Aronson R. The Whole Pregnancy Handbook. New York: Gotham Books, 2005.

Gaskin I. Ina May's Guide to Childbirth. New York: Bantam Dell, 2003.

Green J, Coupland V, Kitzinger J. Expectations, experiences and psychological outcomes of childbirth." Birth 1990;17:15–24.

Greene E, Goodrich-Dunn B. The Psychology of the Body. Baltimore: Lippincott Williams & Wilkins, 2004.

Hastings-Tolsma M, Vincent D, Emeis C, et al. Getting Through the Birth in One Piece: Protecting the Perineum. Am J Matern/Child Nurs 2007;32(3):158–164.

Hodnett ED, Gates S, Hofmeyr GJ, et al. Continuous support for women during childbirth. Cochrane Database of Systematic Reviews 2007;3 Art. No: CD003766. DOI:10, 1002/14651858.CD00376.pub2.

Jones C. Mind Over Labor. New York: Penguin Books, 1987.

Midwifery Today e-news, April 14, 2004, vol 6, Issue 8. Available at www.Midwifery today.com. Accessed May 3, 2009.

Ricci S. Essentials of Maternity, Newborn, and Women's Health Nursing. 2nd Ed. Baltimore: Wolters Kluwer Health/Lippincott Williams & Wilkins, 2009.

Sakala C, Corry M. Evidence Based Maternity Care: What Is It and What It Can Achieve. Milbank Memorial Fund. New York. Available at http://www.childbirthconnection.org/article.asp?ck=1057. Accessed July 1, 2009.

Shea M. Biodynamic Craniosacral Therapy Vol. One and Two. Berkeley: North Atlantic Books, 2008.

Simkin P. Just Another Day in a Woman's Life? Women's Long-Term Perceptions of Their First Birth Experience. Part I. Birth Dec. 1991;4:203–210.

Simkin P. The Birth Partner. 3rd Ed. Boston: Harvard Common Press, 2008.

Simkin P, Ancheta R. The Labor Progress Handbook. 3rd Ed. Oxford: Wiley-Blackwell, 2011.

Simkin P, Bolding A. Update on Pharmacological approaches to relieve labor pain and prevent suffering. J Midwifery Womens Health. 2004; 49(6):489–504.

Tornetta G. Painless Childbirth: An Empowering Journey through Pregnancy and Birth. Nashville: Cumberland House Publishing, 2008.

Tully G. SpinningBabies.com: Easier childbirth through fetal positioning. Available at www.spinningbabies.com. Accessed May 3, 2009.

Upledger J, Vredevoogd J. Craniosacral Therapy. Seattle: Eastland Press, 1983.

For additional resources, please visit http://thePoint.LWW.com/Osborne-Pregnancy2e!

6

Postpartum Perspectives and Techniques

Learning Objectives

After study of this chapter, you should be able to:

1. Explain typical physiological adjustments of the early postpartum period.
2. Describe normal emotional responses to early mothering demands.
3. List five symptoms of postpartum affective disorders.
4. List signs of other postpartum complications.
5. List three major contraindications or precautions regarding safe postpartum massage therapy.
6. List five goals of massage therapy in the first 3 months after giving birth.
7. Describe how pregnancy-related musculoskeletal concerns can affect a woman for many years after giving birth and how you can address those effects.
8. Perform techniques that can reach the goals of postpartum massage therapy.

With her newborn warmly snuggled against her, a postpartum woman moves into the joys and challenges of motherhood. The baby's first smile and early motor skill milestones are thrilling events. An infant is both exhilarating and exhausting, and a new mother must grapple with many changes in the days and months ahead. She must adapt physiologically, emotionally, and structurally to her nonpregnant state. She needs to heal, "get back to normal," feed and care for her infant and for her expanded family (Fig. 6.1).

As a knowledgeable and caring massage therapist, you can enhance a woman's assimilation of these typical changes and her more comfortable adaptations to mothering. This chapter overviews the normal concerns of the immediate and long-term postpartum period and helps you to recognize the signs of complications (see Chapter 7 for when these special postpartum needs arise. You may also want to consult the online resources at http://thePoint.lww.com/Osborne-Pregnancy2e for additional medical charts, terminology, and illustrations of postpartum maternal changes.) You will learn safety protocols for therapeutic bodywork and massage and how to perform essential techniques for effective postpartum sessions. For your clients with older children, you will learn to recognize pregnancy's legacies and how to help resolve residual back, pelvic, and abdominal discomforts of childbearing.

Early Postpartum Maternal Adjustments and Healing

In the first 6 weeks of the postpartum period (**puerperium**), most women cope with common needs and adjustments that your work often can support. These can include:

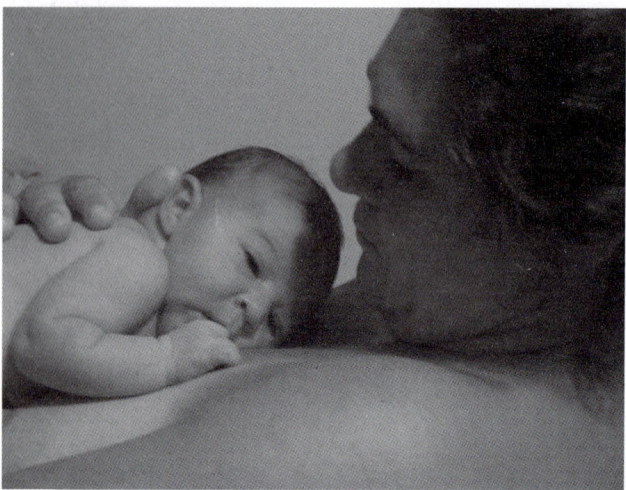

FIGURE 6.1 Good for baby and for mom. Research has confirmed the wisdom of many childbirth practices worldwide: extended skin-to-skin cuddling can help a newborn grow and bond with her mother, whose postpartum recovery can be quickened by this close contact.

- Recovery from labor, including exhaustion, pelvic ligament and joint strain and pain, and epidural and other pain medication after-effects such as headache, backache, or fever
- Pelvic floor tenderness or repair, possible urinary incontinence and/or retained urine, leaving the bladder distended and more prone to infection
- Hemorrhoids and/or constipation
- Two to six weeks of the "afterpains" of uterine **involution** and discharge
- Elimination of excess prenatal and/or intravenously administered fluid, metabolic wastes, and residual medications
- Episodes of shakiness and involuntary vibration, particularly immediately after birth through the first few weeks
- Significant endocrine changes shifting all body systems toward a nonpregnant state, including 2 to 3 weeks to normalize dissolution of blood clots and significantly minimize relaxin's effect on connective tissues
- Mammary changes including milk production, engorgement, and adjustments to nursing, or to the decision to bottle-feed instead
- Emotional adjustments
- 15 to 18 lb of puerperium weight loss, and the shift in center of gravity this creates
- Resolution of residual postural and movement patterns
- Lack of abdominal skin and muscle tone and integrity
- Pain from trigger points and/or tension in the abdominals, iliopsoas, quadratus lumborum, spinal erectors, and other pelvic and posterior areas
- Healing and functional restrictions due to surgery if a cesarean birth occurred
- Strain of childcare on stretched, weak or imbalanced joints and muscles, and on the neck and pectoral girdle (Ricci, 2009)

Goals and General Guidelines for Early Postpartum Massage Therapy

In some cultures, new mothers are massaged daily for weeks to aid their recovery and support them through the physical and emotional stresses of newborn care (Kitzinger S, 1995). Even one to three sessions may help toward these goals. Postpartum massage therapy may also contribute to healthy family development and reduce the likelihood that excessive musculoskeletal pain will distract from motherhood's pleasures (Field 1996). General guidelines to accomplish these goals follow. You will find detailed specific instructions in this chapter's technique manual and the online videos.

My Story

Rhonda began having spasms in the sacroiliac and sacral areas that "took her breath away" during the last 2 months of her pregnancy, and they continued postpartum. She called me when Mackenna was 5 weeks old seeking relief and infant massage instruction. At this point, she was afraid to go upstairs in her own home, needed help with outside errands, and feared dropping the baby when the pain hit. After her first infant massage lesson, I sculpted the tensor fascia lata and all of the other hip muscles, focusing on piriformis, iliotibial tract, and quadratus lumborum, followed by deep fanning to these areas. The immediate relief she experienced lasted for 3 days, then intermittent twinges returned. Our second session was similar, with additional deep work in her upper back and pelvis. She's been pain-free for 6 weeks now, and her confidence and mobility are normal.

—Linda Hickey, Calgary, AB

PROVIDING NURTURANCE AND EMOTIONAL SUPPORT

Some 50% to 90% of postpartum women get the **"baby blues"** and are anxious, sad, moody, and mildly depressed, especially from days 3 through 10 (AWHONN 2007). During and after this time, you can help her adjust hormonally and emotionally. Provide a special time to focus on "mothering the mother" by creating a calming ambience and listening with your hands and your heart. Promote postpartum relaxation with Swedish and Esalen circulatory styles, energy balancing, connective tissue massage (*Bindegewebsmassage*) for the abdomen, breasts and upper body, foot zone therapy, and passive movements performed rhythmically, with fluidity and focus. Soothing scalp and foot massages, the autonomic sedations series 3-1-1, and other techniques from earlier chapters can help to calm sympathetic arousal, possibly helping her to sleep better and heal quicker. A quiet, soothing massage may help satisfy a new mother's yearning for solitude and recuperative rest, and give her the nurturing attention she may long for.

Some therapists like to hear a woman's birthing story and begin her physical healing by working each of her feet while she recounts her labor's ups and downs. Hold her feet, palms to her soles, and follow your foot work with long, superficial inferiorly directed leg strokes. These techniques can begin any necessary "getting her feet back on the ground" and also help her to moderate emotional lability. This may also prompt the unburdening of any negative feelings about the birth and her postpartum life. Listening with a nonjudgmental, supportive attitude can provide just the atmosphere for her to tell her story honestly, including her disappointments, angers, fears, and regrets. Your nurturing support is an example of the oxytocin-based "tend and befriend" response to stress (Taylor 2000). Rather than "getting back to normal," it can buoy her while she gradually establishes her new normal, with this baby integrated into her life.

Most women celebrate a healthy newborn, but many are grieving, too. In addition to the obvious pain of a stillborn or fetal/infant death or injury, women can be grieving loss of the pregnancy experience and the special anticipation of gestation; disappointment when birthing and parenting expectations are unmet; loss of the "dream baby" as she adjusts to the real baby; reduced romance and intimacy with her partner; loss of self-identity or of her own childhood, which is particularly poignant if she was neglected or abused; and loss of her former lifestyle (Kitzinger 1994).

Remember that women who chose to terminate their pregnancies are also in postpartum recovery. If there was considerable conflicting feeling about the abortion, or if it was performed in the second trimester, she may have increased postpartum adjustments to make (see Chapter 7 also). Again, your compassionate ear, coupled with hands that say, "I am here," will be powerful tools in her grief recovery.

Massage may help promote healthy parent/infant bonding, the infant's growth and development, and supportive family

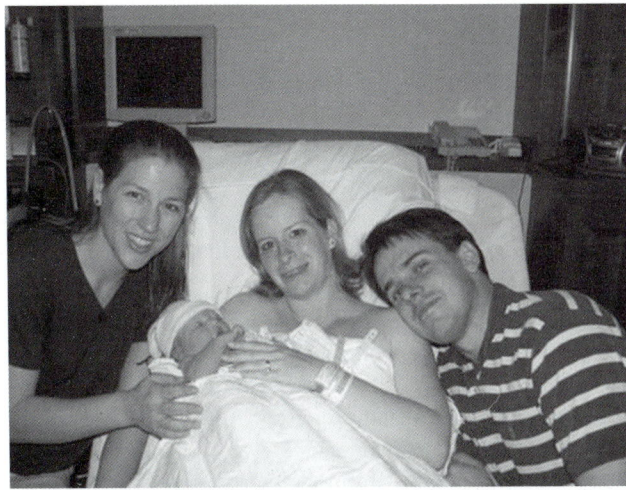

FIGURE 6.2 Transitioning the family. The postpartum period is a getting-to-know-you time, facilitated by a knowledgeable massage therapist. You can encourage the involvement of the baby's partner and any siblings in newborn care, particularly infant massage.

ties (Scafidi 1990; Massaro 2009) (see online resource on prenatal and perinatal psychology and health). You can teach your clients simple effleurage strokes for the baby's legs, arms, and back. Take an infant massage instructor's course to complete your understanding of and ability to teach baby massage (see online resources for suggested programs). Encourage your clients to trade back and foot rubs with their partners and older children. Regular, nurturing touch among family members can help soothe the strain of postnatal adaptations (Fig. 6.2).

HEALING FROM LABOR

Ideally you will work with your clients within their first week postpartum when a complete body session of Swedish and lymphatic drainage is perfect. It may facilitate restoration of normal physiology by opening capillary beds and increasing cellular respiration, cleansing residual metabolic wastes from labor's exertions and any residual anesthesia, and by pumping excess fluids from interstitial spaces into general circulation for elimination (Andrade and Clifford 2008).

Connective tissue massage, zone therapy, and other reflexive modalities also stimulate the body's return to normal energy and hormonal levels (Ezner 2000). Labor creates a surge in adrenalin and oxytocin, resulting in a postpartum euphoria for many women; however, that is shortlived as other changes ensue. Estrogen and progesterone production decrease by 90% within the first 3 postpartum hours; oxytocin and prolactin levels increase, especially if a woman is breastfeeding (Moberg 2003). Adjusting to these hormonal changes, plus a drop in blood sugar and tidal volume in the lungs, also increases exhaustion (Ricci 2009).

Because these vast physiological changes compound labor's emotional intensity, some women may experience a type of nervous system clearing and resetting. Your client may shiver, shake, or sweat profusely during or after a session in the first two postpartum weeks. Keep her comfortable and breathing normally, reassure her of the normalcy and transient nature of these experiences, and encourage her to embrace rather than resist their deeply restorative potential.

> **REMINDER:** *Your work in the first days or weeks after giving birth can significantly help women heal and adjust to being a new mother.*

During labor some women can feel "torn apart," with the pelvic base seemingly left widened and unstable. They appreciate massage therapy and exercise that helps them to regain core stability and integrity. Another way to do this is a wrapping technique modified from the practices of Mexican midwives, which they accomplish by systematically wrapping their *robozo* (shawl) around the new mother (Gonzalez and Vinaver 1997). You may simulate the "closing" effect of this practice by applying firm, sustained, and medially directed pressure bilaterally, working from her head to toe, as though pressing her back together. Another way to do this is to sensitively and systematically wrap her in the bottom sheet over your table, allowing her time to rest in this enveloping, healing cocoon (Fig. 6.3).

● ENCOURAGING PELVIC FLOOR AND ABDOMINAL HEALING

With a vaginal birth, most women experience some swelling, tenderness, bruising, and at least superficial microtears of the vaginal mucosa. Some suffer actual tears of the skin, connective tissue, or pelvic floor muscles. Anywhere from one stitch to, in rare cases, several dozen stitches may have been necessary. About 60% of expectant women are incontinent, but that drops to about 11% by 6 weeks after birthing and remains about the same percentage for a year. Longterm, half of all women who have given birth develop some amount of urinary incontinence in their lifetimes (Thomason and DeLancey 2007).

To aid in the recovery of sphincter control, to help prevent long-term incontinence, and to prevent uterine prolapse, remind her to exercise the pelvic floor (see Chapter 5 online resources). Work on her calcaneus and the dorsal surface of her tarsal bones to reflexively help speed perineal healing. Many women find a warm water sitz bath temporarily soothing, whereas cold packs usually offer more extended relief from perineal pain (Simkin et al. 2010). Remember that clients with pelvic floor trauma and dysfunction may need a physical therapist who specializes in pelvic floor rehabilitation (see online resources).

Many women are disappointed when they don't immediately resuming their prepregnancy figure; instead, usually the abdomen is still enlarged and somewhat pendulous. The skin and the connective tissue are stretched, loose, and often etched with stretch marks. Hypotoned, stretched abdominal muscles are rich in trigger points and weakened by separation. Displacement of the intestines, uterus, bladder, and other abdominal and pelvic organs may persist. She may feel such intense abdominal afterpains of uterine involution that they require focused attention to relaxation and abdominal breathing. This is especially true for breastfeeding women, those who need synthetic oxytocin, and after second and subsequent births (Ricci 2009).

Spending 10 to 15 minutes of each puerperium session on the abdomen, with client's permission, combined with appropriate, gradual exercise can help reduce the jellylike feel of many postpartum bellies (Byrne 2007).Connective tissue massage and skin rolling may be helpful in functionally normalizing abdominal skin and connective tissue. Although they eventually lose redness, a reliable method to erase stretchmarks remains unconfirmed. In this chapter's technique manual and the online videos, you will find specific instructions for basic positioning and massaging of the postpartum uterus, and for adapting common abdominal massage techniques for postpartum needs. Remember to modify for postsurgical discomforts and precautions that are covered in more detail later in this chapter.

In the perinatal period, the stretched rectus abdominus separated at the strained, softened linea alba. As a result, it failed to maintain spinal and pelvic alignment. Be alert to these effects on postpartum postural dysfunctions, lack of balance, musculoskeletal pain, and diminished self-image. Help her determine whether she has a separation and measure its extent. Then guide her to abdominal strengthening while supporting any diastus (see online resources for assessment

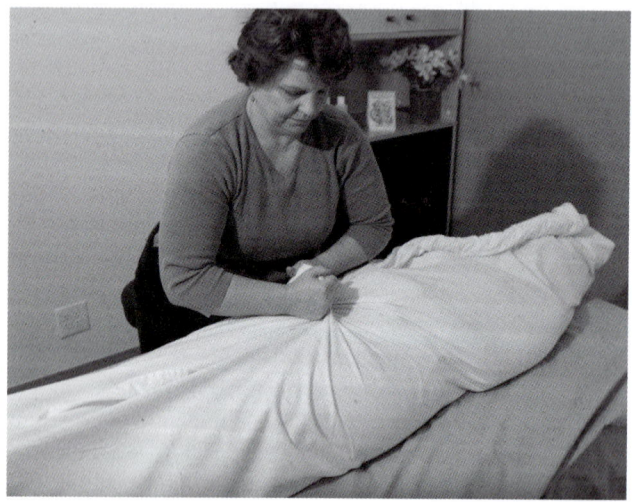

FIGURE 6.3 Wrapping for closure. Use either the bottom sheet or an additional flat sheet that you placed prior to your session to gradually enclose your client. Beginning at her head and finishing at her feet, bring each side over her, twisting it gently yet firmly to compress her toward her midline. Hold at each point, particularly where she feels most "open" before moving along. Give her a breathing space in the sheet if necessary so that she can breathe easily throughout. After a satisfying rest period, slowly unwrap her from head to foot.

and exercise). Remind her to roll onto one side when rising from a reclining position and to avoid jack-knife-like movements, which further strain this vulnerable area.

● SUPPORTING SATISFYING BREASTFEEDING

Feeding her newborn is often one of a mother's greatest pleasures; however, if a mother breastfeeds, changes in her breasts may initially create discomfort. Her nipples can become sore, cracked, and become blistered. Perinatally the breasts began secreting colostrum, and then by 72 hours after birth, her breasts begin to swell with milk. This breast engorgement continues until the baby's demand for milk regulates the supply, though long intervals between feedings may still result in engorgement.

Warm showers, heat, and massage can ease engorgement, help prevent blockage of milk ducts, help avoid breast infections (**mastitis**), and may improve overall breast health (Simkin et al. 2010). She may need you to show her how to use cold packs or towels wrapped around each breast to reduce swelling. If breastfeeding is problematic, she may want to seek advice from a lactation consultant or her local *La Leche* League (see online resources).

A rested, relaxed mom usually has an easier, more satisfying breastfeeding experience. Use all your skills of relaxation and autonomic sedation. Increase circulation in her chest with Swedish massage and by passive and active stretching of the pectoral girdle, particularly opening it from anterior rotation, from collapse of the chest and other remnants of pregnancy's postural compensations. Myofascial and deep tissue relaxation of the pectoralis major and minor is particularly important.

Despite the overwhelming benefits of breastfeeding (see online resources), some women will need to or prefer to bottle-feed, or a sudden change to bottle-feeding becomes necessary. Most women terminate milk production and reduce breast engorgement with ice packs to the breasts and a tight binder or bra. If she is bottle-feeding, breast massage may be a very important self-care practice to help compensate for the loss of breastfeeding's benefits to long-term mammary health (Curties 1999). Just remind her to wait to do preventative breast massage or even breast self-exams until her milk has completely dried up.

If a mother is breastfeeding, she may spend 40 hours a week in that activity alone. Many parents spend hours each day cradling their baby, mesmerized by gazing into the soulful eyes and inviting face of their "little miracle." Unfortunately, this side-bending, forward-tilting posture of the neck and head, coupled with the mostly static use of the upper back muscles for holding, creates an overuse syndrome, "new parents' neck" (Fig. 6.4). Encourage regularly switching sides and periodically lifting and straightening out the neck. Show her how looking behind each shoulder periodically while she nurses makes the opposite and balancing movement. When not holding the baby, she can perform shoulder rolls, arm stretches, and imagining the area behind her ears lifting skyward, to help to relax and stretch these muscles.

To reduce strain during feedings, parents need back support, chairs with low arms, if possible, and sufficient pillows supporting the baby to relax the shoulder. The breastfeeding mother should bring the baby to the breast rather than hunching and sidebending her torso. This can help her to maintain good wrist alignment as she feeds, helping prevent wrist and hand pain such as **deQuervain's** and carpal tunnel syndrome from developing. Most women suffering prenatal carpal

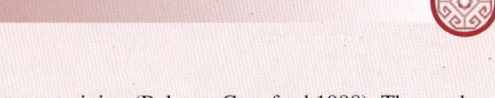

Points of View: Breast Massage

Many educators acknowledge the potential benefits of breast massage, including improved circulation, healthier breast tissue, more ease with screening self-examinations, as possible care to prevent a range of abnormal breast conditions from fibrocystic changes to breast cancer, and to help recover from treatment from breast diseases and surgeries if they occur (Curties 1999). Pregnant and lactating woman who have regular breast massage report that it improves milk production, eases breast discomforts, reduces engorgement and prevents mastitis, enhances her emotional responses to breast changes, and increases her ability to handexpress her milk.

Where many professionals disagree is whether the therapist or the woman should perform breast massage. Arguments against therapists working in this highly sensitive area include legal restrictions, heightened possibility of misunderstood intention, crossing of professional boundaries, and injury due to lack of or inadequate training (Polseno-Crawford 1998). Those who teach and include therapeutic breast massage as a session option advocate for its benefits. Generally, they see a need for improved instruction and availability in the necessary anatomy, physiology, and technical knowledge and skill. They also acknowledge how important learning clear client communication, informed separate consent for breast massage, possible psychological and emotional reactions to breast massage, and precise draping is to its appropriate inclusion in some women's sessions (Fitch 1998).

Your clients may be keen to learn breast self-massage. This is often an acceptable and highly beneficial alternative to doing it yourself. See the online resources at http://thePoint.lww.com/Osborne-Pregnancy2e for instructions for teaching and for important distinctions between breast self-massage and self-examinations.

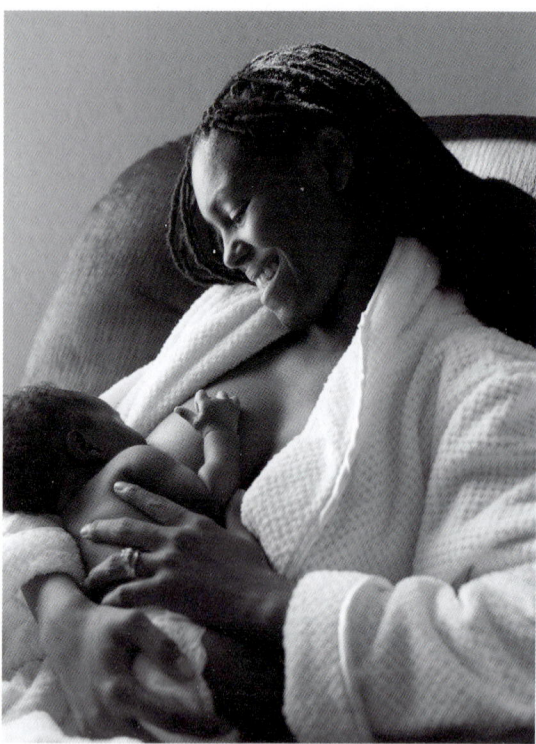

FIGURE 6.4 "New mother's neck." Extended static neck flexion while sidebending can create pain and tension in the sternocleidomastoid, scalenes, trapezius, levator scapulae, and supraspinatus, among other neck and pectoral muscles. (Photo courtesy of Kharisma Studios.)

> **My Story**
>
> As a self-employed massage therapist, I had planned to return to work when my baby was 6 weeks old. With my first two children, this would not have been a problem. With my new career, the strain of holding a newborn's head to my breast exacerbated the weakness in my forearm flexors, and I developed tendonitis in my wrist. There was no way I'd be able to return to work unless I received some serious bodywork. I visited my massage therapist, who did some deep tissue on my forearm. Only one session was necessary to comfortably get back to work, and breastfeeding became easier as well.
>
> —Karen Salas, Salt Lake City, UT

tunnel syndrome will experience relief perinatally; however, older mothers of two or more children tend to develop wrist pain while breastfeeding (Blake Gleeson and Pauls 1993).

Since many mothers may bring the baby to bed for nocturnal feedings, encourage her sit up completely, with pillows supporting her lumbar spine, under her knees, and under the baby. She may prefer to lie on her side, again well supported at her back. This sidelying position is both structurally more comfortable for the mother, and she is less likely to spasm her neck if she jerks awake after dozing. When she is sidelying, she should pull the baby's arm that is against the bed forward toward her breast to encourage him to roll to his back should he also doze after nursing, thus supporting safer "back to sleep" habits (American Academy of Pediatrics 2005).

● REDUCING RESIDUAL PELVIC AND BACK PAIN

If your client had an epidural or a spinal, you many need to pay specific attention to the administration site, usually at L3 or L4, during the first month postpartum. It is frequently tender, eliciting a psychological protectiveness that immobility and positioning during administration or injury to the spinal cord membranes may have caused. Work initially on her back with broad, sweeping, superficial strokes, progressing to deeper, more specific work. Use craniosacral and connective tissue techniques. Position her with feet and hips slightly higher than her head if she has a spinal headache. Work head and neck reflexes on the plantar creases of her big toes, and gently reduce tension and trigger points in the head, neck, and back.

Almost as many postpartum women develop peripartum pelvic pain syndrome (PPPPS) as develop similar pain during the second trimester (Howard 2000). Deep tissue sculpting and postural guidance facilitate healing of these strained pelvic joints, release of chronic muscular tension and of shortened posterior fascial planes. Awkward, sustained labor positions can result in mild to severe lumbar, hip, sacral, or pelvic pain. A woman's pelvic size and shape and their relationship to her baby's head size and position also affect the degree of pelvic ligament strain incurred during labor. Pay particular attention to the sacroiliac, lumbosacral, symphysis pubis, and coccygeal joints. If she had severe injury, these joints may take some time and treatment to heal, and she may need to see a physical therapist or other provider for treatment (Ricci 2009).

Physical therapy studies indicate that strengthening exercise for the smaller pelvic girdle muscles followed by the more global muscles is more effective for reducing PPPPS (Stugea et al. 2006). Likewise, you should first balance the gluteus medius and other hip movers, the quadratus lumborum, and the iliopsoas. Next, focus on the erector spinae, lumbodorsal fascia, latissimus, and gluteus maximus. All of these contracted soft tissues also may harbor trigger points. Use neuromuscular therapy, rhythmic and positional movement techniques, and deep tissue methods to extinguish these referral points. (See technique manuals in Chapters 4 and 6 and online video.)

> **REMINDER:** Abdominal work, with your client's permission, can help to reduce back and pelvic pain, to prevent and decrease pain from infant care activities, and to promote abdominal recovery.

● ENCOURAGING STRUCTURAL INTEGRITY

Guide her standing, seated, and carrying postures to reestablish effortless, graceful alignment and to reduce musculoskeletal strain. Help her to correct the typical anterior tilting pelvis and increased lumbar curvature (see Figs. 4.21–4.23.) The iliopsoas is often not capable of maintaining pelvic alignment throughout the pregnancy. By the postpartum period, it becomes hypertonic and spasmed. Strain may have produced myofascial trigger points referring pain into the lower back, and it may need stretching. Alternately, it may be hypotonic if it was prenatally incompetent. Some iliopsoas strengthening occurs when the postpartum woman repeatedly reduces the lumbar lordosis by tilting her pelvis posteriorly, using the iliopsoas rather than the gluteal, leg, or upper abdominal muscles. As in pregnancy, active and passive pelvic tilts also help relieve lumbar pain (see Chapter 4 technique manual).

As both pelvic stabilizer and one of the primary hip flexors, the psoas muscle is integrally involved in gait. Ideally one psoas initiates leg flexion on the pelvis, followed by contraction of the rectus femoris and other quadriceps group muscles. Simultaneously, the weight-bearing and contralateral psoas stabilizes the pelvis to avoid excess pelvic rotation and tilting. These two psoas functions become increasingly compromised perinatally. The continuous anterior uterine weight contributes to disuse of the normal psoas functions for walking. Instead, the hip joints begin to externally rotate, and the hip rotators rather than the psoas initiate each step. The resulting "duck walk" or "sailor's roll" is characteristic of both the third trimester and the postpartum period. Use imagery and sensitive deep tissue work to guide the mother in regaining psoas use and strength and to increase her awareness of this important postural muscle. Extinguish trigger points and chronic tension in the hip movers. (See specific techniques for these areas in the Chapter 4 technique manual and later in this chapter.)

REMINDER: *The iliopsoas needs considerable postpartum attention to restore and improve its function as a major postural muscle.*

My Story

A new client who was 11 days postpartum greeted me at the door bent over and walking like she had been "in the saddle" for months. I immediately taught her a pelvic tilt without clenching the gluteals and abdominals, as she had been doing. Hip, abdominals, and low back deep work were gratefully received, but more than that, the information I had to share was like a lifeline to her. She had been desperately asking every woman she knew "why do I hurt so much, and why can't I stand straight?" She had enough college anatomy training to understand my descriptions, and, when I isolated the psoas muscle for her, it was like a light going on. She got off my table standing 100% better, but it wasn't just my work. It was the relief that she now understood what was going on, and she had a tool to deal with it.

—Deborah Donaldson,
Framingham, MA

● PREVENTING STRAIN AND PAIN FROM CHILDCARE ACTIVITIES

Infant care is usually a love-filled, if sometimes tedious task. Diapering, consoling, carrying, and interacting with her baby often involves repeated extreme forward bending, a movement a new mother has not done for many months. When performed incorrectly, these repetitive actions contribute to lumbar, thoracic, and cervical pain. As the baby grows, its additional weight exacerbates back strain. Remind her to get assistance in these tasks and to observe proper body mechanics, especially immediately after the birth. The new mother, her partner, and any other caregivers will benefit from lessons in how to lift, hold, carry, and bend over. Teach them prenatally if possible because you often won't see them in their earliest infant care days.

Instruct parents to lift their baby as any object should be lifted: protect the spine by bending the knees; lift from the legs by straightening the knees rather than lifting with the back or pectoral girdle; when possible, avoid lifting and twisting the spine simultaneously. Scooping a baby up at his bottom is both better for the mom and for the baby's developing motor organization. By not lifting under the baby's arms, she avoids wrist and thumb strain. The baby's reflexes keep him or her upright, and torso musculature begins to rapidly strengthen (Creager 2010).

She should carry her baby close to the center of gravity and under his bottom whenever possible. Show parents alternatives to holding him upright on the upper chest, propped looking over one shoulder. In this common carry, a parent frequently leans posterior, painfully compressing the lumbar spine and tenses the carrying shoulder. Guide her to drop the carrying shoulder to a more relaxed level and to maintain the spine's vertical alignment.

As the baby gains head and torso control, the hip carry is common. Although most mothers' hips are wide enough,

> **My Story**
>
> Andrea had Connor by cesarean after an unsuccessful, ultrasound-assisted version to move him out of breech. Her hip that we had worked with at 36 weeks was occasionally painful, but her left pectoral girdle was most problematic from carrying him while attending to other tasks and her three-year-old. Before she undressed, we worked with her standing alignment and alternative ways to carry Connor. In sidelying position, rhythmic passive movements and positional releases began to loosen the shortened and spasmed pectoral girdle structures. Deep tissue sculpting and cross-fiber friction, both to the area and to the paravertebral muscles, further lengthened fascial planes, reduced fibrous buildup, and increased circulation. She reported the pain completely gone after I extinguished a very tender trigger point at the rib cage rectus attachment. We finished this session on her feet after gentle abdominal work, including a plan to begin progressive scar work at our next session.
>
> —Carole Osborne, San Diego, CA

many will sling the carrying hip laterally. This provides additional support for the baby, but it can contribute to excess tension and trigger points in the quadratus lumborum, erector spinae, and oblique abdominals. Occasionally, scoliosis of the spine results from this posture.

If the parent cannot maintain spinal and pelvic alignment, facing the baby outward at waist level is a good alternative. One forearm supports under his base, and he leans forward onto the other forearm. This carry is easier on the parent's structure, as long as she does not lean posteriorly at the waist. The "football carry," with the baby prone on the forearm, is another possibility, and dads often particularly like it. Both of these carries have the additional advantage of stimulating head and torso strength while providing the baby an alternate worldview (Creager 2010).

Even better: once her baby has head control, encourage her to wear her baby on her back, low to her center of gravity. Many women discover musculoskeletal relief, increased mobility, and a more content infant by using a sling or other cloth carrier. In addition, studies show that, much like infant massage, this helps promote healthy infant growth and development (Albright 2009). (See online resources for more information on "baby wearing" and other childcare activities.)

> **REMINDER:** Encourage women to carry their babies close to their own center of gravity.

How she gets her baby in and out of cars, carries awkward, heavy car seats and diaper bags, and the heights of her baby furniture, stroller and bath can all affect musculoskeletal comfort and health. Both preventative ergonomic instruction and massage therapy techniques are helpful in reducing pain created by these childcare tasks. Focus deep tissue sculpting, passive movement, stretching, and trigger point therapy on sternocleidomastoid, the suboccipitals, splenius capitus, levator scapula, supraspinatus, rhomboidei and other scapula stabilizers, and quadratus lumborum. Then work with the trapezius, latissimus dorsi, and erector spinae group. Reflexively reduce strained and painful areas by stimulating the related zones of the feet for the back, neck, and shoulders.

● PROMOTING HEALING FROM CESAREAN SURGERY

The woman who has given birth operatively has further needs. After all, she is recovering from major abdominal surgery. Her need for therapeutic massage can be greater, because she is likely to experience most of the following difficulties, particularly in the first few days to a week or more of her puerperium:

- Swelling, numbness, and/or or pain surrounding the incision
- Severe abdominal and subscapula pain from intestinal gas and air trapped under the diaphragm during surgery, and more painful contractions of uterine involution
- Extreme fatigue, especially in the first few days
- Pain when rising to stand, and simply walking and/or lifting and holding the baby
- Guarding tension throughout her trunk and hips that can become a long-lasting habit

Some postcesarean mothers feel very disappointed, and typical postpartum feelings can be more intense after cesarean than after vaginal birth. Emotional intensity is usually more dramatic with an emergency cesarean because of the fear and an overwhelming sense of loss of control associated with unplanned cesareans (Simkin et al. 2010). If she labored, then had a cesarean, she might discover a need to finish the

> **REMINDER:** Remember that whenever any complications result in restricted activity, especially extensive bed rest, take precautions related to higher risk of thrombi and pneumonia.

incomplete labor phases. As you address abdominal and pelvic recovery, encourage her to move, grunt, and bear down if she expresses that urge. Be prepared for some emotional release and relief as well.

As after a vaginal birth, nurture her and help promote her overall recovery with this chapter's techniques. To reduce additional gas pain and improve lung health, encourage and help her to breathe deeply, sometimes with a forced exhale. Address pain from gas, constipation, and the incision initially through corresponding zones on her feet. Perform abdominal massage as described and limited in this chapter's technique manual. Early, thorough scar work can prevent or reduce fascial shortening and adhesion formation that can lead to visceral dysfunctions and other long-term postural imbalances (Chikly and Chikly 1997; Pirie and Herman 2003) (Fig. 6.5).

One general surgical study showed the possible benefits of postcesarean massage therapy. In this small study, the patients receiving massage experienced short-term decreases in pain intensity, unpleasantness, and in anxiety. Their pain intensity and unpleasantness decreased faster during the first four postoperative days than the control groups. This study did not show any significant long-term differences, nor in length of hospital stay, complications, or opiate use (Mitchinson et al. 2007). In Europe, physicians commonly prescribe lymphatic drainage for their postsurgical patients to enhance circulation, immunological functioning, and parasympathetic stimulation. With a planned cesarean birth, presurgical work is beneficial, and postsurgical full-body lymphatic drainage techniques can facilitate postoperative recovery (Chikly and Chikly 1997).

The possible improvements listed above in a family's critical first few days can be essential for long-term emotional health. The first 30 to 60 minutes after birth has the highest sensitivity for bonding to begin. Attachment between the infant and its caregivers, progresses over time, particularly

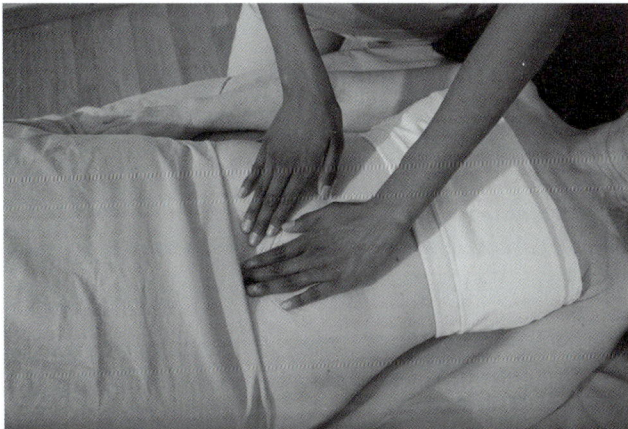

FIGURE 6.5 Postcesarean scar massage. Progressive and sensitive massage of the skin and the underlying fascia of the linea alba can help the body lay down more organized scar tissue, free of adhesions and other fascial restrictions, from superficial to visceral.

What Would You Do?

You are a staunch supporter of natural childbirth whose client managed to arrange to have a cesarean birth so that her out-of-state mother could better schedule to be there and to help her afterward. Within the first week postpartum, she calls for you to come to her home to help her with severe headache and back and abdominal pain. What postpartum complications should you be alert for? What further information do you need from her or her doctor? How will you manage your "I told you so" attitude regarding her preference for an operative rather than vaginal birth?

in the early days and months of infant care. This process can be delayed or hindered when women are exhausted, in pain, dealing with an unwanted outcome, the effects of anesthesia, or lack of adequate support system (Ricci 2009). Given the special attention and benefits of postsurgical massage therapy for these women and their families, postcesarean women especially deserve massage therapy!

Guidelines and Precautions for Postpartum Massage Therapy

Most women can benefit from massage therapy immediately after birth; however, they usually are more eager to bond with their newborn, to begin reconfiguring their family, and to rest. Begin postpartum massage therapy as soon as the mother desires after birth, if no complications have occurred. Ideally, you will see her in the first 24 hours to a week. Most new mothers would benefit from three to five sessions within their first three to six postpartum months. Therapists report that, if clients return for postpartum massage therapy, about 66% of them schedule within the first 3 months (Osborne 2010). Regardless of when and how many times you work with her, your work needs to adapt to the baby, positioning and equipment needs, physiological contraindications, and the implications of any complications that may have occurred.

● INFANT CARE

Both you and your client will be more responsive to maternal needs without the baby present. Though some newborns sleep throughout a session, their squirming, grunting, and other infant behaviors are inevitably distracting. With the baby securely in another's care, the mom more effectively lets go of all but her own concerns, and you can focus on attending to her. Suggest that a caregiver accompany her to her session, taking the baby out for a walk during your session time.

What Would You Do?

Your client returns for her first postpartum session with her daughter along. She is obviously beaming with pride and love for her newborn. She also comments on how needy she feels for a thorough massage therapy session. How can you interact with her and keep the focus on her care rather than becoming distracted by her adorable baby? What possibilities can you think of for continuing your work on her if the baby remains awake and continues to need attention?

If the baby must be there, she may be on the table too. This works best with your client in a sidelying position. Some babies can be content for a while carried on your back if all concerned are comfortable with trying that. Floor play on a blanket also works until the baby is more mobile. With a fussy infant, use this as an opportunity for body mechanics guidance as she comforts the baby. Work on her feet, legs, or head while she sits holding her baby. Convert to a lesson in simple infant massage if necessary. Be flexible to create a productive session.

● POSITIONING AND EQUIPMENT

All positions for receiving postpartum massage therapy are safe options, but some will be more comfortable. Most women need accommodations for breast tenderness, particularly when prone. Sometimes using additional breast supports can take pressure off of her breasts. Try additional chest and/or abdominal pillows, or use a bodyCushion™ with larger breast recesses.

Sidelying positioning is often the most comfortable for posterior work. The sculptured torso cushion of the Sidelying Positioning System is particularly effective in cradling not compressing tender breasts. Remember to lift her ceiling-side arm off of her breast with a pillow or a bolster at her chest. All the other supports and guidelines for safe and comfortable sidelying positioning explained in Chapter 3 still apply, except you can eliminate the belly pillow once her uterus has completely involuted.

Because they are concerned about milk leakage, and to be more comfortable, most women prefer to keep their bra on during a massage. Thoughts and sounds of their baby actually cause the hormonal changes that make milk flow, not pressure. Nevertheless, both you and she can feel assured that you have protected your table if you place a thick towel over the head end. Until lochia flow has ended, she will probably keep her panties on, as well. Work around her underwear, or ask permission to temporarily unhook her bra when you need access to her back.

The supine position is ideal for postpartum abdominal work. Use high knee bolsters to mechanically reduce any excess lumbar lordosis. If she is still edematous, level her calves with her knees, as well. Until clotting factors normalize (see explanation below), this will help prevent venous pooling that could lead to thrombi development. You may need to avoid supine position until any tenderness around the epidural site has dissipated.

● CIRCULATORY CONTRAINDICATIONS AND PRECAUTIONS

The circulatory system undergoes dramatic postpartum changes. The heart can drop to its normal position as the uterus shrinks. Blood volume decreases rapidly, reaching normal levels within 4 weeks, but cardiac output only gradually reaches nonpregnant levels over 3 months. Pulse and blood pressure begin to normalize after pregnancy and labor's exertions; they are watched carefully as signs of possible uterine hemorrhage or preeclampsia.

Blood clotting factors will stay elevated for 2 to 3 weeks to favor closure of the placental attachment site and prevention of excessive bleeding. Other factors can continue to increase clot formation in the legs and lungs, including reduced activity or vessel damage (Ricci 2009). Continue all prenatal contraindications concerning circulatory massage therapy methods on the legs and pelvis for as long as 8 to 10 weeks postpartum. The more sedentary the new mother is, the more prudent this more conservative precaution becomes.

Technique precautions are the same as in pregnancy. Be particularly light in the medial leg, and avoid jiggling and percussion techniques anywhere on the legs. Remember that many leg thrombi are asymptomatic, without the characteristic swelling, discoloration, or heat that some clots create. Symptoms of pulmonary thrombi involve changes in heart rate, chest pain, coughing, and anxiety. Muscular weakness or numbness could be associated with a clot in her brain (stroke). Refer clients with these symptoms to their healthcare providers for evaluation prior to massage therapy. (See further explanation of this risk in Chapter 2 and guidelines for working with postpartum complications in Chapter 7.)

> **REMINDER:** *Work with women who have postpartum complications only after these have resolved or with her healthcare provider's consultation and release.*

Although many types of abdominal massage are beneficial, carefully avoid pressure in the inguinal area, especially in the first week, as clots are common in the femoral and iliac veins. Be especially cautious when symptoms of thrombophlebitis occur. Women who underwent cesarean section births have a two to three times higher risk of thromboembolism than those who birthed vaginally. Postpartum operative procedures such as **hysterectomy** and **tubal ligation** also tend to foster elevated clot development (Jefferies and Bochner 1991). While a woman is on bed rest, eliminate all leg massage until her healthcare provider has released her from maternity care. Modify or delay most abdominal techniques for postcesarean women, unless working directly under medical direction, until her incision is closed and she receives a release (see Chapter 7 for further guidelines).

● **OTHER POSTPARTUM COMPLICATIONS**

In addition to these postcesarean and thrombi complications, other postpartum complications include hemorrhaging; hypertension; uterine, breast, incision, kidney, or other infections; and mental illness. Warning signs of these complications are usually identifiable. Systemic, pitting edema is characteristic of increased blood pressure. Evaluate her headache symptoms for an association with preeclampsia or eclampsia, which can develop postpartum. When maternal complications requiring restricted activity and additional bed rest have occurred, risk of pneumonia also escalates to two to three times higher (Ricci 2009).

Uterine infections will result in fever and a peculiar color or odor to lochia. If the lochia becomes bright red (except for immediately postpartum or immediately after extended periods of lying down or increased activity) and abdominal pain (beyond tenderness) occurs, hemorrhaging is suspected. A flaccid uterus that does not firm up with fundal massage is often associated with postpartum hemorrhage. Refer any woman with any of the above signs to her physician or midwife. Waiting until these complications have resolved or working only with consultation and release from her healthcare providers is the most prudent policy.

An unusual increase in urinary frequency or burning during urination may signal a urinary tract infection. Whenever a woman has back pain in the kidney area, determine whether she has other signs of kidney infection. If pain near the posterior distal ribcage persists regardless of her activities or position, her backache is not likely to be from musculoskeletal causes.

Breast infections usually result in tender, inflamed lumps in the breast and flulike symptoms, including chills or fever. Although reflexive work on her feet may promote healing in these areas, refer her for medical treatment for these symptoms before performing massage therapy.

> **REMINDER:** Depression and other affective disorders are the most common postpartum complication. Stay alert for signs of their development with your clients.

As many as 28% of American mothers develop postpartum depression (AWHONN 2007). Other postpartum affective disorders discussed in Chapter 7 occur with less frequency. Help prevent these conditions by increasing your client's relaxation so that an uninterrupted 4 to 5 hours of restorative sleep a few times a week is more likely. Be alert to any indications of severe emotional distress including the following: difficulty in getting out of bed or severe sleep disturbances; rapid weight gain or loss and altered eating habits; sustained use of alcohol, sedatives, or other medications; serious accidents related to fatigue, inattention; an inability to think clearly; planning or attempting injury to herself or others; and uncontrollable crying and mood shifts (Dalton 2001). Refer women with these and any symptoms of other postpartum complications to their physician or midwife and ask them to provide written release for massage therapy. (Chapter 7 includes suggestions for working with women experiencing any postpartum special situations.)

The Later Months and Years of Postpartum Massage Therapy

A doctor or a midwife's release from maternity care signals the end of puerperium care; however, most women will continue their maternity recovery for as long as 9 months to a year or more, in some cases. An appropriate truism is that it takes 9 months to make a baby and at least equal time to recover from the gestation. Your work during this time can include some of the previous approaches, and other work might also be helpful.

Pelvic ligaments can be particularly slow to recover. Use cross-fiber friction throughout the posterior pelvic ligament architecture if she has chronic pelvic pain. Over these months, she can gradually regain muscle strength in her abdominals, psoas, and pelvic floor—the core of postural integrity. If she hasn't already done so, encourage her to check into beginning a progressive sequence of toning exercise targeted to all of these important postural muscles (Byrne 2007). Many exercises are great fun for the baby and mom if she incorporates play with her infant as she exercises. Carrying and caring for a baby also require upper body strength and endurance. A baby's increasing weight provides a perfect graduated weight-training tool. Older babies love to be lifted and swung as the mom tones her leg and arm muscles. Remind her how easy it is to incorporate pelvic floor exercise into feeding and holding times (Creager 2001).

Extended static postures of holding and carrying can strain muscles and joints and contribute to trigger point development. Interrupt and reduce habitual holding and reintroduce movement to rigid joints and soft tissue with subtle, rhythmic movement and deep tissue techniques. When head, neck, and arm pain occurs, check for trigger points in torso and pectoral girdle muscles, and include passive and active stretches in your sessions. Encourage daily stretching, easily incorporated on playground equipment and while playing on the floor with her baby.

Emotional adjustments to mothering take some time, too. After the baby blues/hormonal rollercoaster of the first week, most women move toward a more even keel; however, contrary to the romanticized view of motherhood, most women have ambivalence about mothering's demands. They need time and experience to balance out the baby's, other family members', and their own needs. Relationship adjustments with partners, other children, grandparents, friends, and coworkers are sometimes slow. These difficulties can be hard to discuss with those closest to her and most affected by her feelings. Be alert to her need to share not just the pleasures but the difficulties of her ongoing commitment to her baby. Offer her the compassionate, listening ear and heart she seeks, and remember that depression and other affective disorders can develop during this time too. (See online resources for emotional support activities)

Many women suffer pregnancy-induced back and neck pain far beyond the postpartum period. Unresolved trigger points, restricted posterior structures, and unhealed diastasis recti can lead to chronic back pain. Strained joint structures, particularly in the sacroiliac, lumbosacral, and symphysis pubis joints, lead to PPPPS that can persist for years (Howard 2000). Effective massage therapy in the first 1 to 3 months after birthing, as detailed above, may help her to avoid this problem; however, if she only begins receiving massage many months after the birth, childcare strains may have worsened or created pelvic and back pain. Comfort her immediate pain, but you will need to address the source issues. Focus on deep tissue, neuromuscular, and other myofascial work to the abdominal attachments, the iliopsoas, all pelvic ligaments, and the lumbodorsal structures. Evaluate the integrity of her linea alba, guiding her to protected abdominal toning, if needed (Byrne 2007). For fully restoring and improving structural integration and function, the postpartum period is an excellent time to undergo a complete series of Rolfing or other structural balancing work based on the principles of Ida Rolf or sequential Aston Patterning sessions. (See online resources).

"Once a mother, always a mother" can ring painfully true in some women's back and pelvis. Women with chronic back pain, who were pregnant years or decades ago, may still be feeling pregnancy, labor, and childcare effects. Adhesions in their cesarean scar many contort their posture and dull their pelvic awareness. Although their "babies" might be 30 years or more old, these women often benefit from sessions of postpartum techniques. Choose techniques designed to address these long-standing dysfunctions such as those in the postpartum technique manual that follows and online videos.

> **REMINDER:** *Regardless of her age, if any female client who has been pregnant has back pain, postpartum abdominal and back techniques can be helpful.*

Technique Manual of Postpartum Massage Therapy

This section includes detailed instruction in how to perform selected, specific techniques for postpartum women. As in previous chapters, each technique box breaks down into the following segments:

- **Intention:** The intended outcome or purpose of the technique
- **Procedure:** Precise instructions in how to accomplish the technique
- **Hints:** Ways to make it easier or more effective or to vary it for individual needs
- **Precautions:** Adaptations and contraindications to remember to safely use the technique

See online resources at http://thePoint.lww.com/Osborne-Pregnancy 2e for videos of selected techniques.

Foot Reflexology (Zone Therapy)

Intentions

To create parasympathetic stimulation that promotes systemic relaxation; to promote metabolic functioning by reflexively stimulating the sensory cortex; to reflexively facilitate postpartum recovery, especially musculoskeletal strain and organic dysfunctions.

Procedure

This procedure may be performed in any position.

1. Massage the reflex zones in the feet using tiny, precise movements that compress the skin and undifferentiated nerves of the feet between the bones of the client's feet and your finger bones.
2. Focus on the following postpartum complaint areas: musculoskeletal strain in the neck, upper back, spine, pelvis, and sacrum; headache; constipation; uterine pain; bladder pain; and breast pain. (See Fig 4.50 for map and consult Lett 2000 for other specific postpartum sequences of zone therapy.)

Abdominal Massage

Intentions

To facilitate organic healing through increased circulation and normalization of organ spacing; to reduce abdominal gas and constipation by stimulating peristalsis; to impart a kinesthetic sense of nonpregnancy; to stimulate muscle tone; to facilitate uterine involution and help prevent hemorrhaging.

Procedure

All procedures are best performed in the supine position with knees up or well bolstered.

Kneading (Fig. 6.6)

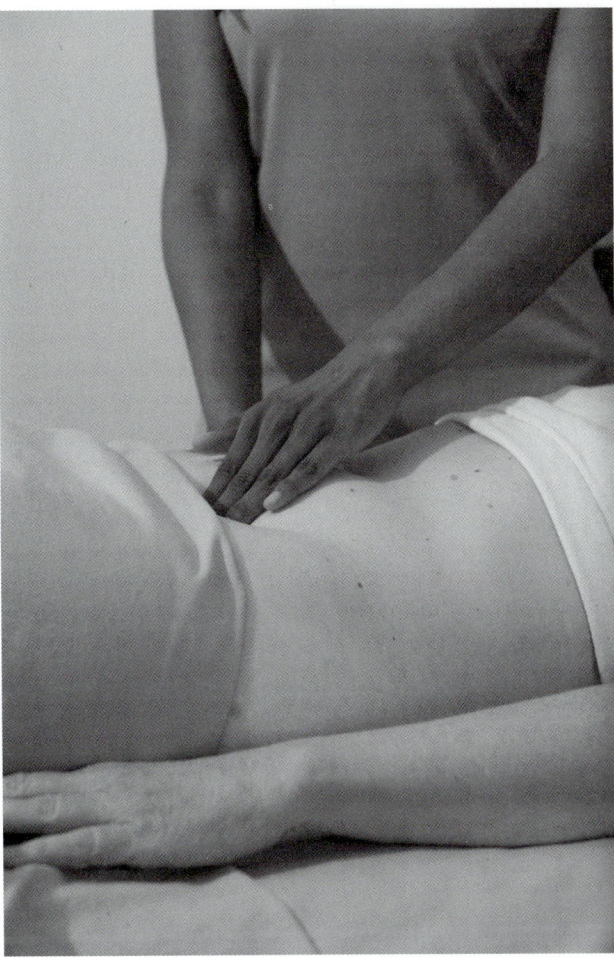

FIGURE 6.6 Abdominal kneading.

1. Stand at pelvic level facing the client's head. Use the heels of your hand and/or fingertips to knead the abdomen in the direction of peristalsis.
2. Especially focus around the perimeter, scooping toward her navel, and at its flexures, particularly deep to the anterior edge of the ribcage.

Uterine Positioning (Fig. 6.7)

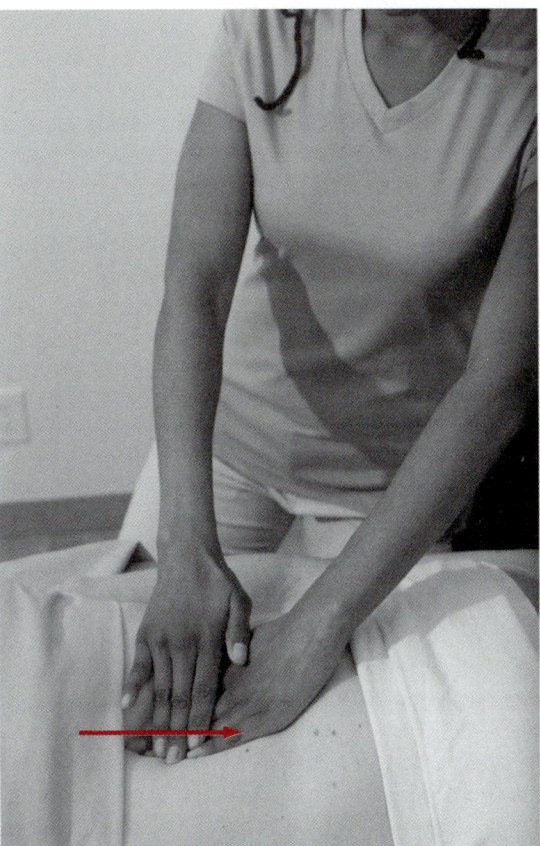

FIGURE 6.7 Uterine positioning.

1. Reposition the uterus and bladder in their fascial matrix with kneading if it is off the midline.
2. If these organs are beginning to prolapse, use myofascial lifting. Stand facing her pubic bone. During the client's exhale, use flattened distal fingers just superior of the pubic bone at the midpoint and sink to bladder level. Without sliding on her skin, shift your body weight toward her head to create a pull on the fascial tissue around the bladder and uterus. Hold for 5 to 10 seconds as she holds her breath, and then release when she inhales again.
3. Repeat two more times.

Vibration (Fig. 6.8)

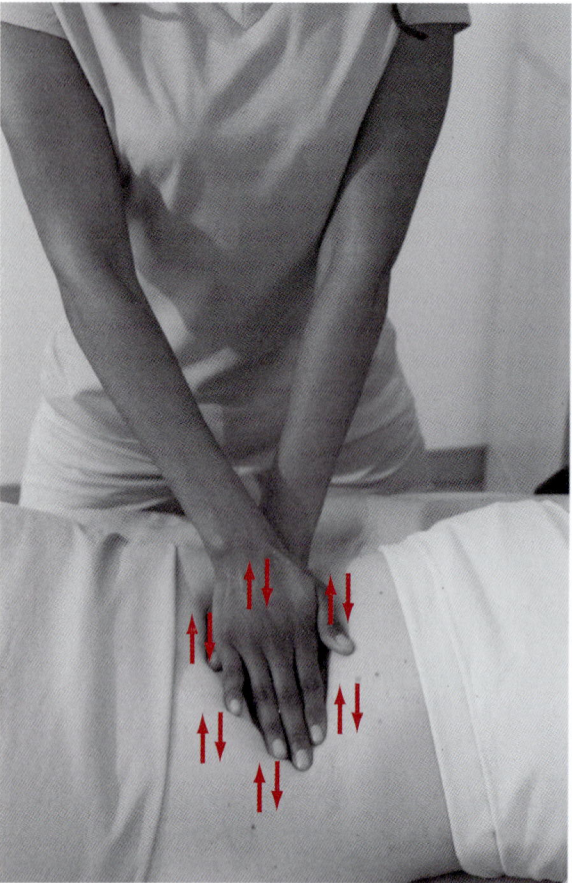

FIGURE 6.8 Abdominal vibration.

1. Place your nondominant hand palm down on the abdomen and your dominant hand directly on top.
2. Initiating movement from your shoulders, create a deep, high-frequency vibration that penetrates to the spine and stimulates deep healing.
3. Relocate your hands and repeat until you have vibrated the entire abdomen.

Fundal Massage (Fig. 6.9)

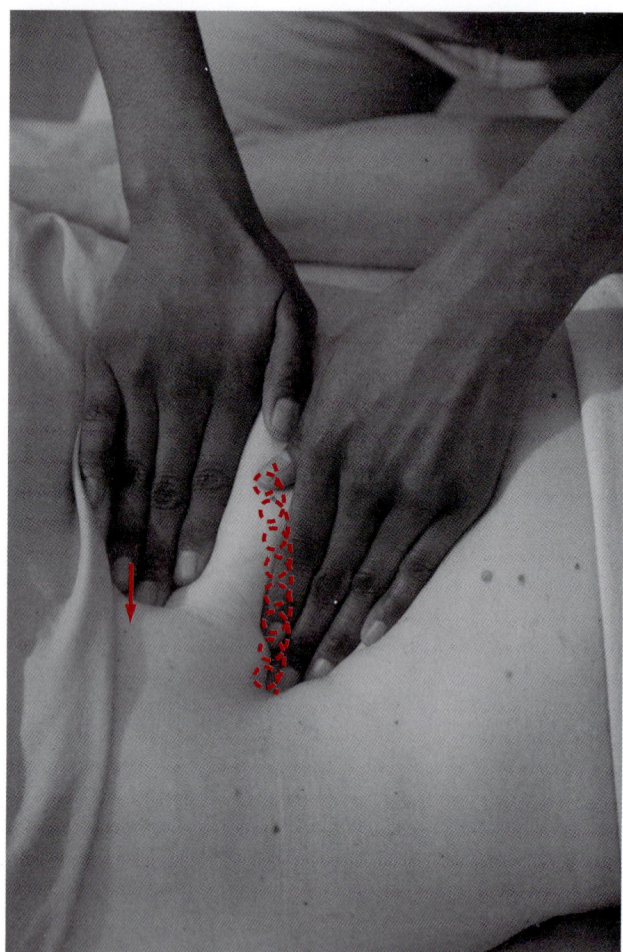

FIGURE 6.9 Uterine involution and fundal massage.

1. Place one hand just superior to pubic bone sinking to bladder level. Maintain a superiorly directed pressure throughout the following steps.
2. Place fingertips of other hand at or just above umbilicus level if performed immediately after giving birth and closer to the pubic bone if 1 to 2 weeks later; this is not beneficial after 2 weeks.
3. Sink to the organ level, making contact with the rounded top of the uterus. Perform circular kneading strokes deeply to the fundus until you feel it harden and/or client reports uterine contractions.

Tapotement (Fig. 6.10)

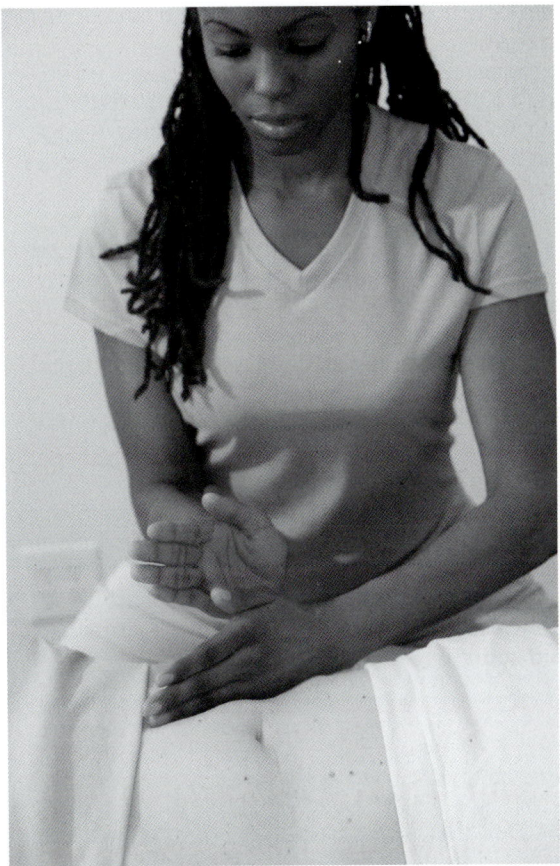

FIGURE 6.10 Tapotement.

1. Tap or hack gently on the lateral edges and on the belly of the rectus abdominis to activate proprioceptors and begin toning these slack abdominal muscles.
2. Repeat for 10 to 20 seconds until you can feel the abdominal muscles reflexively tightening under your tapotement.

Hints

1. All abdominal procedures are most comfortable if the client has an empty bladder. Often this means sequencing them toward the beginning of a session.
2. With fundal massage, expect some pain and some increase in vaginal bleeding during or right after massage.
3. Teach the client to perform fundal massage on herself every 4 hours daily for up to 2 weeks or until the uterus has involuted back to the pubic bone level.

Precautions

1. After cesarean birth, use caution with all four procedures and perform only after postoperative release. Be gentle and careful with the direction of your pressure, avoiding inadvertently tugging on the scar until she receives a medical release several weeks later.
2. Avoid kneading in the inferior inguinal area of the abdomen until 8 to 10 weeks postpartum, after blood clotting has completely normalized.

Abdominal Trigger Points

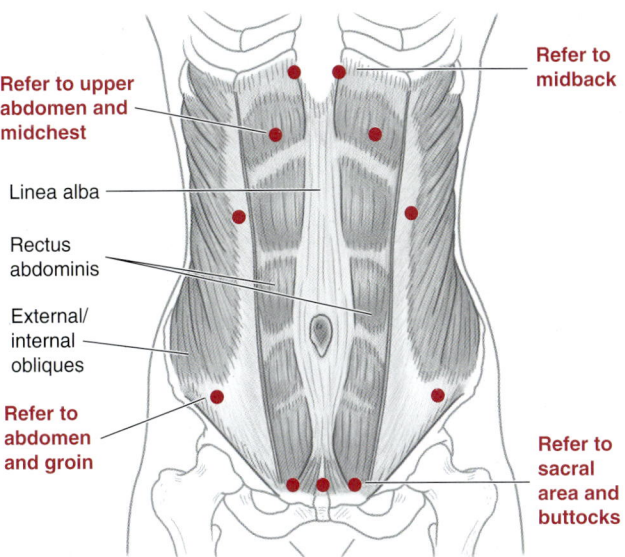

FIGURE 6.11 Abdominal trigger points.

Intentions

To reduce referred pain in the abdomen and back by locating and extinguishing trigger points in all abdominal musculature.

Procedure

This procedure is best performed in supine position.

1. Stand at the pelvic level, facing the client's head.
2. Ask the client to report any tenderness or painful sensations in her anterior or posterior torso as you friction in the abdominal muscle attachments.
3. Use several fingertips to create a sawing motion to check in the locations indicated in Figure 6.11. These include the following:
   - 1 to 2 inches below the xiphoid process
   - Superficial to ribs 8 to 12 and just below the costal border of the ribs
   - Medial to the ASIS
   - Along the anterior pubic bone, avoiding the symphysis
4. Seek to identify any areas eliciting a jump response from the client.
5. Moderate your pressure on the point until the pain is no more intense than pleasure on the borderline of pain.
6. Request client feedback on changes in pain intensity. Once her pain has dissipated, continue to compress for 7 to 20 seconds.
7. If possible, stretch the trigger area for 30 to 60 seconds or perform localized thumb fanning type strokes over the point.

Hints

1. Confirm that any pain in the soft abdomen, off of the bony attachments, is actually a muscular trigger point and not organic tenderness. Check by having the client lift her head and/or torso, activating

the muscle group. If pain increases with contraction, the point is a trigger point; proceed with extinguishing. If pain decreases, the pain is likely organic in nature and will not respond to trigger point treatment, so release pressure.
2. Remember that most abdominal trigger points refer to organs, except the rectus points, which refer to the midback and sacrum/buttocks.

PRECAUTION

Wait until the cesarean scar heals, and after postoperative release.

CESAREAN SCAR MASSAGE
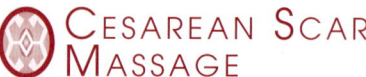

INTENTIONS

To prevent or reduce adhesions; to improve circulation, reduce swelling, and support healing; when performed on older scars, to dissolve any adhesions that may have formed; and to reduce any postural, visceral, or other imbalances that have resulted. See Fig. 6.5.

PROCEDURE

All procedures are best performed in the supine position with knees up or well bolstered. Proceed at the client's speed, and expect to accomplish these steps over an extended time rather than in one session. Perform each step directly to the visible scar, whether horizontal, or in some cases vertical, except Nos. 6 and 8.

1. Initially, have the client carefully place her hands over the bandages, directing warmth and healing intention to the incision.
2. For the early weeks after surgery, teach her to move localized edema near the scar toward the inguinal nodes with feather-light fingertip vibration, moving from midscar out laterally.
3. After the scar is closed, no longer oozing, place your hands lightly and use warmth, intention, and vibration to the level of client tolerance physically and emotionally. Create no pain.
4. Once she has postsurgical release, with any staples removed and the skin closed, begin using a light fingertips circling to gently move the visible scar on the superficial fascia below it. Add pressure to progress to gentle movement of the scar and superficial fascia on the muscle layers beneath.
5. Locate any immobile or rigid areas. Create a tensile stretch in multiple directions, holding each stretch for 30 seconds minimum.
6. Once the superficial layers are mobile, progress to deeper fascial levels. Most cesarean surgeries are horizontal "bikini-line" incisions superficially, with deeper tissues severed vertically at the linea alba (refer back to Fig 5.8). At this tissue level, circle from the center of the scar moving up toward the umbilicus, holding tensile stretch on any immobile area for at least 30 seconds.
7. Return to a superficial level to apply fingertip cross-fiber friction. At any point of rigidity, compress the scar against underlying tissue and perform brisk stationary friction for 3 to 5 minutes.
8. Moving vertically from the midline, as in step 6 above, perform friction to deeper fascial layers when the skin level is no longer rigid.
9. Using your thumbs and fingertips, lift the scar and gently roll the skin in one long stroke or in sections and in all directions. If there are rigid or restricted areas, roll back and forth through that tissue, holding a tensile stretch if needed.

HINTS

1. Describe the work, discuss its benefits, and get her permission for it before beginning.
2. Some women may only tolerate brief, very gradual work. Physically, the scar can become tender; emotionally, she may be flooded with feelings. Monitor her responses carefully and sensitively. Allot 5 to 15 minutes of each postpartum session to this work, and progress through the steps above at her comfortable pace.
3. Some women will feel motivated to work on their scar more frequently. Teach her to perform the appropriate steps of these procedures at convenient times, such as when watching television or while breastfeeding.
4. Some women will experience numbness at the incision site and as high as the umbilicus for 6 months or more. Be sure to err on the side of superficiality and light pressure if she is numb.

PRECAUTIONS

1. Perform on scars where the skin is closed and the staples have been removed, except for steps 1 and 2. Impeccable hygiene is also an absolute necessity to further ensure safety.
2. Create realistic expectations of this work, reminding her that the scar will not disappear but will become more pliable from this work. **Keloid scars** will become softer and less raised.

STRUCTURAL BALANCING FOR ILIOPSOAS
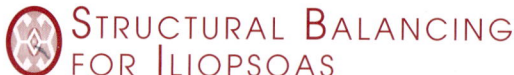

Adapted from Maupin 2005 (Fig. 6.12).

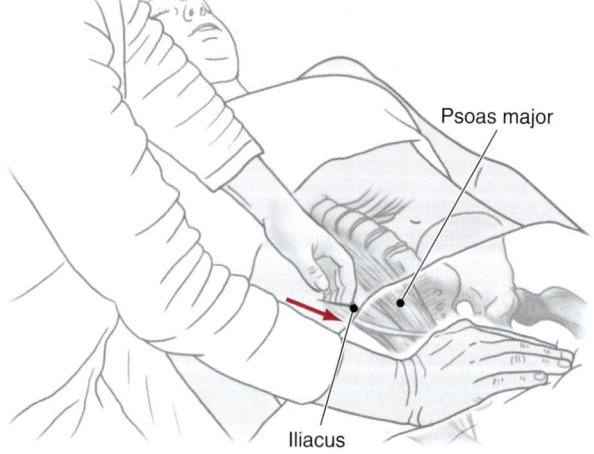

FIGURE 6.12 Structural balancing for iliopsoas.

INTENTIONS

To reduce iliopsoas spasm, to activate and strengthen iliopsoas awareness and tone, to reduce back pain from improper spinal and pelvic alignment

Procedure

This procedure may be performed in the sidelying or supine position; it is described in the supine position.

1. Stand at the pelvic level facing the client's feet. Place your outside hand supportively on the anterior upper thigh. Straighten your inside hand; then, leading with your little through middle fingers, use the edge to gradually sink into the pelvic bowl just medial to the ASIS, sliding down the medial ilium as the tissue softens.
2. Continue to compress into the abdominals. If release allows you deeply enough to contact the iliopsoas, continue in an inferior direction releasing any stringiness, bunching, or tenderness in the myofascia.
3. Maintain a melting compression for at least 30 to 60 seconds.

Alternative Procedure

1. Teach your client to activate the iliopsoas using imagery that encourages lengthening of her lumbar spine against the table and/or flexion of her thigh on her pelvis.
2. For lengthening, try the monkey tail imagery (see Chapter 4 technique manual) Repeat for as many as 12 times. Coach her to coordinate the movement with exhaling breath, if possible.
3. For hip flexion, have her imagine a string tied to her upper thigh (place your flat palm over her anteromedial thigh, just inferior of her inguinal ligament). The string continues up toward the ceiling. Have her imagine that a giant puppeteer pulls the string, lifting her upper thigh slightly from the table while her lower back lengthens toward the table. After imagining that movement several times, ask her to initiate that movement. Coach her to coordinate her movement with her exhaling breath if possible.
4. After she can adequately do one of the movements above, sink gradually into the iliopsoas and then ask her to imagine and do the movement. During each activation of the iliopsoas, maintain your compression. Coach her movement until you can confirm activation of the iliopsoas under your fingertips. As the tissue softens and lengthens, follow the tissue changes.
5. You can similarly release more superior segments of the iliopsoas, if necessary. Work in the midpsoas, entering at the lateral edge of the rectus abdominus at umbilicus level. Sink in just medial of the costal edge of the ribcage, avoiding pressure on the xiphoid process, just where the rectus abdominus crosses the ribcage toward its attachments. In these upper areas, the pelvic tilting rather than the hip flexion will be the most productive movement to work with.

Precautions

1. Expect tissue dysfunction and possible protective responses that may prevent entry to the iliopsoas level. Proceed slowly at the speed of tissue release, extinguishing any trigger points. Sometimes, you will need several approaches over several sessions to sensitively reach this deep intrinsic muscle complex; don't force your way painfully in.
2. By entering at the ASIS, keeping the palmar side of your fingers against the flat of the ilium and reducing pressure if painful, you will avoid any pointed or excessive pressure on vulnerable abdominal organs.
3. Be especially sensitive and avoid working beyond the client's experience of pleasure on the borderline of pain.
4. Do not apply direct pressure in an inferior direction on the inguinal ligament, as it may be weakened, thereby causing a hernia.
5. Wait until after blood clot dangers have passed to work in the inferior section; superior work may be performed after involution is complete.

6. Wait until postoperative release, monitoring carefully for painful pulling on a cesarean scar. You may have to loosen and soften it first before attempting this technique (see the scar work above).

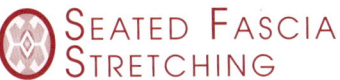 Seated Fascia Stretching

Adapted from Maupin 2005 (Fig. 6.13).

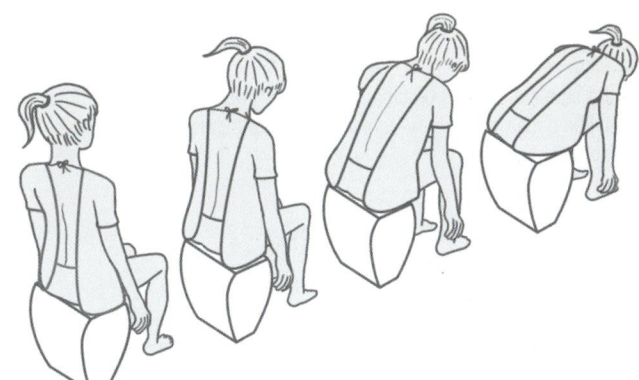

FIGURE 6.13 Seated fascia stretching.

Intentions

To elongate myofascial tissue and fascial planes and to reduce back pain by reeducating spinal alignment and normalizing curvatures.

Procedure

This procedure is performed with the client seated on a sturdy stool or backless chair, adjusted to a height so that her thighs are parallel with the floor, with feet flat on the floor.

1. Drape the client to modestly cover her breasts, but leave access to her bare back from top to panty line; a hospital gown or a robe worn backward works best.
2. Instruct your client to perform the following movements shown in Fig. 6.13: sit upright with the back of your neck elongated, arms at your sides. Begin to move your torso toward your thighs by first dropping your chin to your chest. Gradually roll forward and downward from the top, one vertebra at a time. When your torso reaches your thighs, or you cannot roll down any further, reverse to erect your spine in the opposite order. Allow your foot to push into the floor as your sit-bones press into the chair. Let your sacrum and waistline move back first as a base to erect your spine vertebra by vertebra from the bottom to the top. Finally, bring your head up and lift through the crown of your head.
3. Observe fluidity and range of client's movement. Note where spinal segments are moving as a unit rather than as vertebrae individually articulating.
4. Explain that she will repeat this movement while you use your fists to stroke deeply down both sides of the paravertebral musculature and fascial planes. Stand behind and place your gently fisted knuckles near C7. Direct your pressure caudally and medially. As the client rolls her spine down, let her movement glide you down her back. Proceed paravertebrally to the coccyx, if possible.

5. Allow the speed of her movement to guide your speed and intensity as you stroke down.
6. When she reverses her movement as in step 2 above, help guide more differentiated movement of the vertebral elements by tapping gently on each consecutive vertebra to call her attention to individual movement that stacks her spine from the bottom up.
7. Repeat using your elbows for a narrower, more medial stroke.
8. Repeat using your one or two knuckles into the laminar groove, if possible.

Precautions

1. Do not perform on any client with spine injuries or diseases. Take extra care when there is a scoliosis.
2. Be sure the client is breathing normally throughout this procedure.
3. If she becomes dizzy or light-headed from this technique, discontinue it.

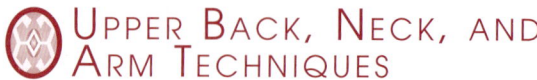

Upper Back, Neck, and Arm Techniques

Most postpartum sessions need to include a considerable amount of work to reduce the strain of childcare activities on the upper body. See the section "Reducing Upper Body Discomforts" in the Chapter 4 technique manual for relieving tension, trigger points, and other sources of pain in the neck, upper back, and pectoral girdle structures.

CHAPTER SUMMARY

No part of a woman's childbearing experience is more neglected in Western cultures than the intense and trying early months with a newborn. (See online resources for traditions of extended postpartum care in other cultures.) After 9 months of being the center of attention, postpartum women are easily sidelined as the infant takes center stage. Most medical care focuses on uterine involution, whereas the many other physiological and emotional experiences of the puerperium make a more daily impact on women's lives. A mother's love affair with her baby, or the seeming lack of one, impacts that baby's and the family's development. Most women are unprepared for the ferocity and gentleness that mothering inflames. New mothers and their families need reliable, sustained care for many weeks or months to maximize postpartum recovery and foster family development. Unfortunately, fragmented extended families and inadequate social policies often leave mothers and their newborns isolated, with minimal attention to their many postpartum needs. By providing postpartum massage therapy, you can give one-on-one, focused care to a new mother's body and emotions. With caring, knowledgeable hands, you can help ease women into the magical and the mundane realities of mothering, truly nurturing her birth and growth as a mother.

Test Yourself

For answers, visit the website at http://thePoint.LWW.com/Osborne-Pregnancy2e!

1. List three major physiological adjustments of the early postpartum period.
2. What are three normal emotional responses to early mothering demands?
3. What are five symptoms of postpartum affective disorders that you should be alert to in your clients?
4. What other symptoms should you be alert to that might be related to other postpartum complications?
5. List three contraindications or precautions to ensure safe postpartum massage therapy.
6. List five goals of massage therapy during the first three postpartum months.
7. How can pregnancy affect women's musculoskeletal health many years after giving birth?

REFERENCES

Andrade C-K and Clifford P. Outcome-Based Massage: From Evidence to Practice. Second Edition. Baltimore: Lippincott, Williams and Wilkins, 2008.

Albright L. Kangaroo Mother Care: Restoring the Original Paradigm for Infant Care and Breastfeeding. Accessed at www.llli.org, July 20, 2009.

American Academy of Pediatrics. Policy Statement of Task Force on Sudden Infant Death Syndrome. Accessed at http://www.aap.org/healthtopics/Sleep.cfm, June 16, 2010.

AWHONN. Conquering postpartum depression. Nurs Womens Health 2007;11(4):422–423.

Blake Gleeson P, Pauls J. Carpal tunnel syndrome: during pregnancy and lactation. Parenting Today Mag, September, 1993:52–54.

Byrne H. Exercise after Pregnancy. 2nd Ed. Oakland: BeFitMom, 2007.

Chikly B, Chikly A. Applications of pre- and post-surgical lymphatic drainage therapy. Massage and Bodywork, Summer/Fall 1997: 64–67.

Creager C. Bounce Back into Shape after Baby. Berthoud, CO: Executive Physical Therapy, 2001.

Curties D. Breast Massage. New Brunswick, Canada: Curties-Overzet Publications, 1999.

Dalton K. Depression after Childbirth. 4th Ed. New York, NY: Oxford University Press, 2001.

Ezner S. Reflexology: A Tool for Midwives. Pymble, Australia: Suzanne Ezner, 2000.

Field T, Grizzle N, Scafidi F, Shanberg S. Massage and relaxation therapies' effects on depressed adolescent mothers. Adolescence. 1996;31:903–911.

Fitch P. The case for breast massage. Massage Ther J, Winter 1998; 36–4:64–78.

Gonzalez H, Vinaver N. Massage Techniques from Mexico. Workshop Presentation at Midwifery Today Conference, March, 1997.

Howard F. Pelvic Pain: Diagnosis and Management. Baltimore: Lippincott Williams & Wilkins, 2000.

Jefferies J, Bochner F. Thromboembolism and its management in pregnancy. Med J Aust, August 19, 1991;155:253–258.

Kitzinger S. The Year after Childbirth. New York, NY: Charles Scribner's Sons, 1994.

Lett A. Reflex Zone Therapy for Health Professionals. London: Harcourt Publishers, 2000.

Massaro A, Hammad T, Jazzo B, Aly H. Massage with kinesthetic stimulation improves weight gain in preterm infants. Journal Of Perinatology: Official Journal Of The California Perinatal Association [serial online]. May 2009;29(5):352–357. Available from: MEDLINE, Ipswich, MA. Accessed October 30, 2010

Maupin E. A Dynamic Relationship to Gravity, vols 1 and 2. San Diego: DawnEve Press, 2005.

Mitchinson A, Kim H, Rosenberg J, et al. Acute postoperative pain management using massage as an adjuvant therapy. Arch-Surg 2007;142(12):1158–1167.

Moberg KU. The Oxytocin Factor. Tapping the Hormone of Calm, Love, and Healing. Cambridge: DeCapo Press, 2003.

Noble E. Essential Exercises for the Childbearing Year. 4th Ed. Harwich: New Life Images, 1995.

Osborne C. Pre-and Perinatal Massage Therapy: Survey of Massage Therapists, 2009. Available at www.bodytherapyassociates.com. Accessed June, 2010.

Pirie A, Herman H. How to Raise Children without Breaking Your Back. Cambridge: IBIS Publications, 2003.

Polseno-Crawford D. Why don't we do breast massage? Massage Ther J 1998;36-4:95–106.

Ricci, S. Essentials of Maternity, Newborn and Women's Health Nursing. 2nd Ed. Baltimore: Lippincott Williams & Wilkins, 2009.

Simkin P. The experience of maternity in a woman's life. J Obstet Gynecol Nurs 1996;25; 247–252.

Simkin P, Whalley J, Keppler A. Pregnancy, Childbirth and the Newborn. Fourth Edition. New York: Simon and Schuster, 2010.

Stugea B, Holma I, Vollestada N. To treat or not to treat postpartum pelvic girdle pain with stabilizing exercises? Man Ther 2006;11:337–343.

Taylor S, Klein L, Lewis B, et al. Biobehavioral responses to stress in females: tend-and-befriend, not fight-or-flight. Psychol Rev 2000;107:411–429.

Thomason A, DeLancey J. Urinary incontinence symptoms during and after pregnancy in continent and incontinent primiparas. Int Urogynecol J Pelvic Floor Dysfunct 2007;18(2):147–151.

For additional resources, please visit http://thePoint.LWW.com/Osborne-Pregnancy2e!

Clients with Special Needs

Learning Objectives

After study of this chapter, you should be able to:

1. Recognize warning signs of the most common prenatal complications.
2. Adapt your prenatal massage sessions appropriately when medical complications develop.
3. Provide safe and effective massage therapy sessions to women who are on bed rest for prenatal complications
4. Adapt your prenatal massage sessions appropriately when your clients have a higher risk of developing prenatal medical complications.
5. Be aware of and adapt to prenatal situations requiring special sensitivity, such as after fertility treatments, with diverse parents, and with depressed, abused, and other challenged women.
6. Provide safe and effective care when complications and special needs arise during labor.
7. Assist women in recovery from traumatic or complicated birthing and when tragic outcomes result.

The previous chapters have focused on developing your understanding of what to normally expect when clients are expecting and on increasing your skill in meeting their needs. This chapter begins to prepare you for the more unexpected: illnesses, pregnancy losses, worrisome medical conditions, and the possible results of riskier lifestyles. This chapter introduces you to a diversity of possible clients, in addition to the norm of a woman and her husband who conceived through sexual intercourse.

You will learn to adapt and effectively respond to labors that slow, stall, charge forward, or need medical management. This chapter also prepares you for when postpartum emotional or physiological complications occur. You will learn skills to deal with grieving parents when outcomes of a pregnancy are less than optimal or tragic. It points you in directions for further study and resources if you wish to specialize in high-risk and complicated prenatal and perinatal massage therapy.

When Pregnancy-Related Complications Develop

Doctors consider about one in four pregnant women at high risk for developing medical conditions that may result in negative outcomes for the mother, the fetus, or both (Ricci 2009). Sometimes, even without these higher-risk factors or unhealthy lifestyles, for no predictable reason, the strain on maternal body systems overwhelms basic health and well-being, and medical complications can result. You don't need to have a medical education to be prepared for these women; their doctors or midwives will carefully monitor, screen, and diagnose these conditions. Sometimes, though, you will work with a woman before her healthcare provider confirms her condition. For this reason, you should be alert for the signs and symptoms of a likely complication that are summarized in Box 7.1. Your work with a woman with

Box 7.1

Summary of Warning Signs of Prenatal Complications (listed in bold italic)

- Bleeding, vaginal discharge, gush or slow leakage of amniotic fluid, low back and/or pelvic pain, cramping, contractions, pelvic or thigh pressure: ***miscarriage; trophoblastic, ectopic or tubal pregnancy; cervical insufficiency; premature labor; premature membrane rupture; placental abnormalities***
- Severe nausea, weight loss, dehydration: ***hyperemesis gravidarum***
- Low weight gain, decreased fetal movement: ***intrauterine growth restriction (IUGR) or small for gestational age (SGA)***
- High blood pressure, protein in urine, rapid weight gain, systemic and pitting edema, violent headaches, severe vomiting, visual disturbances, upper midback pain especially on right, convulsions: ***gestational hypertensive disorders***
- Heat, swelling or pain in the calves, particularly unilateral: ***thrombii***
- Excessive hunger and thirst, frequent urination, sugar in urine: ***gestational diabetes***
- Any abnormal results of blood and other laboratory tests, fetal and maternal monitoring procedures: ***any of the complications above***.

---

high risk and medical needs has great potential to help her secure the best possible outcomes despite the difficulties she faces (Fig. 7.1).

> **REMINDER:** *One-quarter of your pregnant clients are at higher risk for developing a pregnancy-related complication.*

Below, we consider some general guidelines for dealing with prenatal complications as they arise. Then, each of the following sections will present a specific, more common complication that your clients may experience in pregnancy. You will also find and will also give you some strategies to engage therapeutically with your clients when these situations occur.

● GENERAL GUIDELINES

Whenever your client reports or you notice a sign of any possible prenatal complication, there are several immediate responses you should make:

- Assess for any other signs of complications by asking further questions, palpating, or observing her.
- Do not add to her stress with an alarmist response to her symptoms or high-risk condition. Talk about your concerns calmly, professionally, and with a positive intention. Examples: "You know, whenever I have a client with bleeding and back pain, etc. happening, I like to run that by her midwife before proceeding, just in case there is something more going on that I am not qualified to assess." Or "Most likely this fluid, swelling, shortness of breath, etc. is not indicative of a problem, but I like to be sure. Can you discuss this with your doctor before our session, and let me know what she says?"
- Inquire as to whether her doctor or midwife knows of this occurrence.
- If not, have her inform her healthcare provider immediately of any worrisome observations.
- If a complication is already established, consult with the doctor about how to proceed and adopt his or her level of concern, from none to detailed treatment parameters. If she is hospitalized, secure necessary permissions if she'd like you to see her there.
- Secure your client's permission before engaging in phone, internet, or written communication about her care. If she'd

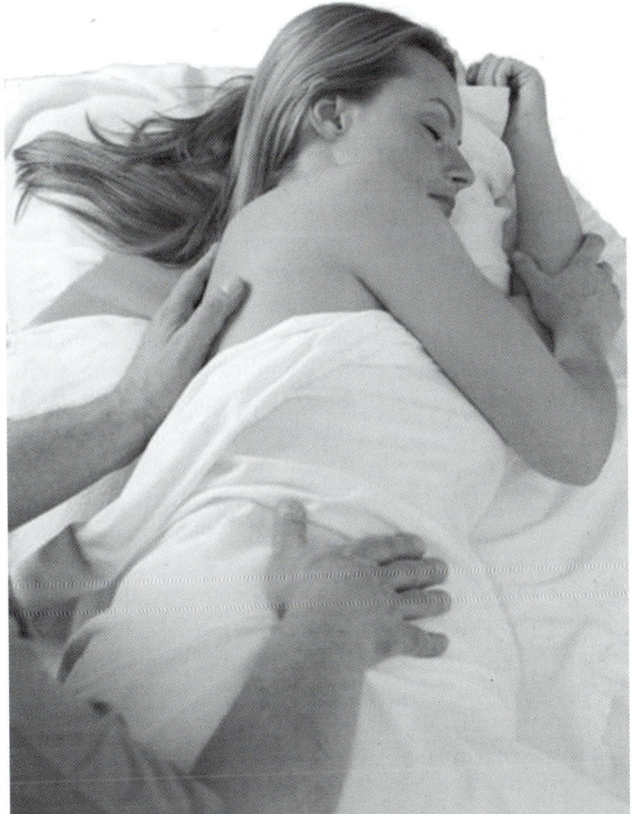

FIGURE 7.1 Reducing the stress of medical complications. Improving your client's breathing capacity and reducing joint and myofascial pain are direct ways you can help women cope with the additional worries and difficulties of medical complications. With many conditions, you may be limited to working in left sidelying position.

prefer, ask her to discuss with her doctor or midwife if and how to proceed with her massage therapy.
- Ask for the date and the result of her most recent visit with her midwife or doctor.

Once your preliminary assessments and communications are complete, keep these general guidelines in mind as you proceed into sessions with her:

- Whenever in doubt about positioning, or without specific instructions, use only left sidelying.
- When a client has any given condition, carefully consider the intention and the effect of your positioning and every technique for its implications, positive and negative. If in doubt, err on the side of caution, and you will do no harm.
- Take thorough health histories and perform verbal, visual, and palpatory assessments and update at each session. When you identify a higher-risk factor, review the possible complications and their typical signs. Assess carefully for them, without conveying unnecessary anxiety.
- Since many such situations potentially involve threatened placental problems, miscarriage, and prematurity, consider the possible liabilities associated with abdominal massage and any techniques that directly impact her abdomen such as the baby lift. Instead of direct abdominal contact, use breathing, visualizations, and reflexive techniques.

> **REMINDER:** *When working with high-risk clients or those who develop complications, consultation and medical release improve client care and reduce liability implications for therapists.*

In addition to following the guidelines above, you should also be prepared for when your clients' healthcare providers place women with complications or who are in high-risk categories on **bed rest**. This can mean either total inactivity or reduced mobility with long rest periods each day. They may prescribe several restricted days or weeks or many months, depending on the woman's condition. Most of these women are monitored at home, while others require hospitalization.

With these restrictions and the concerns that prompt them, women often experience a variety of physical and emotional side effects, many of which you can help to minimize (see online table at http://thePoint.lww.com/Osborne-Pregnancy2e for detailed categories and other support resources). When you work with women whose doctors prescribe bed rest, consider the following guidelines:

- Wait until after consultation and receiving release from her doctor to begin your work.
- Depending on your client's level of restriction, perform the massage at your office, in her home, or her hospital room.
- Position her in a left sidelying position to maximize fetal circulation. Prevent back strain when leaning over her bed by positioning her safely near the edge and raising her bed if it is adjustable. Better yet, use your therapy table if she has permission to transfer to it.
- Ask her healthcare provider's permission to use right sidelying or semireclined position to better relieve typical compression and pain from the prescribed extended periods on her left.
- Focus on relaxation, helping her to manage and reduce any negative thoughts and feelings.
- Address discomforts caused by inactivity: sluggish circulation, constipation, heartburn, edema, muscle strain and atrophy, cramping, and stiffness.
- Improve circulation by focusing Swedish and lymphatic drainage work on the torso and arms since all but the most superficial of leg strokes are more risky, due to increased risk of clots.
- Reduce her musculoskeletal pain with appropriate myofascial, passive movement, stretching, and trigger point techniques. In particular, mobilize, stretch and release spine and pectoral girdle tension and guide her breath deeper into her abdomen toward her baby (Fig. 7.2) (see other chapters' technique manuals and online resources).
- Soothe, center, and nurture her with focused, gentle touch, selected craniosacral or other relaxing techniques performed with a calm, positive intention and demeanor.
- Perform gentle foot, head, and neck massages for relaxation, but avoid zone therapy on the feet of those with high risk of deep vein thrombosis (Ezner 2000).
- If she has doctor approval to gently stretch and exercise in bed, reduce myofascial restrictions that make these activities more difficult or painful.
- Allow generous session time if she has feelings to share or companionship needs you can professionally meet.
- Encourage her to use this "time out" to tune in to her baby, to have her physical and emotional needs fully met, and to read, relax, meditate, or pray.
- Teach her family and friends simple massage techniques.

> **REMINDER:** *Remember precautions to protect from thromboembolism with bed resting clients: only the most superficial of leg massage unless working under direct medical supervision.*

Because chronic stress is a contributing factor to most complications, you can be a critical part of prevention and management of these conditions. Make parasympathetic arousal a prominent therapeutic intention, using environment, relationship, technique, and education to sedate her nervous system. The autonomic sedation series 3-1-1 is particularly effective for these women. Teach the three simple strokes to family members so that they can help with daily massages for her. Women with high-risk pregnancies, complications, or on bed-rest experience so much more scrutiny and are

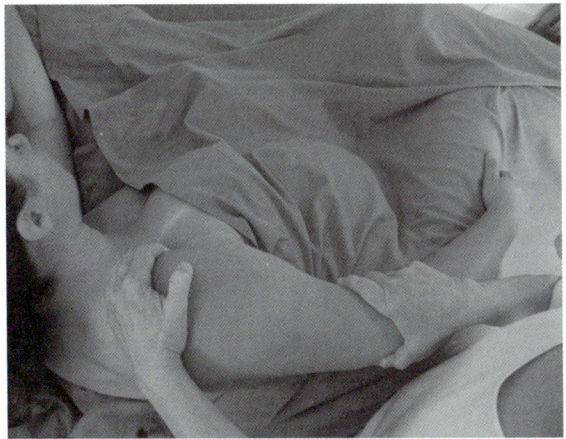
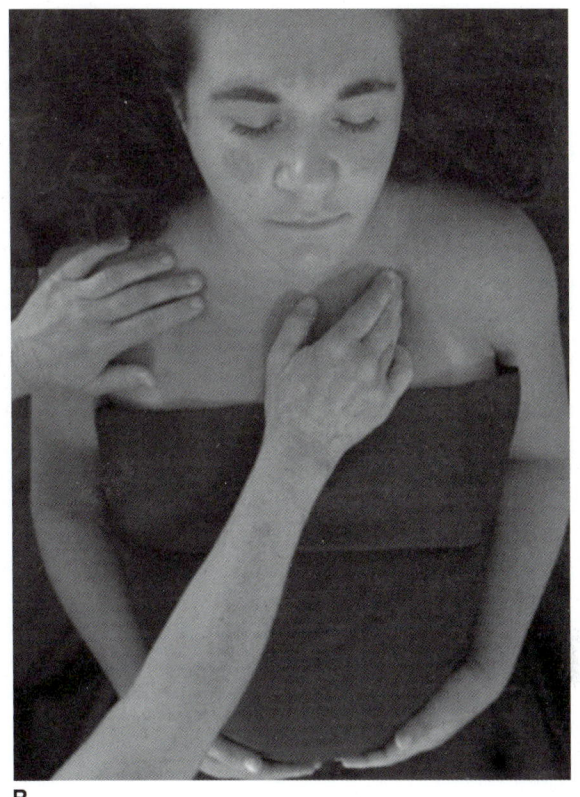
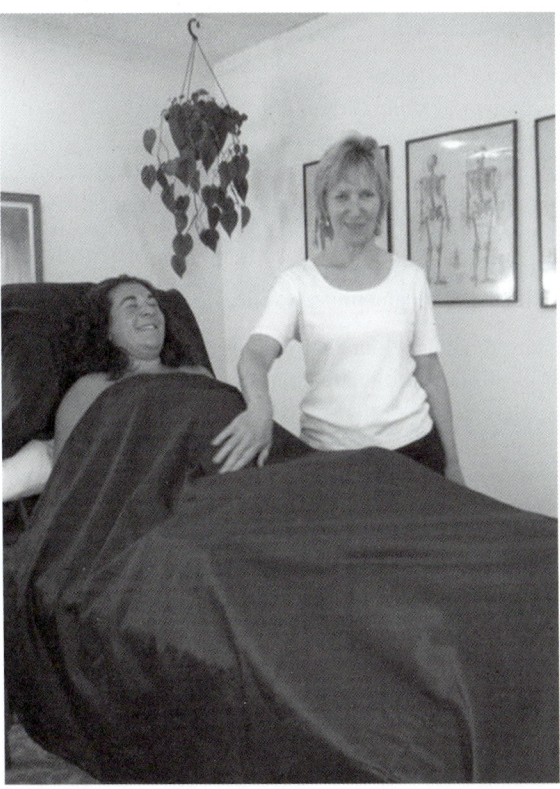

FIGURE 7.2 Upper body techniques for clients on bed rest. **(A)** Undulate and mobilize the pectoral girdle and release tension in the pectoral muscles to **(B)** reduce shoulder and neck tension. **(C)** Help her to connect with and enjoy her baby with relaxed, focused breathing.

subject to more tests and appointments. Your soothing touch will be a welcome change from the poking with needles and prodding with instruments she receives. With the increased precautions, it is hard for them to feel normal, and your work can help normalize their experience, making them some of the most gratifying and appreciative clients. (See Chapter 4 technique manual for specific relaxation techniques.)

● ANTEPARTUM BLEEDING

Vaginal bleeding, from light staining to profuse hemorrhage, can occur at any time before labor. It has many possible causes and one usual maternal response: fear. About 20% of expectant women have vaginal bleeding during the first trimester, but only about half of these women actually have a pregnancy loss. (Gilbert and Harmon 2003). (See Chapter 2 for bleeding associated with miscarriage and prematurity. See online medical glossary for other causes of prenatal bleeding.)

> *REMINDER:* In every case of bleeding or other special needs, make parasympathetic arousal a prominent therapeutic intention, using your environment, relationship with the client, specific technique, and targeted education to sedate her nervous system.

Whenever a pregnant client has bleeding, with or without pelvic, back or abdominal pain, attempt to determine if any pain is musculoskeletal in origin or referred from uterine contractions of threatened miscarriage or premature labor. Regardless of the cause, women experiencing bleeding often require your special emotional and physical support. She will especially appreciate stress reduction while awaiting test results and/or while on restricted activity until bleeding has resolved. Sedate the autonomic nervous system and deepen her breathing. Guide her in visualizing nurturing light, energy, or protection around her growing baby. (See Chapter 4 technique manual and online resources.)

With a threatened miscarriage, offer her water before, during, and after her session. Eliminate all abdominal techniques, and be very sure to avoid deep and specific pressure over points with the potential for stimulating uterine contractions. It is at these times, when her physiology may be on the verge of initiating contractions, that these points may be their most potent. Whatever the cause, if a pregnancy loss results from bleeding, these women need not only regular postpartum care but also assistance in their grieving process (see Chapter 6 and later sections on grieving).

> **REMINDER:** *If your client shows signs of threatened miscarriage or early labor, be extra cautious on or near labor-stimulating points.*

● GESTATIONAL HYPERTENSIVE DISORDERS

Gestational hypertension—or high blood pressure during pregnancy—is among the most common of prenatal complications, occurring in as many as 12% to 20% of pregnancies. It is also the second most deadly, after thromboembolism. Its frequency has been increasing steadily since 1990 in all groups, and particularly in women younger than 20 or older than 40 years. Other women at highest risk for preeclampsia and eclampsia are those

- Having their first baby
- With congenital anomalies or chronic stress
- With multifetal pregnancies
- With familial or personal history of preeclampsia
- With underlying diabetes, hypertension, or **renal diseases**
- With poor nutrition
- In lower socioeconomic groups
- Of African American ethnicity (Ricci 2009)

Confusion about labeling this condition is often the result of both multiple and outdated classifications that define the varying degrees of hypertensive disorders. The more outdated terms include *toxemia of pregnancy* and *GEPH* (gestational edema proteinurea hypertension) disorder. The most current labels for severity of gestational hypertension or pregnancy-induced hypertension, in order of less severe to most severe, are mild preeclampsia, severe preeclampsia, and eclampsia (Box 7.2). Gestational hypertension occurs when blood pressure exceeds 140/90 mm Hg on two occasions at least 6 hours apart. Although the cause of gestational hypertension is still

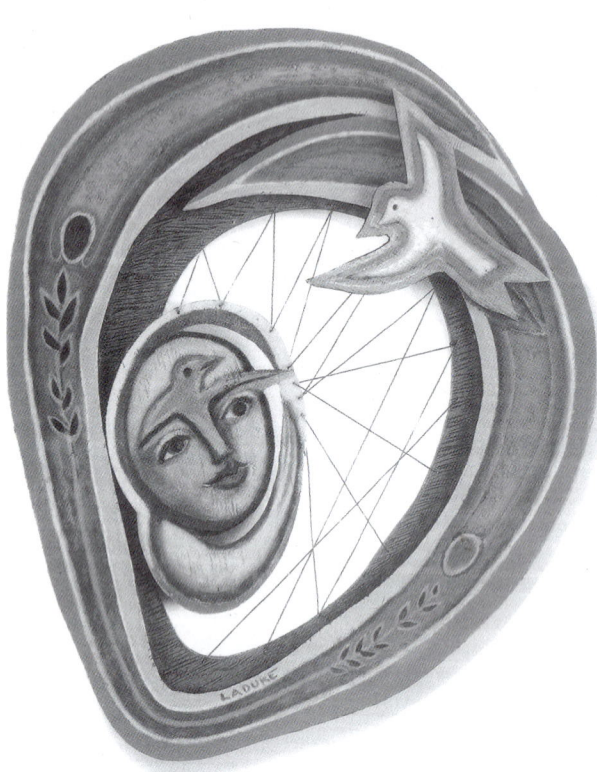

Child Within Betty La Duke

(c) Betty La Duke. Used with permission of the artist.

Box 7.2

Degrees of Prenatal Hypertension

Mild Preeclampsia
Blood pressure >140/90 mm Hg after 20 weeks' gestation, slight proteinuria, mild facial or hand edema, weight gain

Severe Preeclampsia
Blood pressure >160/110 mm Hg, medium proteinuria, hyperreflexia, headaches, visual disturbances, systemic, pitting and pulmonary edema, epigastric or right upper quadrant pain, HELLP (hemolysis of red blood cells, elevated liver enzymes, and low platelets)

Eclampsia
All of the above and seizures, coma, severe headache, cerebral hemorrhage, renal failure

unclear, in addition to the increased systolic and diastolic blood pressure, the easily recognized signs and symptoms of preeclampsia include the following:

- Protein in the urine
- Systemic edema (not just in the legs and feet)
- Rapid weight gain of retained water evidenced by swelling in the face, hands, and feet
- Pitting edema (small depression remains after pressing into swollen area) (Fig. 7.3)
- Shortness of breath (due to pressure of retained fluid in the lungs)

High blood pressure decreases blood flow to the brain, liver, kidneys, lungs, and placenta. When the liver and the kidneys malfunction, you might confuse the resulting referred pain with musculoskeletal pain. Note that a change in activity or position will not bring significant relief to this type of pain. Carefully interview all women with the following types of pain to discover any other warning signs of gestational hypertension:

- Severe midback to shoulder pain, especially on the right side (due to malfunctioning liver)
- Pain mimicking heartburn (due to malfunctioning liver)
- Pain in the lower back (due to kidney malfunction)

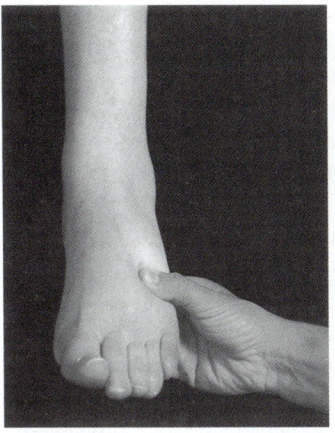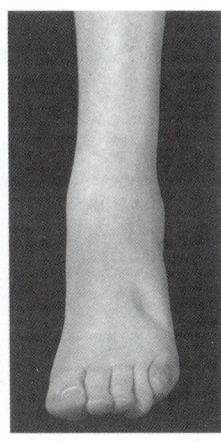

FIGURE 7.3 Pitting edema. Assess all clients for signs of gestational hypertension by noticing how quickly fluid refills into where you press. With pitting edema, that spot will blanch and take longer than 10 to 30 seconds to fill in.

At its most severe, eclampsia of pregnancy also involves neurological symptoms from lack of blood in the brain. These include the following:

- Violent headaches and vomiting
- Visual disturbances of spots and flashing light
- Convulsions

Points of View: Edema

Edema (also known as *lymphostatic edema* or *nonpitting edema*), particularly in the lower legs and feet, is a normal result of prenatal hormonal and circulatory system changes, mechanical constriction of pelvic vessels, and women's activity levels. Perinatal massage therapy instructors generally agree that this type of edema that is secondary to a healthy pregnancy responds well to techniques *generically* called *lymph drainage techniques*. These are superficial rhythmic strokes, primarily directed toward the heart, performed on proximal areas before moving further distally. Some emphasize a critical first step of stimulating the lymph nodes throughout the body, whereas others think that only the inguinal nodes must be prepared for assimilating the fluid load from the legs.

There are considerable differing opinions about whether to begin or end with this lighter work. Both those advocating beginning superficially and those preferring to finish in this way make the argument that other deeper techniques will compress lymphatic channels, thus obstructing fluid flow. Applying this reasoning, deeper work followed by more superficial techniques would seem to make the lighter strokes ineffective; lighter work followed by deeper is believed to cause the lymphatic channels to compress again, contributing to a rapid return of excess fluid.

As a result, some educators warn against deep pressure on any part of an edematous limb at any time during prenatal massage. When working with women with a lymphodynamic edema caused by dysfunction in the kidneys, heart, or liver due to underlying medical conditions or, more commonly, due to preeclampsia or eclampsia of pregnancy, there's agreement that the maternity healthcare provider should evaluate and make individual recommendations. Certainly, when lymphedema resulting from tissue damage or organ malfunction occurs and when hypertension is untreated and/or uncontrolled, superficial pressure is particularly warranted if massage is recommended by a physician. A well-trained and certified manual lymph drainage specialist may be best for working with these cases.

Of course, attempting to force fluid through edematous limbs is counterproductive. On the other hand, some women with little or normal prenatal swelling have a greater need for relief of muscular tension, fascial restriction in the extremities, and joint restrictions in the extremities. Eliminating all but the most superficial techniques might deprive these women of the possible relief created by deeper Swedish and deep tissue techniques and selected myofascial work. These methodologies are otherwise safe on healthy women's legs, except on the medial aspect and including the other limitations described in Chapter 2. When other contraindications to deep leg work occur, such as severe varices, bed rest, or elevated thrombi risks, then deep pressure should be avoided for those reasons. Remember, optimal pelvic alignment helps to open the anterior torso so that fluid can more easily flow past the inguinal ligament. Less stress and pain and, in most cases, more activity also help relieve and prevent edema. Your work should focus on those intentions throughout your client's body. As with many debates in perinatal massage therapy, each educator is applying her best knowledge and reasoning to a situation in which little actual data are available (Stager 2010; Stillerman 2008; Yates 2010).

Women with these severe symptoms need immediate medical care to prevent permanent organ damage, premature labor, fetal damage or loss, or death.

Decreased placental blood flow associated with hypertension results in intrauterine growth retardation, premature placental separation, and lack of fetal oxygenation. These developments mandate increased caution to position these clients for maximum fetal circulation, that is, the left sidelying position. Often, they are started on a week of monitored bed rest as a first defense to lower pressure, reduce stress, and maximize fetal oxygen and nutrients. At its most extreme, women are hospitalized so they can be constantly monitored, medications to prevent seizures and lower blood pressure may be administered, and the mother and the fetus prepared for an imminent birth to protect one or both of them if pressure cannot be managed successfully. Gestational hypertension can come on gradually or increase very quickly over a day or several hours. Sometimes labor brings it on. When preeclampsia is severe or eclampsia occurs, the birth of the baby is the only cure. An induction or a cesarean birth is quickly completed.

> **REMINDER:** *Gestational hypertensive disorders are the most common of prenatal complications and the second most deadly.*

If prenatal exams reveal elevated blood pressure or protein in your client's urine, you can easily assess if she has other signs of more severe preeclampsia, such as systemic or pitting edema. Refer women with symptoms of hypertensive disorders to their maternity healthcare provider for further evaluation and treatment, and then follow all of the general guidelines listed above if you work with her. In addition, with edema related to hypertension, leg work, if recommended at all by her physician, should only be superficial (see Points of View discussion).

● GESTATIONAL DIABETES

Diabetes precipitated by the physiological stresses of pregnancy is a metabolic disorder affecting approximately 8% of pregnancies, most often developing in the second trimester. These women are excessively hungry and thirsty, urinate more frequently, and have sugar in their urine lab tests. Women of color (African, Hispanic, or Native American descent) are at higher risk, as are those with previous pregnancies involving congenital anomalies, larger babies (over nine pounds), gestational diabetes, or unexplained fetal demise. Women over 35, a history of skin, genital, or urinary tract infections, those with hypertensive disorders, who are overweight, or with diabetes or a family history of it are also at greater risk (Ricci 2009).

Pregnancy tends to increase the need for glucose to ensure a constant supply to the fetus. Both estrogen and progesterone stimulate increased pancreatic insulin secretion to transport glucose to the cells. In the second and third trimesters, the pregnancy hormone, human placental lactogen, and cortisol also assist in regulating blood sugar. These increased demands and the actions and interactions of these hormones can result in either the inability of the pancreas to produce sufficient insulin or the inefficient use of available insulin. Gestational diabetes is different from several classifications of diabetic conditions that may develop in childhood, adolescence, or adulthood, and which are unrelated to pregnancy.

Gestational diabetes increases the likelihood of excessive amniotic fluid and can lead to additional complications, including gestational hypertensive disorders, premature membrane rupture, and stillbirth. As such, your work with these women will follow similar general guidelines as previous complications. Left sidelying position, unless you receive permission for other alternatives, will be your only positioning option. Although chronic stress doesn't appear to contribute to the development of gestational diabetes, women often become stressed by the diagnosis, the increased need for prenatal visits, and daily monitoring of blood sugar, nutrition, and exercise. Include relaxation as a primary goal in your work.

Often, doctors and midwives recommend at least three exercise sessions lasting longer than 15 minutes each week to lessen insulin needs. The more pain-free you can help a client to be, the deeper her breathing, and the more energetic she is, the more likely she will accomplish this level of exercise, or more. Reduce musculoskeletal and swelling pain with postural guidance, myofascial and deep tissue techniques at pain sites, trigger point therapy, and other joint techniques. Take extra care with pressure on the extremities until glucose metabolism is stable, avoiding deep tissue techniques and any other deep compression. Help to maintain kidney and bladder health by teaching her to stimulate these organs' zones on her feet. (See Fig. 4-50 for locations.)

● HYPEREMESIS GRAVIDARUM

Morning sickness is a normal reaction to pregnancy. Persistent, uncontrollable nausea and vomiting beyond the 20th week of pregnancy (**hyperemesis gravidarum**) are not. Severe vomiting can cause weight loss, dehydration, and

---

> *My Story*
>
> *I was initially alarmed when I developed gestational diabetes, but my therapist helped calm me. She taught me to breathe more deeply, and I was better able to tune into my body signals. That helped me to better notice blood sugar fluctuations and to eat according to my nutritionist's guidelines.*
>
> —Andrea

serious imbalances for the mother that requires hospitalization. The resulting decrease in placental blood flow, growth restriction, and tendency toward preterm labor threatens the fetus.

Although the cause of hyperemesis is unclear, what is known is that those more likely to develop this condition include very young mothers, those who experienced problems in earlier pregnancies and in tolerating oral contraceptives, first-time moms and those with multiple gestations, obese women, and those with heartburn and hyperthyroidism. Medical treatment aims to help reduce and resolve dehydration, decrease nausea with medications, prevent malnutrition, and rest the entire body and the gut, often in the hospital (Ricci 2009).

In working with a client with this condition, use the left sidelying position to counteract decrease placental blood flow created by the hyperemesis. Some women are least nauseous in the semireclining position, as this takes pressure off of her stomach, so check with her doctor to see whether this is an acceptable position. Autonomic sedation is highly effective for such clients. (See Chapter 4 technique manual.)

The most specific technique to use is acupressure to the *Neiguan* point on the wrist (Fig. 7.4). Both perform and teach this technique to her and her family members (Ricci 2009). Help counteract dehydration by offering water before, during, and after your session, but only if she can tolerate it. Remember the connection between strong odors and nausea, and avoid them on you, your equipment, or in your work environment. Eliminate any rocking techniques, and tone down any other techniques so that you are not inadvertently rocking her. Keep a trashcan and a wipe-up towel accessible to her in case she does need to vomit. Some women need a nasal feeding tube to assure adequate nourishment; just work around the equipment, taking care not to disturb ports and tubes.

AMNIOTIC FLUID IMBALANCES

In less than 10% of pregnancies, fetuses float in either more or less amniotic fluid than the healthy ideal. Too much fluid (polyhydramnios or hydramnios) can be indicative of some type of fetal development anomalies. These fetuses are more likely to be born early, malpresent for birth, and have **umbilical cord prolapse**. Too little fluid (oligohydramnios), more common in weeks 32 to 36, can be the outcome of fetal kidney malfunction, a potentially life-threatening fetal condition. This also puts the fetus at greater risk of cord prolapse (Ricci 2009).

Left sidelying position is usually the safest massage therapy position when there are amniotic fluid imbalances. Because of the potential for preterm labor, avoid abdominal work and be especially careful to avoid any labor stimulation points. Performing a baby lift would be ill-advised with the increased possibility of cord prolapse. Be especially alert for any signs of preterm labor. Follow the other previous general guidelines.

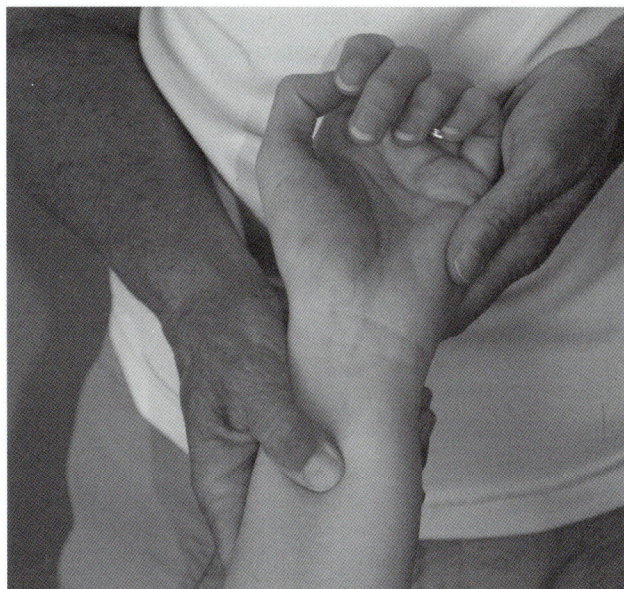

FIGURE 7.4 Acupressure relief for hyperemisis gravidarium. Locate the *Nei Guan* or PC-6 point that is between the flexor carpi radialis and the palmaris longus muscle tendons on the anterior surface of the forearm, 2 inches proximal to the wrist crease. Apply deep, rhythmic thumb or fingertip pressure to this point on each forearm four times daily for 10 minutes each application. Studies suggest that this can help to reduce severity and frequency of nausea.

ABNORMAL FETAL GROWTH OR MOVEMENT

About 10% of infants are large for gestational age (LGA or macrosomia), and another 10% are born small for gestational age (SGA). These deviations may be the result of genetic predisposition, or these newborns have perhaps developed above or below the norms due to maternal illness or other gestational conditions. Those who suffered **intrauterine growth restriction (IUGR)** had shortages of oxygen, nutrients, water, or other building blocks for growth result in smaller-than-expected fetuses (Gibbs et al. 2008). This stunting of growth can be due to placental insufficiencies, hypertension, poorly controlled insulin-dependent diabetes and other disease processes, or lifestyle choices such as tobacco and alcohol use.

In pregnancies involving twins or other multiples, it is common for one or all of the fetuses to be significantly smaller than normal. A smaller-than-normal fetus can also suggest that the growth of his body systems is not proceeding well. These smaller babies are at higher risk for premature birth, a more tenuous temperature and oxygen balance, and an infant more at risk.

Smaller fetuses often move less to conserve energy. Although their growth may remain normal, other babies indicate distress by reduced intrauterine movement. This distress could be the result of maternal use of medications, kidney and other fetal malfunctions, or just their own sleep cycles. Many women note that intrauterine movement typically stops during a fetus's 20 to 40 minutes sleep cycle and gradually increases at night. The quality and quantity of fetal movement is a general indicator of fetal well-being, so women often learn to attend closely to the swirling in their bellies.

The most important massage therapy adaptation for you to follow with abnormal fetal size or movement is the strict use of left sidelying position, unless you specifically discuss alternatives with her healthcare provider. The slight increase in fetal blood supply when lying on the left side is significant with a compromised fetus.

Sixty-seven percent of surveyed prenatal massage therapists reported their clients noticing a change in fetal activity during their sessions. Three-quarters of these therapists said there was an increase in kicks and squirming rather than a decrease (Osborne 2009). Likely this is less an actual increase in movement and more an example of the increased bodily awareness fostered during a focused session. Those who notice a decrease often interpret the stillness on the massage table as the baby relaxing too. Although this is certainly less than conclusive information to drive practice guidelines, you might want to consider the advisability of massage and be sure to consult with her healthcare provider for individualized guidance with SGA pregnancies.

It seems more likely that, in general, countering the effects of stressful factors on the expectant mother would be a healthy contribution to these pregnancies. Remember that under stress, blood supply to the baby can be as much as 65% less than when she is relaxed. (See Chapter 1 for full discussion of the autonomic nervous system during pregnancy.) Facilitate deep, relaxed breathing patterns and help to ground her in her physical experience. Offer her your respectful, knowledgeable, and compassionate ear, and a shoulder if needed. Don't forget that one of the stressors that your work can be most effect in directly reducing is pain, from whatever musculoskeletal source. By nurturing the mother, you can potentially help foster the normal growth and development of her baby.

● PREMATURE RUPTURE OF MEMBRANES

When the amniotic sack breaks prior to true labor, the fetus loses some or all of its watery cushion. In addition, an environment develops for the umbilical cord to prolapse, compressed between the mother's pelvis and the fetus, or for infection or placental abruptions to occur. "Broken waters" is most commonly associated with preterm births, and sometimes occurs even before 37 weeks, when it is officially called *preterm premature rupture of membranes* (PPROM) (Ricci 2009).

Once again, as a parasympathetic stimulator extraordinaire, you can help a woman to cope with the worry and fear a premature rupture usually creates. If the rupture occurs after 37 weeks, then consult with her healthcare provider about the advisability of helping to more naturally initiate labor through deliberate work on the labor-stimulating points. (See the section later in this chapter on overdue babies.) If prior to 37 weeks, then very diligently avoid any touch that might activate these points; avoid abdominal massage techniques (legal precaution), and do not perform the baby lift to avoid risk of umbilical cord prolapse. You may want to use additional towels or waterproof covering on your table just in case further leakage occurs during your session.

● PREMATURE LABOR

Chapter 2's precautions regarding abdominal massage should give you the guidance you need to work with women whose pregnancies are threatening an early end. In addition to those liability precautions regarding abdominal massage, remember to carefully avoid the labor-stimulating points, particularly on the feet and calves. Of course, you need to know not just about what not to do, but also what to do: help reduce the stress of a threatened early birth with parasympathetic arousal, deep relaxation breathing, and focused, caring nurturing (see Chapter 4 technique manual).

● GENETIC CONCERNS

Other than stress-reducing, relaxation techniques, no other specific massage therapy will be of notable benefit or harm when blood incompatibilities or other genetic concerns put a pregnancy at higher risk of complication. Follow the general recommendations made earlier in this chapter that apply to all prenatal medical conditions. Consult the online medical glossary for more examples of these conditions.

Women with Health Conditions that Increase Risks

> **REMINDER:** Although a woman may have a high-risk condition, in most cases she is still more likely to have a normal pregnancy than not.

Physicians consider a pregnancy to be high risk when there is a greater than average likelihood of increased complications, injury (morbidity), or death (mortality) for the mother, the baby, or both. Fortunately, the usual incidence of prenatal complications is generally low; therefore, even a woman at higher risk is still quite likely to have a normal pregnancy and a normal baby. Of course, the more of these conditions that a woman manages, the higher her risk becomes, and the more helpful nurturing, therapeutic massage might be (Fig. 7.5).

When you identify a higher-risk factor or that a woman is in a more vulnerable group, review the types of complications

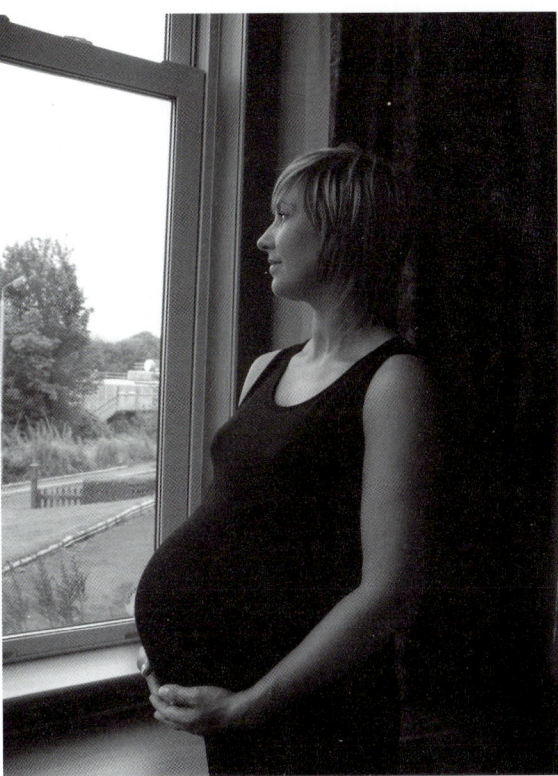

FIGURE 7.5 Coping with high-risk conditions. Taking time for reflection, journaling, recreation, and massage therapy may help women manage the additional stress of a pregnancy at risk for developing complications.

that might occur and their typical signs and then be extra alert for them. Work conservatively with those managing riskier conditions and situations because of the greater likelihood that a complication may occur. If you have any doubt about a woman's prenatal health, then modify your work as described in this chapter as if the complication has occurred. These high-risk and vulnerable group categories include maternal health conditions as well as the psychosocial, sociodemographic, and environmental factors listed in Box 7.3. The online medical resources include definitions and more detailed descriptions.

> **REMINDER:** Asthma is one of the most common and potentially serious medical conditions that might result in complications to a pregnancy.

Of course, every woman will uniquely respond to the pleasures and problems that her pregnancy brings. Not every teen or employee of a chemical company will develop medical complications, but the possibility is higher. Being aware of these increased risks, your work can help reduce the odds of complications through stress reduction and other appropriate somatic work. See online resources at http://thePoint.lww.com/Osborne-Pregnancy2e for some particular massage therapy approaches for women with these situations.

What Would You Do?

You have been working on a low-risk, no-complications client regularly throughout her pregnancy when she calls to tell you she's been on bed rest for the last 2 weeks to hopefully control her increasing blood pressure. Her doctor recommends her spending only 2 to 4 hours total each day up. She is in her 32nd week, and she has been having more headaches than normal for her. She is also starting to experience some sinus congestion, heartburn, and, of course, generalized achiness due to lack of activity. What other information and communications do you need prior to working with her now? On what areas of her body will you now need to take additional precautions? What types of modifications? How will you position her for her massage?

My Story

Because I was carrying triplets, I was on total bed rest from week 22 until their birth at 35 weeks. I got so stir-crazy and was either in pain or generally achy all the time. The last weeks I got by with my massages—they were the highlight of each week. I never would have carried my babies as long without it; massage helped me maintain the pregnancies and my sanity.

—Kristen

Situations Requiring Special Sensitivity or Consideration

Although some pregnancies are difficult due to medical complications or the threat of those developing, other women also need special considerations when they are pregnant. These women are those who have not conceived through sexual intercourse, have physical limitations, traumatic childhoods, or less common family structures. Women from some religious and ethnic groups have expectations and limitations that you need to be sensitive to, as well.

● WORKING WITH WOMEN UNDERGOING INFERTILITY TREATMENT

Technological advances have made pregnancy possible for the 6 million **infertile** American men and women of reproductive age who previously had to accept childlessness. Male and female fertility drugs, in vitro fertilization, egg and/or sperm donation, surgery and other technologies (see online

Box 7.3

Factors Placing a Woman at Risk During Pregnancy

Note: the following content is adapted from Ricci 2009, p. 527.

Biophysical Factors
Genetic conditions, chromosomal abnormalities, multiple pregnancy, inherited disorders, blood incompatibility, and hematological disorders such as iron deficiency anemia, thalassemia and sickle cell anemia, cardiovascular disease and disorders including congenital heart disease and dysrhythmias, chronic hypertension, renal and thyroid diseases, large fetal size, medical and obstetric conditions, preterm or post-term labor, placental, cervical and uterine abnormalities and fibroids, infections such as urinary tract infections, cytomegalovirus, rubella, herpes simplex virus, hepatitis B, varicella zoster virus, paravirus B19, group B streptococcus, and toxoplasmosis, HIV/AIDS and sexually transmitted infections, diabetes, maternal collagen and connective tissue disorders such as rheumatoid arthritis, multiple sclerosis, systemic lupus erythematosus (SLE), scleroderma, thrombophilias, and other diseases, asthma and other respiratory diseases and infections, inadequate nutrition, food fads, overeating, eating disorder, underweight or overweight status.

Psychosocial Factors
Smoking, caffeine, alcohol, many prescription, over-the-counter, and recreational drugs, victims of falls and vehicular accidents, inadequate support system, situation crisis, current or history of violence or childhood sexual abuse, emotional distress, depression or other prenatal affective (mood) disorders, unsafe cultural practices or risky or unhealthy lifestyles.

Sociodemographic Factors
Poverty, lack or accessibility of prenatal care, age under 15 or over 35, all first pregnancies and more than five pregnancies, unmarried, nonwhite ethnicity, victims of natural disasters and warfare.

Environmental Factors
Infections, radiation, pesticides, industrial or household pollutants and chemicals, and other substances that can cause physical defects in utero (**teratogens**), second-hand cigarette smoke, personal stress.

---

medical glossary) can help women to successfully conceive and birth longed-for babies (Ricci 2009).

While your client is undergoing treatment in hopes of conceiving, you can be a valuable complementary part of her healthcare team. The emotional, time, and financial investment that she and her partner, if there is one, make can be enormous; the stress and exhaustion that result can significantly increase her need for relaxation and reassurance.

Below are some suggestions as to how you can help such clients:

- Help her to learn to relax and breathe deeply into her abdomen, focusing on reducing soft tissue restrictions on her breathing and posture, and engage her inner sensitivity and body awareness.
- Perform abdominal and pelvic techniques that reduce myofascial restriction and congestion in these areas (see Chapter 6 technique manual and online resources).
- Time your use of these deeper abdominal techniques to the 10 to 14 days of her cycle after her period has begun, and before her expected ovulation time.
- Between anticipated ovulation and conception or her period, it is best to not massage the abdomen at all, to avoid any possible liability implications.
- If she has a history of miscarriages, avoid abdominal work of any type, but only for liability reasons. Be extra vigilant near and on labor-stimulating points.

● SURROGATE MOTHERS

In vitro and other fertility methods have made possible the gestation of a baby within the uterus of a woman other than the biological mother (surrogacy). Women agree to offer their healthy bodies to a woman or couple who cannot successfully carry to term, sometimes with financial compensation and sometimes as a generous gift. Working with these pregnancies requires a delicacy of relational finesse and emotional awareness. Striking the balance between her connection with the pregnancy and a frequently expressed need to keep some emotional distance for the baby she will not raise can be challenging. Use your active listening skills to learn how she is feeling about the pregnancy. Take your cues from her about how much or little she prefers to connect with the fetus. In some cases, you will interact with or perform massages for both the biological and the surrogate mother. In that case, it is helpful to clearly determine upfront who your client is: surrogate, biological mother, or both.

My Story

I have found that it is really difficult following an unsuccessful in vitro or early miscarriage for women to return and be in my treatment room with the baby and pregnancy images I have all around. I have given women the option to use another treatment room until they felt ready to come back to my room. Even with these sensitive options offered, it is often emotionally difficult for them to return the first time.

—Linda Hickey, Calgary, AB

BEING RESPONSIVE TO DIVERSITY

Today's families are less exclusively the nuclear unit of a wife, husband, and their children living together that they were 50 years ago. Unmarried, separated, and same-sex couples and single women are having babies with greater frequency, although they are still less than 50% of expectant women. As you intake your prenatal clients, learn who is in her circle of support and what their roles are. Tailor your verbal interaction to use appropriate references to these people. "Friends" and "family" can work with single women, and "partner" is usually a safe term to use in reference to a significant other until you hear her use a different label. If you find that you have irreconcilable difficulties with providing positive support to one group of partners or another, be sure to refer these women to another therapist for their massage therapy (Pepper 2005).

Avoid stereotyping your clients, but be alert to cultural differences in addition to personal styles and preferences. For example, women of some cultures are often more accustomed to labor support from other women, particularly their own mothers. Some cultures prize a quiet stoicism with respect to labor pain, whereas others are more accepting of loud expression during labor. Many cultures have prohibitions on body exposure and touch, particularly when males are present, that can influence your client care with these women (Kitzinger 1995) (see online resources for how cultural beliefs can affect maternal health).

Women who are offering their newborns for adoption require similar delicacy as surrogate mothers. Seldom do they make this decision casually or easily. They often have deeply conflicted feelings about their pregnancies. Their desire to do what is best for their child often leads to the adoption decision, but that same instinct can make it hard to nurture themselves and their fetus without becoming too painfully attached. Again, you will need to take your cue from her body language and her words as to how to walk the thin line between celebrating the pregnancy and making its outcome more difficult for her.

What Would You Do?

You are considering volunteering at a facility that serves unwed teenage mothers. What risk factors and special needs are you likely to encounter in this situation? What types of technique and positioning modifications might you make in response to those concerns? What can you do to connect with her fetus in a welcoming, reassuring way, while respecting your client's situation if she is considering putting the baby up for adoption?

MOTHERS WITH DISABILITIES AND OTHER CHALLENGES

Women with joint injuries and inflammation, especially those with rheumatoid arthritis, have special prenatal needs. Although at least half of pregnant women with rheumatoid arthritis have less severe symptoms than when nonpregnant, their options for pain management through usual medications are limited (Gibbs et al. 2008). You can help to maintain more comfortable joint spaces in arthritic or damaged joints by reducing soft tissue restriction around these joints. Use localized heat or cold applications for painful or swollen joints, taking care with heat especially in the first trimester. A woman with excessive ligamental laxity may have similar problems prenatally, though she needs joint compression rather than distraction and stretching when you work with her joints.

All of these conditions might limit some women from labor positions such as squatting due to joint restrictions. As an alternative, suggest assisted squatting on a birth ball and/or apply the pelvic press to help widen the pelvic outlet. Other spine and pelvic dysfunctions require special attention to labor positioning too. For example, those with lumbar or thoracic disc herniation fare best semireclined with lumbar support or sidelying rather than squatting, with their knees to chest or on hands and knees as these positions tend to flex the spine, putting pressure on vulnerable disc areas (Boissonnault 2002).

Your work with women with **cerebral palsy** and other neurological challenges proceeds well in the sidelying position. The flexed position helps to reduce spasticity, and deep tissue sculpting works well for those areas. Joint mobilizations need to be extremely subtle and slow to avoid triggering muscle spasm. Firm, slow Swedish work is good, too. These women benefit from breathing practice and directed breathing activities from early in their pregnancies on. They may need more assistance getting on and off your table and for rolling over; often they do best going to hands and knees to change to the other side (Checca 1998).

When depressed or anxious women become pregnant or develop these mood disorders prenatally, a cloud hangs over their pregnancy. Depressed mood dampens the joy and excitement of a new life, increases her fatigue, and can make it difficult for her to care for herself and her fetus appropriately. Anxiety commonly accompanies depression, creating excessive worry about negative outcomes that can lead to elaborate routines to attempt to manage the anxiety. These women are more likely to use drugs and have poorer nutrition (Gibbs et al. 2008). They are more likely to be nauseous, and their babies are often born small and early (Li et al. 2008).

Your work with an anxious and/or depressed expectant woman can help to ease some of these negative effects. Focus on reducing pain and promoting parasympathetic arousal. Help her to breathe deeply and fully. Postural guidance can be more difficult as slumped posture is a natural expression of suppressed mood; nevertheless, help her to see how a more vertical, spacious posture can potentially help to lift her mood.

One study of massage with depressed second trimester women documented reduced back and leg pain, lower levels of stress-related neurotransmitters, and less reported anxiety. Their babies were less likely to be premature and scored better on newborn assessment scales than control babies whose mothers were also depressed but only received relaxation guidance prenatally (Field et al. 2004).

● SURVIVORS OF CHILDHOOD SEXUAL ABUSE

Women who survive **childhood sexual abuse** usually experience lifelong impacts of this type of violence. Pregnancy and birthing trigger many possible reactions. One woman might finally feel normal and relish the nurturing and closeness pregnancy can bring with her partner and her baby. Another might feel victimized again by her fetus taking control of her body. Very traumatized women who have dissociated from their bodily sensations to cope can be unaware of their pregnancies for many months, or even until giving birth. Many prenatal complications are associated with childhood sexual abuse (Simkin and Klaus 2004).

Engorged genital tissues and enlarging breasts and belly can bring harrowing attention to a woman's sexual organs. The innately sexual nature of gestation, labor, and birth can stir uncomfortable feelings and memories. Childhood sexual abuse survivors can find vaginal exams and other routine diagnostic procedures invasive and reminiscent of the violation. Loss of control in its various manifestations during pregnancy and birthing can be retraumatizing.

On the other hand, pregnancy and childbirth presents an opportunity for a woman to further heal from early trauma. With understanding, supportive caregivers and family, she can potentially reclaim control, pride, and strength in her own body and its resiliency and creative power. She can come from these 9 months with a healthy baby and healthier self-esteem (Simkin and Ancheta 2011).

> **REMINDER:** *Pregnancy and birthing has the potential to retraumatize or promote healing for survivors of childhood sexual abuse.*

When both tissue and feeling need to heal from abuse, you can be an ideal facilitator. Your scope of practice includes respectful, healing touch, education on body structure and function, and awareness of the body and the connection between feeling states, memories, and physical experience

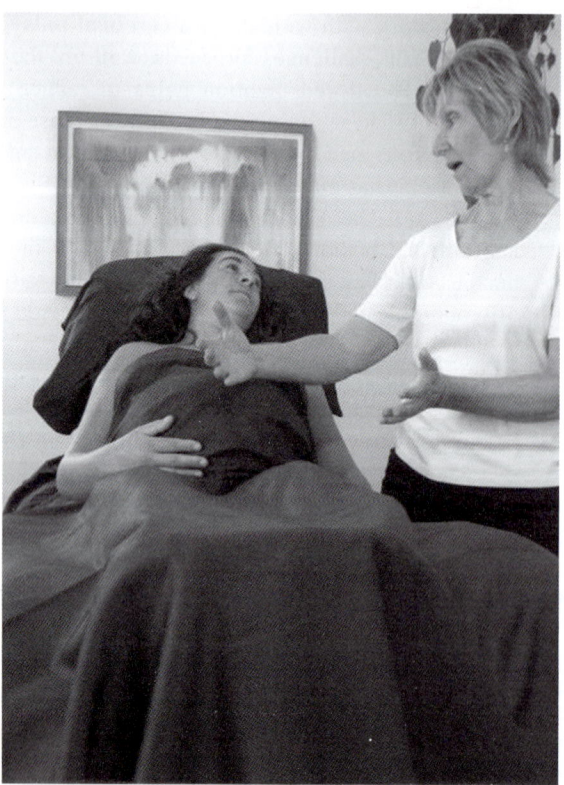
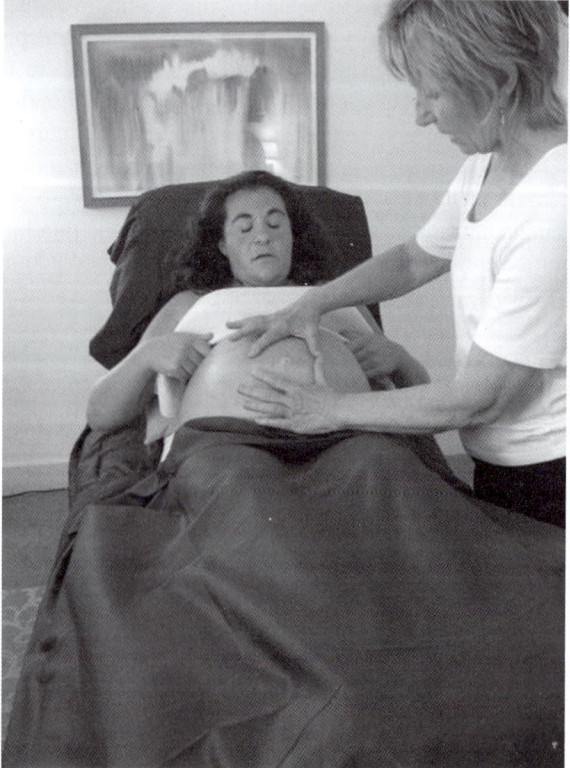

FIGURE 7.6 Education is empowering. When clients are more self-aware and learn about the brilliant adaptations that their bodies make to nurture life, they are often more actively engaged in their own care and their labors.

(Fig. 7.6). Appropriate massage and bodywork can help pregnant survivors to reduce anxiety and pain; reach deeper relaxation states, improve body awareness, and embody positive touch experiences; resolve and discharge unproductive traumatic memories and feelings; and physically and emotionally prepare for childbirth and mothering (Simkin and Klaus 2004).

Many abuse survivors will appreciate your work alone or as an adjunct to other forms of counseling. For best results, you should seek communications with her entire team of healthcare providers (see Chapter 8 and online resources for further guidelines for your work).

Working with Labor Complications

As you nurture your clients through birthing their babies, several complications may develop. When labors stall, massage therapy can help reduce the maternal distress that is frequently at the root of the problem. Women whose labors stall or are prolonged and who are beyond their due date may be advised to consider medical induction and/or augmentation procedures. Massage therapy offers a viable complement or alternative to pharmacological interventions, and it may help women to cope with the intensity and stress these procedures may create (Simkin and Ancheta 2011). At the opposite extreme, when a labor proceeds exceedingly rapidly, your work can help her to manage the intensity and speed of this type of labor experience. In either case, you will need to work closely and cooperatively with her and her partner and her doctor or midwife regarding how to help her get the best outcome possible.

● LABOR DYSTOCIA

Sometimes, a woman's cervix takes a prolonged time to dilate or it stops dilation in the active phase of labor. In other labors, the pushing phase is protracted or stalled. This is called **dystocia**.

Other terms commonly used to describe when labor progresses slower than "normal" include arrested labor, dysfunctional labor, or failure to progress,.

Regardless of the label given or its cause, these women and their partners usually feel very frustrated and disheartened when this occurs, and they are usually frightened. How a woman handles this difficulty, and your role in that, largely depends on her care provider's approach. Some prenatal care providers are proponents of very active management of women's labors. At the other end of the spectrum, when the mother and the fetus show no signs of distress, others wait to let the natural process unfold (Simkin and Ancheta 2011).

One of your greatest contributions to a labor will be to help maintain and reactivate the natural progression of the birth. Perform the following techniques to assist in this goal, referring to Chapters 4 and 5 for procedural steps for some:

- Use soothing, grounded, centering, and rhythmic touch, and craniosacral therapy to maintain parasympathetic arousal before and during labor.
- Help her maintain deep, relaxed abdominal breathing.
- Help the perineal sphincters to relax by helping her to maintain a relaxed jaw. Use sculpting on the temporalis and masseter, suggest exhaling through her mouth, encourage deep-pitched sounds, and try the toe squeeze.
- Reduce or eliminate painful sensations, and help her conserve energy by encouraging relaxation, and acknowledge her progress.
- Use the labor and relaxation techniques in earlier chapters to counter the fight, flight, freeze response to her distress.
- Intensify the "tend and befriend" response to stress and support oxytocin production by maintaining close, supportive physical contact with the mother, or have her partner do so too, as long as she desires it (Moberg 2003).
- Use zone therapy to the entire foot, pressing deeply into the uterus points on the medial calcaneus, to support uterine contractions.
- Press rhythmically and deeply on the labor stimulation reflex points throughout the body. (Figs. 2.7 and 2.8)
- Try out a variety of gravity-assisted positions, walking, bathing or showering, and rhythmic activities.

● INDUCTION AND AUGMENTATION

Ideally, labor begins spontaneously, and the laboring woman's own physiology energizes and directs the progress to a healthy baby and a satisfied mother. When medical conditions warrant, or sometimes for convenience of mother or staff, nonpharmacological and medical procedures can start and maintain labor progress (see online medical glossary for definitions of common procedures). When labor is started (**induction**) or sustained (**augmentation**) in these ways, other interventions generally are more likely to follow, including cesarean birth, forceps or vacuum assistance, epidural, and admission to the neonatal intensive care unit (NICU) for the newborn (Ricci 2009).

With a client scheduled for induction, check to see if she and her healthcare provider want a trial of nonpharmacological induction methods. In a small pilot study of 142 postdue women, those who learned to massage specific Shiatsu points were 17% more likely to spontaneously begin labor (Ingram et al. 2005). Concentrate on the labor stimulation points from Asian medicine, and teach her where and how she and her partner can work with these several times daily for 2 to 5 days prior to the scheduled induction (see Chapter 5, labor technique manual).

Confirm and improve her ability to breathe deeply to her baby. Encourage or lead her into deep relaxation, visualizations of birth, and clearing of any hesitations or apprehensions (see Chapter 4 techniques on relaxation and nurturing) (Fig. 7.7).

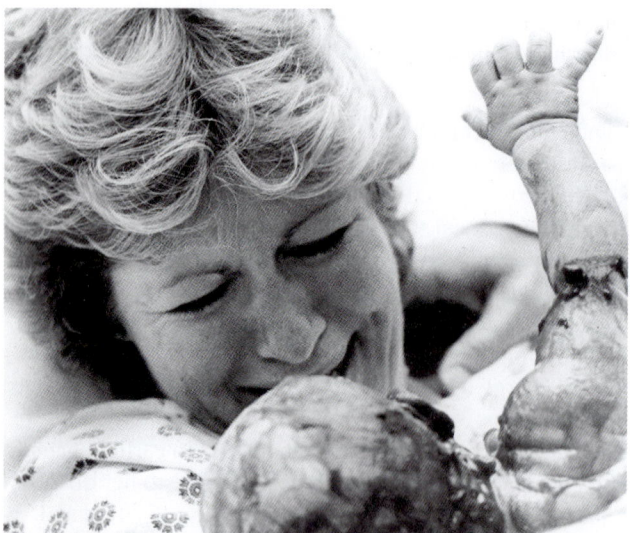

FIGURE 7.7 Welcoming the new mother and baby. Your nurturing care may help a woman triumph over the length and intensity of her labor, and improve her immediate and long-term satisfaction with her birth experience. (Photo used by permission of Harriette Hartigan. www.harriettehartigan.com)

● RAPID LABOR

Some expectant women might think that the perfect labor is one that lasts only 1 to 3 hours (**precipitous labor**). Because this usually happens only when the perineal tissues are soft and readily stretchable, the mother usually fares well physically in such a sprint. However, the fetus has more potential for head or nerve trauma and lack of oxygen due to contractions that are so rapid that the uterus doesn't relax fully between contractions (Ricci 2009).

Moreover, the surprise, intensity, and pain of managing rapid labor, can result in a panicked, discouraged, and/or angry laboring woman. After all, if such painful, fast contractions are what she starts with, thinking of 12 to 18 hours of worsening contractions can make even the most confident woman frightened. Often, her partner or caregivers don't accept that this is the real thing; sometimes, she doesn't either because it is so different from the normal gradual process she has prepared for. One description for this type of labor is that it is like a whole labor of transition phase, with erratic labor patterns, little rest time between contractions, and lots of anxious energy.

A woman in rapid labor needs your focused attention to help her cope, more than helping her relax. You need to think fast on your feet and usually keep your hands on. Because of its rapidity, finding and maintaining a rhythmic ritual for riding the contractions can become a struggle. Penny Simkin describes a "take-charge routine" that is an excellent format for assisting in this and any especially challenging labor situation. Its foundation is firm, calm, confident, and kind guidance that can help her regain a rhythmic response. In some ways, this is the demeanor that you always have with your clients, except in this case your aim is to take charge until she is able to regroup. Stay close and speak and act in a manner that is confident, kind, and optimistic. Gently insist that she open her eyes, and use rhythmic talk or touch to help her pace her breathing and vocalization (Simkin 2008).

Bilateral compression on her feet, legs, or shoulders is particularly effective. Look for where she may be tensing against the pain, and hold there. Pay particular attention to your own grounding so that your pressure comes from the earth through your core. If your touch is disconnected, segmented, and weak from isolated hand or pectoral use, it will not convey the power, stability, and solidity that she needs; remember the laboring mind sensitivity to these nonverbal cues? Shift your weight from your feet into your hands, relax your own shoulders, and deepen your breath. (See Chapter 3 body mechanics) Fluidly undulate your torso or your arm to visually or kinesthetically remind her of her lost rhythm. Between contractions, you might need to suggest a position change to side-lying or some other non–gravity-assisted position to reduce the gravitational and fetal pressure against the cervix.

While not in your scope of practice, be prepared, as a Good Samaritan, for the slim but real possibility that you must assist a precipitous birth. If her partner and medical personnel are not available, call 911 if the birth seems imminent at her home. Enlist other motorists to do so if you are in a car. As you await their arrival, reassure the mother, remain calm, and turn up any source of heat in cool or cold weather. Encourage her not to actively push by panting or blowing lightly with her chin up when she feels the pushing urge, and have her lie on her side.

Wash your hands thoroughly if possible and prepare to safely catch the baby and keep him warm. Wipe his face as it emerges. Tear away any membranes or other tissue that could obstruct his first breaths when the vagina no longer compresses his lungs. If he does not breathe spontaneously within seconds after his birth, wipe him again, rub him briskly, and slap his feet. Get his head a bit lower than his lungs to help drain any fluids, with nothing obstructing his nose or mouth, preferably covered on his mother for warmth. Do not cut or tug on the cord. While it is still pulsing, it is his back-up oxygen source until he starts breathing reliably on his own.

Save the placenta if possible for later medical evaluation. Perform fundal massage (see Chapter 6 technique manual), place the baby to the breast, or have her or her partner stimulate her nipples, all to help the uterus contract and prevent hemorrhage (Simkin 2008).

Postpartum Support for Women with Unexpected Outcomes

Obstetric emergencies, such as **umbilical cord prolapse**, placental abruption, **uterine rupture**, and **amniotic fluid**

embolisms, are fairly uncommon. These conditions pose serious maternal and fetal risks, and they will challenge your support capabilities. More common, but still relatively unusual, babies experience birth trauma resulting in cerebral palsy or other injuries, have congenital abnormalities, are stillborn (**intrauterine fetal demise**), or die within hours or days of their birth.

By some estimates, almost all women are somewhat disappointed with their labor and birth experiences. Thankfully, most of them are not coping with such serious or tragic outcomes to their pregnancies, although miscarriage rates are as high as 20% of known pregnancies. For these mothers, and those who chose to terminate their pregnancies, the following support guidelines are also appropriate.

Whenever an emergency, injury, illness, or death occurs, you should make phone contact with your client at least once. Consider whether a home or a hospital visit seems appropriate, particularly if she is a regular client, and check to see whether she would like a visit. You may not necessarily massage her at that time, but be a comforting and compassionate support for her.

● INFANTS WITH SPECIAL NEEDS AND FETAL/INFANT DEATH

Injury, illness, prematurity, low birth weight, or congenital abnormalities usually mean a stay in the NICU. A mother whose infant needs intensive care anguishes over her fragile newborn fighting for his life. She may feel shocked, guilty, and torn between bonding with him and distancing herself, hoping to minimize her pain if he dies. Hopes for his survival and worries about whether he will be normal turn what she anticipated as a joyful time into an anxious ordeal. Often, she is grieving over the loss of the ideal infant she dreamed of and suffering separation from her infant. She may struggle relentlessly to protect and save him, often ignoring her own postpartum care. These women need safe, supportive situations in which to express these feelings and meaningful help and information from others (see support agencies in online resources at http://thePoint.lww.com/Osborne-Pregnancy2e).

The unimaginable is a horrific reality for those 15% of women who have stillbirths, or whose infants die shortly after birth, or within the first year (Gilbert and Harmon 2003). These women, as well as those who lose their fetuses to spontaneous abortion, and even many of those who choose abortion, often grieve long and deeply over their losses while still physically coping with postpartum recovery.

Postpartum massage therapy techniques can assist a woman with a sick infant or a loss as she adjusts physiologically and emotionally. Full-body sessions of Swedish or passive movement methods can convey a sense of wholeness, as do craniosacral and other energetic work. Focus on the same types of physiological recovery as those mothers with healthy infants. Devote yourself to nurturing her, easing postpartum pain, and building her strength and stability through reorganizing and reinforcing her postural and functional integrity. If you can facilitate her rapid physical recovery, she can focus on her emotional process. (Chapter 6 technique manual)

One technique that can bridge physical and emotional recovery is the wrapping technique described in Figure 6.3. Be extra alert for an emotional response to this technique if some unexpected outcome occurred. Massaging a body area where she feels the loss of her baby can prompt her tears and other emotional responses. Common areas are her abdomen, chest, and arms. When this occurs, you must offer her compassionate, caring attention without prying. Because she has experienced such deep loss, her feelings range the spectrum in intensity and texture. Some women completely inhibit their grief, and others delay feeling it to "take care of business," usually another infant or older child.

Appropriate care after emergencies and losses requires great sensitivity and sometimes more time. Be flexible in your scheduling if possible to accommodate her need to talk. When you interact with her, avoid minimizing her grief with well-intended, but insensitive, comments such as "It was meant to be" or "You can always have another." Here are some alternatives: attentive silence; a heartfelt, "I'm so sorry," with a comforting touch; holding her as she talks and/or cries; "What can I do to help you?"; encouraging her expression without prying; or reflecting back to her what you are hearing her say (Gilbert and Harmon 2003). Many women have a deep need to tell and retell their labor and birth story, as though repeating it can make some sense of it. Another way to provide ample time for this is to continue your work on areas such as her feet or hands while she talks. Focus on helping her to feel more connected and grounded, in addition to soothing her through the pleasure of a foot massage.

Each woman, her partner, and their family will grieve in their own individual way. Her cultural and spiritual beliefs will also determine how she responds and copes. Despite these individualities, the typical path in grief recovery moves through denial, sadness, anger, and reconciliation. As her massage therapist, you are an ideal professional to nurture, soothe, and support her as she navigates that journey. Try to identify where she is in this process, and match your care of her to the phase. Respect her need to "keep a stiff upper lip," with quiet nurturing. Help her to open her throat and her breath for full expression when she is seething with anger. (See active listening and somatoemotional integration techniques in Chapter 4's online technique manual.) Consult the support agencies listed in the online Resources.

● POSTPARTUM AFFECTIVE DISORDERS

Mental health disorders are among the most common postpartum complications (Dalfen 2009). The potential negative

> **My Story**
>
> *I first came to my massage therapist, Nanci, after an unexpected 2nd trimester pregnancy loss. I was devastated and felt totally out of sync: body, mind, and spirit. Through massage, Nanci used her healing hands to bring me back to a hopeful place. She helped to cleanse the stress and grief out of my body and to cope with the hormonal changes that affected me physically and emotionally. My muscles relaxed, my circulation improved significantly, and I was able to slowly emerge from a deep depression. When I became pregnant again, I was very anxious. Thankfully, Nanci was there for me throughout the entire pregnancy, knowing how to work through the usual aches and pains, but more importantly, offering her healing touch to control my stress and to help make me strong and resilient. Nanci's massage therapy brought me a stronger sense of connectedness to my pregnancies and to all the changes I experienced."*
>
> —Anonymous Mother

impact on mothers, babies, families, and society is far reaching. Time with an infant should be among the most wonderful in a woman's life, despite the expected ups and downs. When it isn't, women need support, options for treatment, and strategies to help cope and heal. Prenatal and postpartum massage therapy can be an integral part of that support. One small study suggests that even pregnant women diagnosed with major depression who received weekly prenatal massage had reduced depression prenatally and postpartum. Their newborns were also less likely to be born prematurely and low birthweight, and had better neonatal adjustment (Field et al. 2010). To provide appropriate care, you need a basic understanding of the various conditions, heightened awareness of the symptoms, and techniques and strategies for helping these clients to recovery.

Physicians consider postpartum mental illnesses to result from hormonal influences on neurotransmitter uptake in the brain's nerve synapses. This imbalance in brain chemistry makes a woman more susceptible to the difficult effects of psychological stresses, lack of support from family or friends, disappointments, the stresses of infant care and normal life challenges, or unrealistic expectations of birth and postpartum life with her baby. She is especially vulnerable if she has a history of chronic or recurring depression, bipolar disorder, or anxiety disorder, or was depressed during pregnancy. Young maternal age, the baby's health, family history of mental disorders, and her own history of premenstrual syndrome correlate as well. Women with a tendency toward negative, absolute, anxious, and perfectionist thinking are more vulnerable, as are those with a history of physical or emotional abuse (Dalfen 2009).

Postpartum depression, anxiety disorders, posttraumatic stress disorder, and psychosis are the main categories of affective disorders. The distinction between the "baby blues" and postpartum depression has been discussed in Chapter 6. Depression is a more common condition than the other disorders covered below. Anxiety disorders result in new moms who excessively worry about everything or have panic attacks, with terrifying physical symptoms such as pounding heart and shortness of breath. A small percentage of new mothers attempt to manage their anxiety with repetitive actions and thoughts and develop obsessive-compulsive disorder. If her labor was fraught with danger and she feels disempowered from the events, this trauma can lead her to nightmares and flashbacks, as well as avoidance of her baby. The most severe of mental health emergencies only occurs in about 1% of postpartum women. Suicidal or homicidal thoughts, mania, and losing touch with reality are the rare but disastrous result.

Be alert and responsive to any indication of severe emotional distress in your clients. Warning signs of postpartum mental illness include the following:

- Difficulty in getting out of bed and accomplishing normal tasks
- Rapid weight gain or loss
- Sustained use of alcohol, sedatives, or other medications
- Lack of involvement, attention, and pleasure in caring for their infant
- Serious accidents related to fatigue or inattention
- Planning or attempting injury to herself or others
- Uncontrollable crying and mood shifts (Dalfen 2009)

Advise women with any symptom of postpartum complications to consult with their physician or midwife. Ask them to provide written release for massage therapy. Make resources in your community and reference books on mental health routinely available to all of your maternity clientele. (See online resources at http://thePoint.lww.com/Osborne-Pregnancy2e for books and agencies to recommend.)

Massage therapy has great potential for mothers suffering postpartum affective disorders. It can provide meaningfully nurturing time away from the stresses of daily life. It calms and soothes through parasympathetic stimulation. She may learn how to tune into her body more, and you can guide her to focus on pleasurable and positive body sensations. Less physical pain lessens the difficulties she is coping with. Deep, full breathing is the physiological foundation of mental health and well-being. Teach her simple massage techniques for her baby that she can easily incorporate into other infant care such as bathing and diapering (Fig. 7.8). When depressed mothers massage their infants, they minimize the negative effects of other neglectful care (Field 1996).

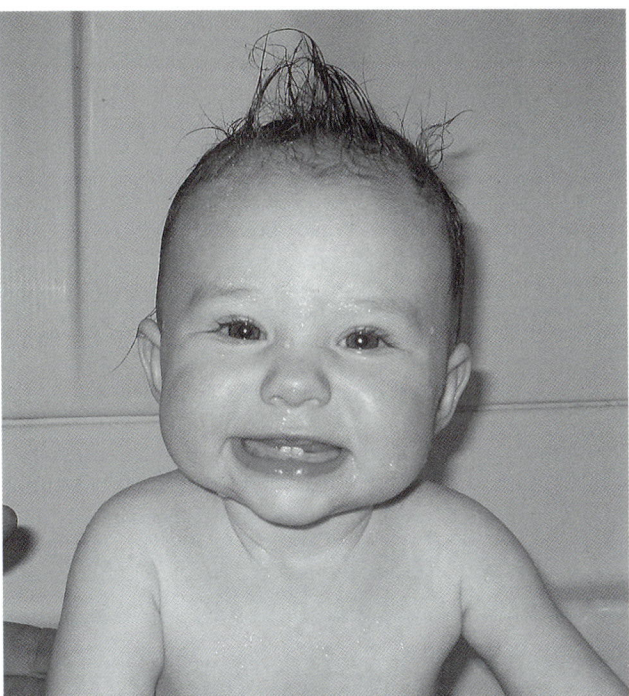

FIGURE 7.8 Overcoming postpartum complications. Massage therapy complements appropriate treatment for women suffering postpartum complications so that they usually can recover and their babies can thrive.

● PHYSICAL POSTPARTUM COMPLICATIONS

Although affective disorders are the most common postpartum complications, the most lethal are physical. Excessive blood loss (hemorrhaging), blood clots, inflamed and obstructed blood vessels, thromboembolisms of the lungs, and various postpartum infections are the leading postpartum causes of maternal death and injury (Ricci 2009). When the uterus doesn't contract and retract to involve normally (**uterine atony**) or retains portions of the defunct placenta, excessive bleeding can result. Placental malattachment can result in postpartum uterine damage and rupture (**placental accreta, increta, and percreta**). Trauma to the urogenital tract during birth and abnormal coagulation are other sources of excessive bleeding. Thrombi can develop in superficial, deep, and pulmonary vessels. Uterine infection and scar infection resulting from cesarean section, episiotomy, or any genital or perineal laceration can also occur. Urinary tract infections and breast inflammations (mastitis) are the most common and, fortunately, the least threatening sources of maternal fevers. Consult Box 7.4 for a summary of postpartum warning signs and see the online medical glossary for further details about each.

Each of these complications necessitates communication with a client's healthcare provider for individualized care,

> ### Box 7.4
> ### Warning Signs of Postpartum Complications
> - Heat, swelling or pain in the calves, particularly unilateral
> - Sudden onset of difficulty breathing, shortness of breath, chest pain, disorientation
> - Excessive, bright red or foul smelling lochia, after the first week
> - Redness, swelling and/or pus at cesarean or perineal stitches
> - Painful, burning urination and/or low back pain unchanged by activity
> - Heat, hyperemia, and tenderness in breast
> - Difficulty with normal life routines, especially sleep and eating
> - Prolonged period of intense sadness, emotional distress or lack of emotion
> - Rapid weight gain or loss
> - Sustained use of alcohol, sedatives or other drugs
> - Planning or attempting injury to herself or others

usually after these conditions resolve. You should not attempt to diagnose or treat any of these conditions. Reflexive work on the appropriate zones of the feet may promote health in these problematic areas, and you can best use them preventatively. Teach her to work the breast zones while she is feeding and to perform daily breast massage to prevent milk duct infections (see Chapter 6 for instructions).

If a client shows signs of possible uterine hemorrhage, have someone immediately call her doctor or 911 while you begin massage of the uterine fundus (see Chapter 6 for instructions). Continue this massage until you feel the uterus firming up against your fingers. Continue to check it periodically and massage again if it has become soft until she is in medical care.

CHAPTER SUMMARY

Because you will primarily work with women having normal, uncomplicated pregnancies and more usual conditions surrounding them, this book focuses on those clients. This chapter should serve as a springboard for empowering you to consider clients' special needs and for furthering your understanding of the medical side of childbearing. Consult the online medical glossary and include an obstetrical textbook in your library for when clients have medical conditions. Take childbirth education courses and attend maternity seminars and workshops. By being more fully prepared for these more worrisome and difficult situations, you will be more able to confidently relax and trust that you can care for all of your prenatal and perinatal clients.

Test Yourself

For answers, visit the website at http://thePoint.LWW.com/Osborne-Pregnancy2e!

1. List five symptoms of the most common prenatal medical complications.

2. List three general adaptations to prenatal massage when complications occur, and the most important adaptation for each of the following specific conditions: gestational hypertension, hyperemesis gravidarum, and abnormal fetal growth.

3. List three additional safety precautions when working with a client on bed rest, and three techniques that are likely to be helpful to her.

4. List five of the most common and/or serious risk factors that can increase a woman's chances of developing a medical complication during her pregnancy.

5. Explain three of the possible effects of childhood sexual abuse on expectant and laboring women.

6. What is prodromal labor, and how can you best help prevent and reduce its negative effects?

7. What are the most common physical and emotional complications that can develop postpartum?

8. List five warning signs of postpartum complications.

9. Summarize a research study mentioned in this chapter that offers some validation of massage therapy's usefulness with prenatal and perinatal special needs.

REFERENCES

Boissonnault J. Modifying labor and delivery positions for women with spine and pelvic ring dysfunction. Phys Ther J Sect Womens Health 2002;26:9–13.

Checca J, Appel C, and Frahm J. The Challenge of Labor and Birth in the Woman with a Spinal Cord Injury. JSOWH, March 1998, 22;1:9–17.

Dalfen A. When Baby Brings the Blues: Solutions for Postpartum Depression. Mississauga: John Wiley and Sons, 2009.

Ezner S. Reflexology: A Tool for Midwives. Pymble, Australia: Suzanne Ezner, 2000.

Field T, Diego M, Hernandez-Reif M, et al. Pregnancy massage reduces prematurity, low birthweight and postpartum depression. Infant Behavior & Development [serial online] 2009;32(4):454–460. Available from: MEDLINE, Ipswich, MA. Accessed October 30, 2010.

Field T, Grizzle N, Scafidi F, Shanberg S. Massage and relaxation therapies' effects on depressed adolescent mothers. Adolescence. 1996;31:903–911.

Field T, Diego MA, Hernandez-Reif M, et al. Massage therapy effects on depressed pregnant women. J Psychosom Obstet Gynecol 2004;25:115–122.

Gibbs R, Karlan B, Haney A, et al. Danforth's Obstetrics and Gynecology. 10th Ed. Baltimore: Lippincott Williams & Wilkins, 2008.

Gilbert E, Harmon J. Manual of High Risk Pregnancy and Delivery. 3rd Ed. St. Louis: Mosby, 2003.

Ingram J, Domagala C, Yates S. The effects of shiatsu on post-term pregnancies. Complement Ther Med 2005;13:11–15.

Kitzinger S. Ourselves as Mothers: The Universal Experience of Motherhood. Reading: Addison-Wesley, 1995.

Li D, Liu L, Odouli R. 2008. Presence of depressive symptoms during early pregnancy and the risk of preterm delivery: a prospective cohort study. Human Reproduction Advanced Access published online on October 23, 2008. Abstract available at http://humrep.oxfordjournals.org/cgi/content/abstract/den342v1

Moberg KU. The Oxytocin Factor: Tapping the Hormone of Calm, Love, and Healing. Cambridge:Da Capo Press, 2003.

Osborne C. Pre- and Perinatal Massage Therapy: Survey of Massage Therapists. 2009. Accessed at www.bodytherapyassociates.com, June, 2010.

Pepper R. The Ultimate Guide to Pregnancy for Lesbians (Second Edition). Cleis Press, 2005.

Ricci S. Essentials of Maternity, Newborn and Women's Health Nursing. 2nd Ed. Baltimore: Lippincott Williams & Wilkins, 2009.

Simkin P. The Birth Partner. 3rd Ed. Boston: Harvard Common Press, 2008.

Simkin P., Ancheta R. The Labor Progress Handbook (Second Edition). Oxford, England: Blackwell Science, 2011.

Simkin P, Klaus P. When Survivors Give Birth. Seattle: Classic Day Publishing, 2004.

Stager L. Nurturing Massage for Pregnancy. Baltimore: Lippincott, Williams, and Wilkins, 2010.

Stillerman E. Prenatal Massage. St. Louis: Mosby/Elsevier, 2008.

Yates S. Pregnancy and Childbirth. Edinburgh: Churchill Livingston, 2010.

For additional resources, please visit http://thePoint.LWW.com/Osborne-Pregnancy2e!

Business Considerations

Learning Objectives

After study of this chapter, you should be able to:

1. Plan the who, what, and how foundations of your perinatal business.
2. Determine several appropriate strategies for marketing your prenatal and perinatal massage therapy business.
3. Name some of the obstacles to developing a practice in the perinatal market and develop strategies for how to overcome each of them.
4. Collect and record client heath information and perform an effective client interview.
5. Establish and maintain an effective system for managing your client records.
6. Enhance client education.
7. Expand and diversify your business.

The previous chapters have equipped you with the general knowledge of pregnancy and specific massage techniques that you need to become a skilled maternity massage therapist. This chapter takes you beyond the realms of biology and massage and into that of business, presenting strategies for developing and managing a successful prenatal and perinatal practice.

Specifically, this chapter zeroes in on the practicalities of how to market, run, and grow your *maternity-related* business. After considering the practical foundations of your prenatal and perinatal work, such as **target market** and where and how you will work, you will find many promotional ideas, culled from the experiences of thousands of certified maternity massage therapists. You will find recommendations on how to acquire and record critical health intake information, how to develop educational and support materials, and how to expand and diversify your practice. Moreover, this chapter presents some of the major obstacles you may face in building your perinatal massage business and suggestions to overcome these obstacles. Because most therapists are more likely to be in private practice (Osborne 2009), this chapter focuses on that practice setting. Go to the Professional Resource and Business Center in the Student section of the book's companion website at http://thePoint.lww.com/Osborne-Pregnancy2e for the insights of therapists working in spa, medical, midwifery, and other healthcare settings. That is where you will also find more discussion and helpful resources on communicating with healthcare providers, legal, employment, ethical, and longevity issues.

Marketing Your Private Practice

If you are in business for yourself, either full-time or in addition to any employment, you already know how critical marketing is. To grow a maternity practice, your promotional foundation should be establishing your identity and credibility, developing a success plan, and educating and selling prospective clients and their significant others on the value of this work. Choosing promotional activities, actively marketing, and generating publicity about your work will be an ongoing endeavor. You must address certain obstacles to business success with this clientele to overcome their negative impact on your bottom-line. Fortunately, many practitioners have gone before you, and their wisdom can help guide your business efforts.

● PLANNING YOUR BUSINESS

Here are some basic orientation questions to explore and incorporate into a plan for success in this work.

- **What will you call yourself?** If you intend to specialize in prenatal and perinatal, you may want to emphasize this in your title: Prenatal and perinatal massage therapist? Maternity massage therapist? Prenatal massage therapist?
- **What methods of perinatal work will you do?** Swedish massage therapy or craniosacral work (relaxing effects)? Deep tissue and neuromuscular therapy (musculoskeletal relief)? Other modalities?
- **Who is your target market?** Pregnant women only? Laboring and postpartum women? Surrogate mothers? Consider age, income, and educational level; social, religious, and ethnic group; geographical area; marital status; and occupation (Sohnen-Moe 2008).
- **Who influences and makes decisions for maternity clients?** As you consider selling your services to women, incorporate strategies and approaches to these other important people as well: family, friends, coworkers, other healthcare professionals, insurance reviewers, and other financial and healthcare gatekeepers.
- **What is your credibility? An expectant mother will desire** a therapist she feels safe with. Establish your credibility as a trusted healthcare provider by acquiring and publicizing appropriate education, credentials, experience, and professional affiliations. Also remember how important your appearance, demeanor, communications, public image, and the testimonials of others are to your credibility.
- **What impression do you want to make?** How would you want your clients to describe you? Choose five adjectives to characterize that desired impression, such as knowledgeable, safe, effective, nurturing, and wise. Then, use these adjectives to guide your business efforts. For example, a "knowledgeable" therapist speaks and writes articulately, clearly, and accurately. An orange font or background on your brochure could convey energy and vitality, but, if calm, is one of your adjectives, you may want to reconsider your color choice.
- **How will you introduce yourself?** After considering the points above, see if you can develop a 30-second self-introduction to succinctly introduce yourself to a potential client or a professional you hope to network with. Steer clear of bodywork jargon and complex ideas, choosing words that convey the benefits and what you actually would DO. Here are two examples: "I give pregnant and postpartum women opportunities to relax, feel better, and grow a healthier baby through therapeutic bodywork: deep pressure on painful muscles, soothing strokes for tense spots, and practical body use information." - or- "I massage women throughout their labors, staying present and helping them and their families cope productively with pain so that they can welcome their newborn into the world with the most ease possible."
- **What will you exchange for your services?** Here's where you consider the length and types of sessions you offer: 1-hour prenatal massages? Packages for pregnancy, labor, and postpartum therapy? On-site mini-massages? Labor support instruction for a client's partner? Then, determine what you expect back in exchange for your care: not only in fees (Box 8.1), but in the less tangible but valuable things, such as the joy of donating time to charitable causes and the publicity you may gain from doing so.
- **Where will you provide your services?** Consider a private office (76% of therapists surveyed), spa (13%), or wellness center, obstetrical office, hospital, or other setting (14%) (Osborne 2009).
- **Who will perform the services you are promoting?** Consider collaborating with and helping to promote a colleague to whom you can refer your clients when they want services you don't provide. Or, hire or work on commission with a trusted colleague.
- **How will you finance and execute your promotional plans?** Will you send out a letter or e-mail or make phone calls yourself? Will you hire experts to produce your brochure or web site? Make marketing plans that you can afford to do well and that are in line with your promotional image and target market.

> *REMINDER: Thinking about and writing down your answers to the questions included in this section takes you another step closer to a successful maternity massage therapy practice.*

● MARKETING STRATEGIES

When therapists trained in prenatal and perinatal massage therapy were asked what marketing activities are the most successful for them, 94% of respondents included networking/referrals in their top three. Other popularly successful

Box 8.1

Pricing and Packaging Services

Most therapists don't charge additional fees for their prenatal or perinatal work. However, specialists catering to childbearing women sometimes charge higher rates for the additional specialized services and environment they maintain for their predominantly maternity practices.

Of surveyed therapists, 53% charged between $61 and $85 per session, whereas others charged less and some significantly more. Remember the many factors to weigh in pricing: your overall and maternity expertise and experience, your education, target market, geographic variables, the current economic milieu, and the average fee costs in your market.

Many therapists find packaging their services is economically sound and effective for quality client care. An up-front payment can help ensure that the quantity of sessions merits the discount. With packages of five or more hours, clients often pay full price as they go, and then get a complimentary final session. Here are a few package ideas:

- Three sessions distributed over each of the three trimesters for 5% off usual fee upfront
- Three sessions, the first scheduled in the last trimester, an hour of labor massage or labor massage instruction, and a final postpartum session for 5% off the usual fee upfront
- Five sessions with one in each trimester, an hour massage session during labor, labor massage instruction, or a partner session, and the fifth a postpartum session for 10% off usual fee upfront
- Five sessions with three whenever needed prenatally, a postpartum session, and a lesson in infant massage for 10% off upfront
- 10 sessions scheduled as needed within a year of purchase for the price of 8, or 20% off upfront, or with last 2 sessions "complimentary"

Labor massage therapy is a whole other situation. Most therapists charge their hourly rate for up to a maximum of 8 to 10 hours of labor. She can arrange ahead of time for you to be there for a set number of hours or for the entire labor. With this plan, any additional hours of your care (remember you'll be with her until she no longer needs you after the birth) incur no additional charges. Some therapists prefer to base their fee upon the local norm for maternity care. Determine your fee by first surveying the obstetricians and midwives serving your target market. Considering that their flat fee usually covers all of their necessary prenatal and postpartum visits, charge $\frac{1}{4}$ or $\frac{1}{3}$ the average of these healthcare providers with respect to their level of education. This will be your total fee, regardless of the length of time you stay with the laboring woman.

---

activities were internet-based promotions, using discounts and coupons, and presentations they made (Osborne 2009). As a wellness service provider, marketing is more about showing who you are and educating potential clients than selling. Keep that in mind as we look at some typical promotional activities aimed to marketing a maternity massage therapy practice.

Referrals and Networking

Word-of-mouth referrals and networking is an individualized promotional approach that works exceptionally well for prenatal and perinatal massage therapy. In general, women tend to talk about and share the good things in their lives with others. A more relaxed and pain-free client will likely sing your praises to her family, friends, and coworkers and to the other pregnant women she knows. Expectant women both gravitate toward each other and join together to support their growing families. Prenatal exercise and yoga classes, childbirth education classes, and baby fairs are common structured activities where expectant moms swap stories, tips, and resources. Offer your satisfied prenatal clients a few of your business cards and/or brochures to distribute for you. Be sure to thank them for their efforts; you might even give them a small discount for any of their referrals who have a session with you.

Your current clients are already your most ardent salespeople. It doesn't matter that some of your clients may not be pregnant, might be past the childbearing years, or are men; almost everyone knows *someone* who is pregnant or will be. When you are ready, be sure to announce to all of your clients that you are working with expectant women. Purchase or make gift certificates designed specifically as gifts for baby showers and baby gifts. Display them prominently in your office, on your web site, and mention them on your brochures and in other printed materials.

> **REMINDER:** *Notify your current clients that you are prepared to work with expectant women and include a discount on any gift certificates they purchase for a pregnant or postpartum woman.*

Networking has become one of the most cost effective marketing tools, particularly for service professions. Having an interwoven web of contacts who know and trust in you and your services spreads your message well beyond your own closer circles. Join social meeting groups or online sites to list and interact with other businessmen and women to whom you can link in-person or electronically.

Take the time and care to make connections and develop a relationship with one to three of the following perinatal professionals in your community: prenatal exercise and yoga teachers, childbirth educators, doulas, midwives, birthing centers, obstetricians, family practice physicians, hospitals, lactation consultants, home healthcare nurses,

> **My Story**
>
> *I joined a local online network group. For a small fee, they list me on their site. Mostly doulas, they also have local meetings and monthly Meet the Doula nights. I have set up a table at these events, handed out information, and talked to expecting parents about the benefits of prenatal massage. I have even given coupons for a discount along with my card and have found people are very responsive.*
>
> *I have built my professional reputation by being good at what I do. The word spreads quickly if you're good (or if you are not!) By working with the local birthing centers' midwives and nurses while in the labor room, over the years they have gotten to know me. I am knowledgeable, professional and ethical, and they can see that.*
>
> —Nanci Newton, Hadley, MA

chiropractors, physical therapists, home care–visiting nurses, acupuncturists, and psychologists specializing in childbearing issues. Get to know either them or someone on their staff with whom you can regularly connect. Offer an introductory session so that they know your work from experience. Keep them stocked with your business cards and other promotional materials. Suggest educational presentations that you can make for their staff or clientele that promote your business through information sharing. As early in the reintroduction of massage therapy to perinatal healthcare as 1995, a single physician's letter of recommendation propelled one therapist into a burgeoning practice.

Of surveyed therapists trained in prenatal and perinatal massage therapy, other MTs were their second most productive source of referrals (Osborne 2009). Knowing and being known by other therapists means that they may think of you when they need to refer someone to another therapist. You might be better located, have more skills or education, be more available or financially accessible, or be the "right" gender for a client who isn't quite the best fit for the other therapist. If you do labor massage therapy, many very qualified prenatal therapists who can't do labor massage will be thrilled to know that they can refer to you. Get to know your colleagues through joining and participating in your professional organizations, attending Continuing Education (CE) courses, and reaching out to colleagues who look as though they might complement your talents well.

Internet Marketing

Web sites, especially those linked to others' sites, **social networking** sites, **blogging**, and other electronic medium communications are the cutting edge of today's promotions. Reaching the typical age group of pregnant women means connecting with 20 to 35 year olds. More than half of this age group was born after or grew up when personal computers and the internet were becoming widespread.

To reach this age demographic, you must seriously consider having a web presence. Having a basic web site gives you an electronic brochure to complement your printed brochure. Your site needs at least a home page that quickly represents you, a biographical page to allow potential clients to get to know you, and another that overviews your services, prices, and contact information (Sohen-Moe 2008). You may want to arrange for Internet scheduling and "answering" services to facilitate appointment making for you and your clients. (See online resources list for some URL addresses for some notable prenatal and perinatal massage therapists' sites.)

Although the internet might feel daunting to you as a high-touch, not a high-tech, type person, a web presence is relatively easy to achieve. For reasonable periodic rates, various groups, including several professional organizations and businesses, offer a page on their site to promote your practice. Community colleges and adult education programs hold courses that can bring you up to speed on working, selling, and learning on the internet. They also offer courses to take you step by step through a template that creates a functional and basic web site. If getting a professional site designer seems too costly, look into college and high school programs in which students must create a real-world site to complete their requirements. Consider trading services with a computer-bound techie who needs your help with his neck and forearms as much as you need a web site. How about trading with a young expectant woman who will write a blog taking readers through her pregnancy with you tableside?

> **REMINDER:** Establish an internet presence with a basic web site. Subscribe to as many reputable practitioner lists on other sites as possible.

Brochures and Business Cards

To promote your prenatal and perinatal work, you might want to develop a business card that draws attention to your specialized focus (Fig. 8.1). Choose graphic elements and a design that conveys bellies, babies, and your hands at a glance. Other therapists prefer to simply include "prenatal" in a short list of their services. Remember that marketing experts strongly advise against a laundry list of modalities and client populations on a business card, so limit yourself to two or three such mentions (Sohen-Moe 2008).

Your brochure is the appropriate place for lists and explanations (Fig. 8.2). Either purchase premade brochures (see online resources listing) or take the time and hire the expertise you need to create an attractive, informative brochure.

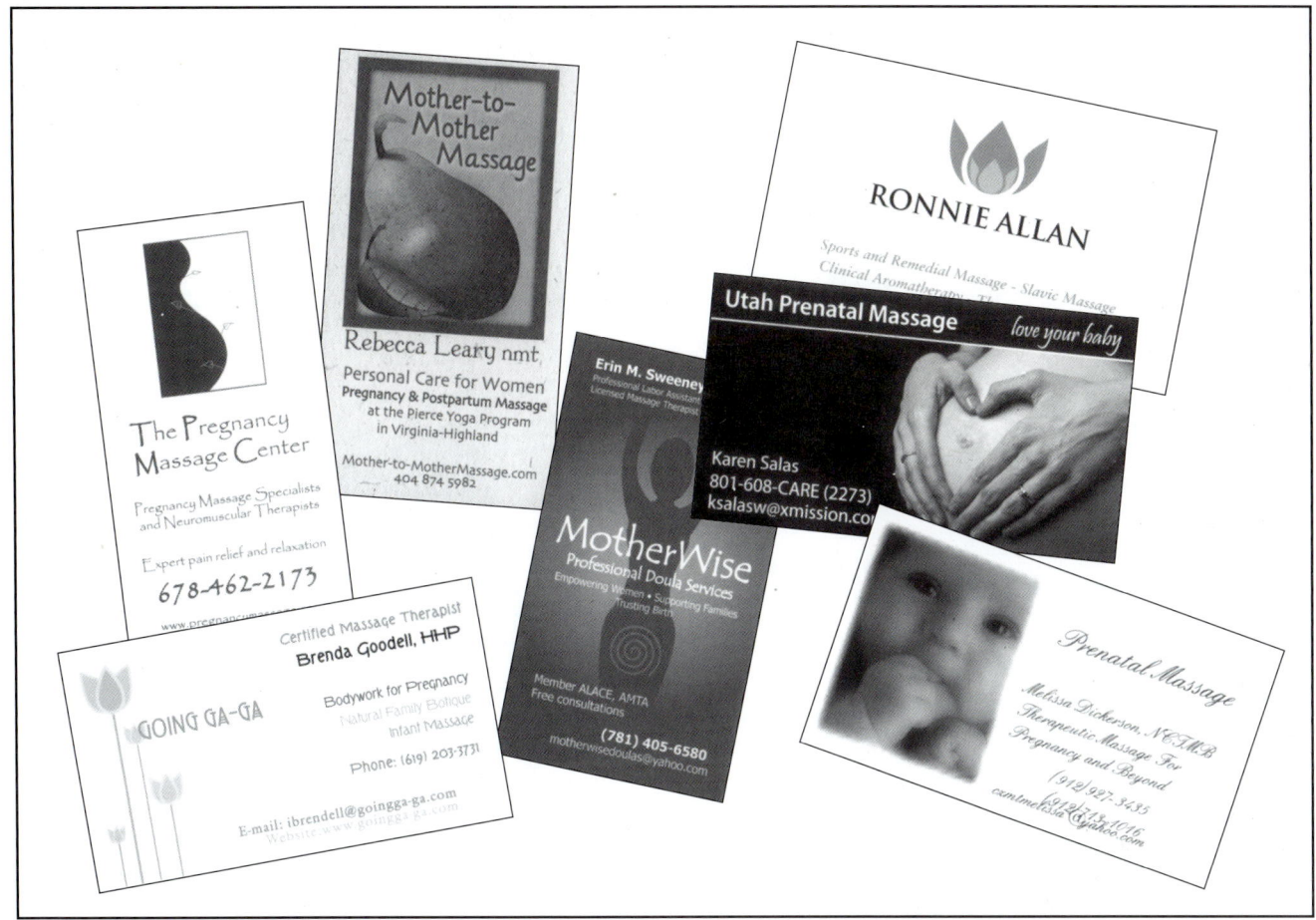

FIGURE 8.1 Sample business cards. Effective business cards are visually appealing and convey basic contact information. These copyrighted materials are used with their owners' permission solely as examples for this publication. They are not to be copied or modified for anyone's individual usage.

Be sure that it includes an overview of you, your services and fees, and your facility and a promotional message that draws your target market to you. When trained perinatal massage therapists were asked what were the three main reasons their expectant clients come to them, lower back pain, relaxation, and upper back, neck, and sacral pain topped the list. Only 4% listed edema relief as a motivator (Osborne 2009). With this in mind, you may want to feature most prominently in your brochure the benefits women seek most. Keep the message brief enough for today's busy women to peruse easily.

Some businesses give calendars, pens, and other items imprinted with contact information to prospective customers. "Pregnatizing" those forms of specialty advertising, you might give candles or small samples of massage oil laced in pink or blue ribbons and a label with your name, phone number, and e-mail address. You might consider developing and distributing an information packet of articles and testimonials. Tailor one for prospective clients, another for doctors and midwives, and yet another for other perinatal professionals.

My Story

Before I worked in a hospital setting, I visited OB-GYN offices in the vicinity and placed materials there, introducing myself to the receptionist. Now that I work in the hospital setting with women on bed rest, I have created a flyer listing the benefits of receiving a massage (even if a patient is high risk). I take copies of these flyers and the magazine Sidelines (a publication for women on bed rest) to the maternity floor. I introduce myself to each of the moms on bed rest, give them the newsletter and flyer, and simply speak with them as I give each of them a hand massage. Most moms on bed rest are feeling restless and alone and that kind of contact is very powerful for them. So far, this approach and word of mouth have been sufficient for generating the number of clients I need to see to keep busy.

—Mia Harper, Annapolis, MD

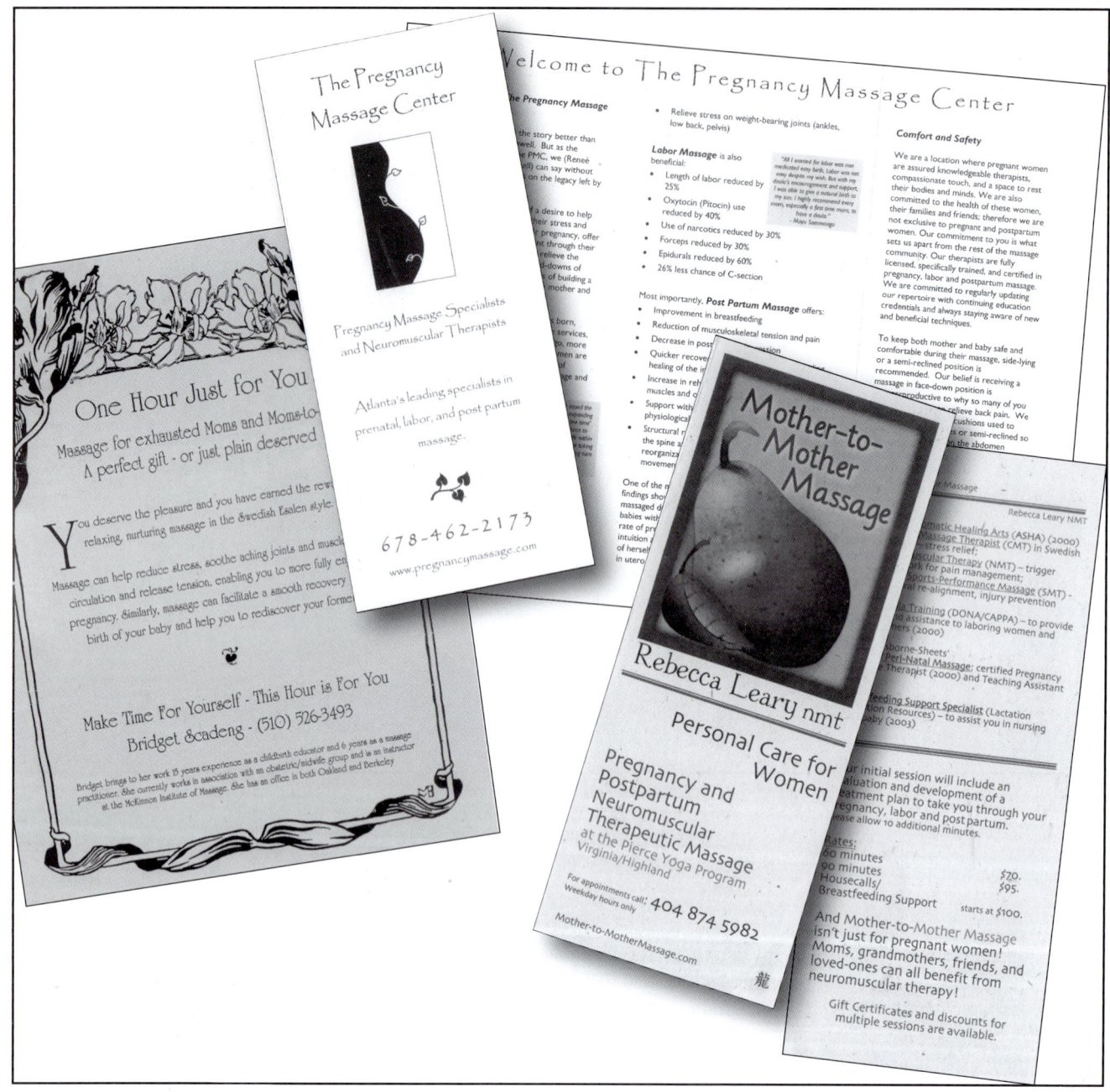

FIGURE 8.2 Sample brochures. Successful brochures establish credibility, focus on the potential benefits to clients, and inspire them to contact you. These copyrighted materials are used with their owners' permission solely as examples for this publication. They are not to be copied or modified for anyone's individual usage.

REMINDER: Purchase or develop a brochure to convey the benefits of your services and a complimenting business card.

Speaking and Demonstrations Engagements

Whereas a card and a brochure are critical printed materials, nothing conveys the feel of what you do and who you are better than an in-person presentation or demonstration. If you are comfortable with speaking to groups, you can present much useful information and promote your business. Include a demonstration if at all possible, and actually touch as many of the audience as is feasible and reasonable. Feeling the warmth, connection, and confidence of your professional touch is worth the proverbial thousand words and a stack of paper products.

Some of your best venues for promoting your maternity work are the obvious: a meeting of doulas, a segment in a

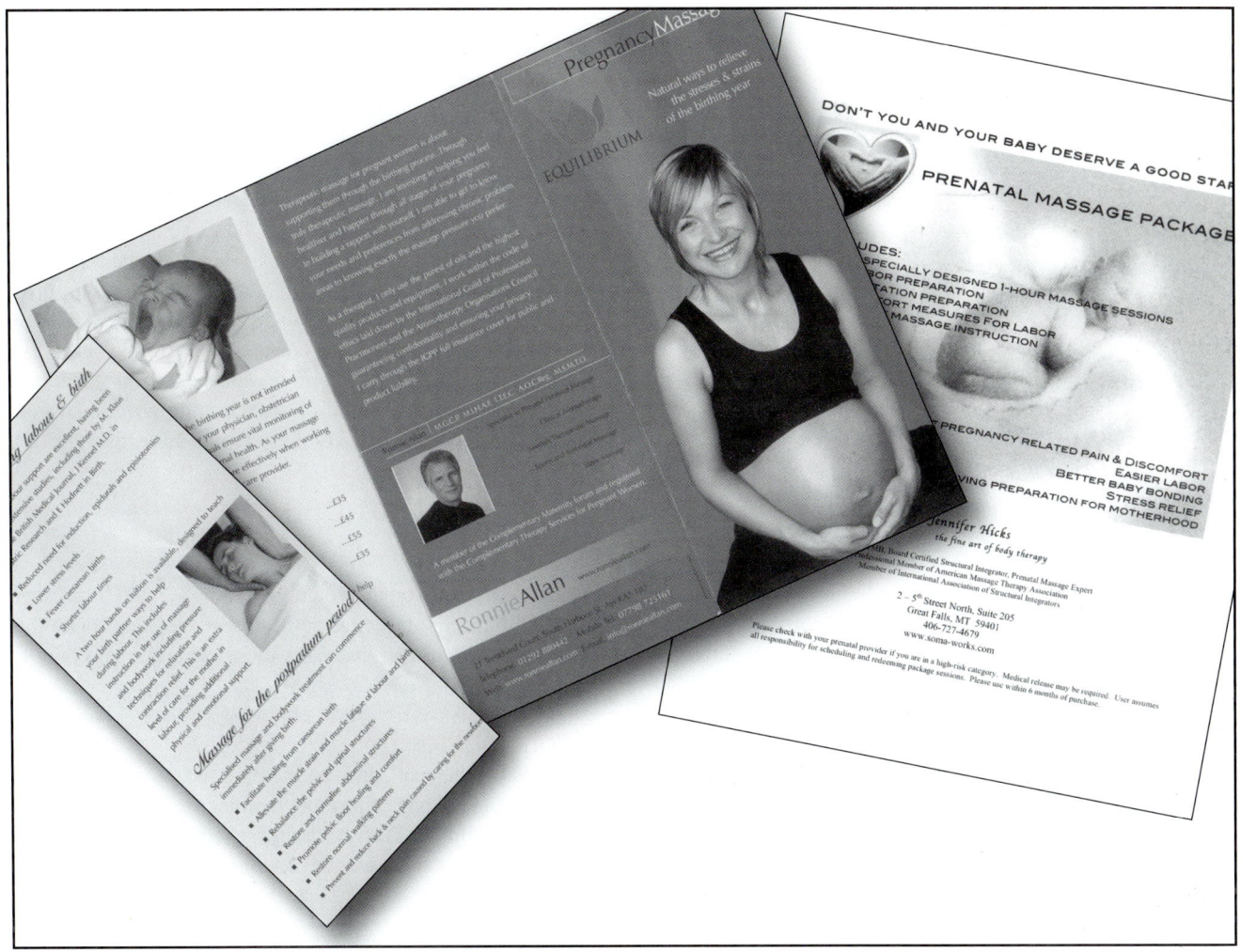

FIGURE 8.2 *(Continued)*

childbirth education class, a lunchtime presentation at an obstetrical or midwifery office (bring a light lunch along, too, for the busy staff), or a presentation following a prenatal exercise class. Other possibilities, less maternity related, include the following: local chapter meetings of American Association of College and University Women (AACUW), other women's service clubs, or at a church, company, or community health fair.

Classes

Speeches and demonstrations usually give you 3 to 30 minutes to educate and sell your audience. When teaching a class for one to several hours, however, the breadth and depth of your knowledge becomes apparent, as does your way of interacting with people, both key factors women consider when choosing a therapist. Keep your focus on informing your students rather than selling your sessions, and you will likely land one or more clients from every course you teach. Some appropriate maternity-related class ideas are: 1 to 3 hours of simple techniques for relaxation to moms and their partners; an hour of self-massage for women's health at a community center; and a short course in an adult education program of "family massage."

Remember to focus on the content, level of complexity, and type of students that you are qualified and prepared to teach. Unless you are also a nutritionist, don't include dietary or supplement advice. If you have no credentials for teaching massage therapists, then don't attempt a CE or core course at a massage school. When you speak at a childbirth education or a prenatal yoga class, complement the instructor's course material rather than usurping or contradicting it. Assure safety by only teaching "lay people" those techniques that an untrained hand and mind can do; omit any techniques requiring advanced anatomical knowledge or refined palpatory skills. Avoid alarmist attitudes, and be sure to inform, warn, and reassure as you give safety precautions and contraindications. (See online resources for labor massage for partners' class plans and tips.)

> **My Story**
>
> I built my professional reputation by writing articles and speaking whenever I could. I have written for the magazine of a local natural birth association that I am a member of, and I spoke at a few conferences they have had. I also spoke at a childbirth educators' conference, labor nurses' professional development day, teachers' professional development day, early childhood intervention staff development day, special needs parents' organizations, etc. Whenever an opportunity came up I said enthusiastically, "YES!"
>
> —Linda Hickey, Calgary, AB

Printed Articles

Just as a class expands your speaking opportunity, writing and publishing a feature article allows you to elaborate your written message. Newspapers, magazines, newsletters, and blogs are just a few of the vehicles available to you if you have any degree of writing ability. Make a list of the perinatal topics that you are most comfortable with and knowledgeable about, and then develop one or several into informative, brief articles. Hire an editor and/ or publicity person to help refine and place your articles in effective publications. (See online resources for sample promotional articles.)

Direct Mail and E-mail Promotions

Sending out brochures, postcards, newsletters, and announcements spreads your message more broadly than when you connect individually with prospective clients. If you have a database of names and contact information of your own clients, you have the beginnings of a direct mail marketing campaign. You also can purchase lists, sorted by almost any imaginable criteria, if you don't have any or need a larger pool of contacts. Choose all the houses within one square mile of your office or all the local childbirth educators, depending on your message and promotional focus. You can reduce postage costs by securing **bulk mailing** rates through a mailing service and getting the tightest target list possible. Postcards require less postage and less material cost than a brochure in an envelope.

It is usually less costly in materials, time, and costs to send e-mail communications. Again, your own list of e-mail addresses is invaluable. Be sure to check with your e-mail service provider regarding regulations to control "spam" or internet junk mail. Several internet businesses specialize in sending **e-mail blasts** of announcements and e-newsletters. They also can help you to enliven your message with graphics and design rather than just text.

Advertising

Print advertising is typically a costly form of marketing. Some exceptions might be inexpensive ads in targeted publications. For example, if your club members are part of your target market, $30 for a quarterly club newsletter ad might make good sense. An inexpensive ad in publications of your local support group for women on bed rest could be feasible. Many therapists find listing in the telephone book Yellow Pages to be worth the expense for the broad exposure plus the accessibility to contact information this creates. As with other forms of promotion, employ the professionals that you need to create an eye-catching ad more likely to create business from your investment. Find an Internet-savvy professional or friend to help you through the complex world of **search engine optimization, banner ads,** and other forms of **electronic advertising**.

● OVERCOMING OBSTACLES IN THE PERINATAL MARKET

Many expectant women would love to have regular massage therapy, but they may face several obstacles that make this difficult. This section discusses these obstacles and how to overcome them.

Financial Stress

Obviously, financial stresses increase when a new family member comes along. With more families needing two incomes for sustainability or lifestyle desires, a reduction in a woman's income means making many spending choices. Ways to make your sessions more affordable include the following:

- Flexible pricing and package discounts (Box 8.1 on pricing)
- Gift certificates (often folks will purchase for a loved one what she won't allow herself to buy) or a special for couples planning a "babymoon," a get-away together before the birth.
- An add-on complementary mini-massage or a package series that includes a massage for the client's partner

Busyness and Not Feeling Well

Of the surveyed therapists trained in prenatal and perinatal massage therapy, 30% considered getting clients in early enough in their pregnancies was their biggest challenge (Osborne 2009). Below are some suggestions for addressing these concerns:

- Offer times when she is less nauseated or tired, has childcare, or is able to get off from work.
- Make home calls to clients with challenges (activity restrictions and new moms).
- Offer a home call for the client's first postpartum session at no additional cost.
- Arrange with a trusted woman with income limitations to provide infant care at your office in trade for session discounts.

> **My Story**
>
> Other pregnancy massage therapists have lamented losing clients once they have given birth. To address this, I offer a package: buy four massages, get one complimentary postpartum massage. Once clients stop associating you only with pregnancy massage, they are more likely to call for a massage at other times. If you get a client early enough in the process, she may accumulate several postpartum sessions. I stress the importance of self-care after the baby is born. I also offer a postpartum home visit, with breastfeeding support (I took a basic breastfeeding support class). I help them with positioning, postural alignment, etc., all of which are essential postpartum.
>
> —Rebecca Leary Atlanta, GA

> **REMINDER:** *Maximize your flexibility in fees, location, and scheduling times to reduce financial and convenience obstacles to your client purchasing perinatal massage therapy services.*

Ignorance of the Safety and Benefits of Massage

Concern for the safety of both the mother and the baby puts hesitation in the minds of women, their partners, and caregivers regarding prenatal massage. By educating your clients, you go far toward easing those concerns. Although massage therapy is one of the fastest growing complementary healthcare options, many people are unaware of the far-reaching benefits of our work. In particular, women, their partners, and their healthcare providers may not think of massage as anything more than a luxury for the rich and famous having babies. Following are some suggestions for overcoming these obstacles:

- Hone your ability to talk and write about the benefits of prenatal massage citing appropriate research studies to document your claims.
- Call or send a card to a client after her due date to congratulate her and remind her how postpartum massage therapy benefits her and her family.
- Display your knowledge and expertise in your printed materials, vocabulary, and credentials.
- Share maternal, medical, and midwifery testimonials with your clients.
- Practice conservatively and convey that standard of precaution.
- Introduce yourself and send an informative packet of materials to local perinatal specialists.
- Consult with clients' doctors and midwives for their expertise and knowledge of the client, and send your brochure along with any necessary forms.

> **REMINDER:** *Educate doctors, midwives, and parents about the potential benefits of maternity massage and your ability and qualifications to safely provide those benefits.*

Outdated Knowledge of Maternity Trends

While you are within the childbearing age group, you will likely stay current with maternity trends. As you grow older, your familiarity with what's fashionable and the newest developments in perinatal healthcare can become outdated. To counteract this, look to staying current and continuing to learn and grow by doing the following:

- Become involved with a young neighbor, friend, or relative as she enters and embraces motherhood.
- Pick up magazines or visit stores or web sites for expectant and new parents.
- Attend a childbirth education class every decade to keep abreast of what women are learning.
- Refresh your reference library every 3 to 5 years with a new book or an updated edition of a favorite title (see online resources for a suggested library list).
- Remember to regularly renew and refresh your massage and bodywork skills.
- Seek certifications from various instructors to broaden your perspective.

Your Own Beliefs, Experiences, and Ethics

Now, turn inward for a moment to consider how you might get in your own way of business success. If the best marketing plan, well executed and adequately financed, isn't producing your ideal appointment load, then consider a few internal things. No one is without beliefs, attitudes, and experiences related to mothering; we have all had a mother, no matter whether we are mothers or not. Ethical conflicts also may sabotage your marketing efforts and your client care. Examine yourself by answering the following questions:

- Do you feel inadequate or distressed if you can't or don't want to have children?
- Have your pregnancies, birthing, and parenting created valuable experience or emotional and mental "baggage" you carry into your therapy room?
- Have you witnessed traumatic births that make you doubt that a baby can be born safely?
- Do you distrust doctors or think midwives are underqualified?
- Do you fear hospitals, think homebirth is dangerous, or loathe any medical interventions?

- What judgments do you have about single moms, husbands, same sex partners, or other individuals who might be a part of a woman's pregnancy?
- Are you comfortable with clients who are often larger than the norm?
- How prepared do you feel to deal with the possibility of perinatal injury or death?

Many unique situations develop in prenatal and perinatal massage therapy that can challenge your and the profession's ethical standards (NCBTMB 2009). Chapter 5 explored some of those ethical concerns inherent in labor work, but there are others to watch for. You can easily wander beyond your scope of practice when a woman asks your advice about a medical procedure. Be sure that you know your jurisdictions' and organizations' parameters. (MTBOK 2010) Boundaries can become nebulous in the fluid intensity of labor massage, and when a very needy woman becomes your client. Managing your therapist relationship is difficult when your client is also your niece. The power imbalance inherent in our relationship can widen as a woman's neediness increases, as can the potential for client transference and therapist countertransference of earlier familial relationships. The easy camaraderie of expectant women can cause you to blunder on confidentiality issues. And finally, there are some situations in maternity care where association ethics and legal parameters clash with clients' legitimate therapeutic needs (Benjamin and Sohnen-Moe 2003).

When you identify any of these obstacles, look to resolving them. Get more education, talk with a counselor or psychologist, or discuss your issues with a friend or practice supervisor. Look for mentoring and/or **supervision** in your bodywork community to help you work your way through these often complex and overlooked issues. (See online resources for further discussion of these ethical concerns and resources for working with them.)

What Would You Do?

Review the obstacles to success with the perinatal market discussed in this chapter. Which of these obstacles are relevant in your practice situation? What strategies can you develop to potentially dissolve those impediments? What are the first three steps you can take from among your strategies?

Male Therapists

Male therapists working with expectant women have some additional situations worth considering. Although some pregnant women are more comfortable with a female therapist during this most feminine of life's cycles, others have no gender preference. In fact, some women prefer a male therapist. On the other hand, some husbands and partners are not so keen to have their wives seeing a male therapist, and that can be the deciding factor in her booking sessions with you. Below are some suggestions for addressing this concern:

- Clearly convey your draping thoroughness and modesty, therapeutic environment, and warm, but clinical demeanor.
- Dress and act impeccably professionally, rather than overly casually.
- Teach partners simple massage early in the pregnancy, including him or her in her massage care.

Having a male therapist offers a healthy way to bring more masculine energy into a woman's prenatal care, particularly in the absence of that, for whatever the reason; however, a client can inappropriately expand her expectations from those of a client to those of a friend, family member, or partner (see online resources about boundary issues). Male therapists need to be sensitive to this possibility and provide professional nurturing and therapeutic care without acting like a substitute partner.

Some men initially feel inadequate or "out of the loop" when entering into this work. Most find that if they call upon their experiences gestating a creative project that consumed their body, emotions, and mind, they can relate to pregnancy and birth. If they have children, their own journey as a father may provide experiential wisdom to help them connect. Extensive reading and viewing of maternity media is a priority, as well. There is no gender-based reason that a male therapist cannot be wildly successful with this population. In fact, there are male therapists whose practice is 50% or more prenatal and perinatal in its focus. (See online resources and Chapter 9 for practice profiles of male therapists.)

Managing Your Prenatal and Perinatal Business

From your first contact to your final session, you will need to adapt and create new strategies for business operations with childbearing in mind. These include your client information and charting, communicating with medical and other healthcare providers, your client policies and procedures, and insurance coverage and reimbursement.

● INTAKE AND CLIENT INTERVIEWS

Intake should begin when a prenatal client schedules an appointment. To determine the appropriateness of your work for her, you need some basic information. Ask her these questions:

- What do you hope to get from a prenatal massage?
- How far along are you in your pregnancy?
- Does your prenatal healthcare provider consider your pregnancy to be proceeding normally and with low- or high-risk factors? If so, what are those concerns?

Strike a balance between what you absolutely must know for safe practice and having her feel interrogated before you have established good rapport with her. As your first opportunity to begin establishing trust and connection, convey your warm receptivity, genuine concern, and knowledge. Listening in a professional manner will set the stage for an effective session.

With these fundamental facts, you can determine whether you need further information or documentation from her, her healthcare provider, or her insurance company before seeing her. Make arrangements to get any necessary paperwork or authorizations (Box 8.2) prior to her appointment or for her to bring them with her. You will have a sense of what her positioning and technique needs might be, and you can better prepare to optimize her session time.

When she comes in for her first session, and each one thereafter, remember how important it is for her to feel cared for. Yes, her swelling belly will draw your attention, but attend to HER; she is your client, and the fetus is only your client by association, so to speak. "Hello, how are you?" rather than "Wow, look at this belly!" is usually a more client-centered greeting. Ask "How are things going for you?" instead of "How's the baby doing?" Shake hands with a new client, resisting your urge to touch her belly; it's best to wait until you have built a relationship than to be overly familiar. Offer

water, immediately ask if she needs the restroom, and provide a stool where she can prop her legs while waiting or for during her intake process.

Once in your office and with some additional rapport, most women feel amenable to providing you with more details about their maternity and general health history. You now know how many factors go into delivering a safe and appropriate session for each individual expectant woman, even if she is only seeking a relaxing, nurturing massage. Solicit these details through oral interviews, taking your own notes as your conversation progresses. This has the advantage of not only getting information, but you will also get all-important impressions about how she is feeling and thinking about her pregnancy. A written intake questionnaire (Fig. 8.3) that she completes prior to your work has the probable advantage of insuring a written record that is not subject to your own interpretations or misunderstandings. Decide which works best for you and your style of practice.

Whether oral or written, you need 10 to 20 minutes to acquire at least the information listed on the basic intake form in Figure 8.3. (You will find some additional sample intake forms in the online resources that you might find more applicable in your circumstances. Also see online discussion of intake and record keeping in other practice settings.) Although some of these questions repeat what you initially asked her when scheduling, she might surprise you with how much more she will share as she begins to feel your professional attentiveness. Sometimes, some critical information doesn't emerge until this point, maybe even not until you are actually into your massage. Of course, if this happens, you may need to tactfully alter your session for a health issue or creatively address a concern she hadn't previously expressed. Don't forget to ask all of the questions that you usually ask of any client such as general health history and activities, intensity and frequency of any discomforts, and whether she has received massage therapy before and with what results.

Attend to how she moves about, her posture, her breathing and her general energy level as she talks with you. Watch her facial expression and hear what's between the lines to get more affective information. As she points out a painful spot, ask whether you may feel there to get a palpatory first impression. Many pregnant women will have a hand over an aching SI joint or under their belly, comforting while unintentionally signaling you about where they hurt. Listen to your intuition and instincts about her and her needs. Consult Chapter 4's overview and guidelines for typical trimester concerns and developments.

In addition to getting information, you need to give her information. She needs orientation to your office, your approach, expectations, and policies. Again, tell her or give her materials to read, whichever seems appropriate for you. Giving her written materials allows her to refer to the information later and to educate and reassure others. It also creates a record that you both can refer to if any misunderstandings or conflicts develop. Be sure to ask her whether she has any questions and what might make her session more enjoyable and effective. After sufficient exploration, let her know

---

Box 8.2

Sample Healthcare Provider Release

To: Maternity Healthcare Providers
Re: Release for Therapeutic Massage During Pregnancy/Postpartum

Your patient, _____, has requested prenatal/postpartum therapeutic massage. Therapeutic massage is provided prenatally and perinatally as adjunctive healthcare by a massage therapist who has met written and practical exam criteria. It is our policy to work with her only if her maternity healthcare provider has reviewed this request with her. In addition, if her pregnancy is high risk, or she has experienced any prenatal or postpartum complications or contraindicated conditions, we require a written release from her healthcare provider stating any specific limitations or precautions that you feel to be appropriate. Please verify your clearance of this request by your signature below. This verification can be modified or withdrawn at any time should your patient's health status change. I welcome this opportunity to work with you in providing prenatal care to your patient. Thank you for your time and assistance.

Patient's pregnancy is (circle one): normal progression   high risk
Specific limitations or precautions:
You may contact me directly for clarification or concerns regarding this patient.   Yes   No
Signature: _____ MD DO Midwife _____ Date: _____
Please print your name: _____
Office phone: _____ (fax): _____ email: _____

Prenatal Intake and Health History Form

Name: _____ Phone: _____

Address: _____

Today's date: _____ Birthdate: _____ Referred by: _____

1. What discomforts, pain, or other needs are you hoping to have addressed through this massage therapy?
   _____
   _____

2. In what week of your pregnancy are you? _____

3. Are you regularly seeing a physician, nurse-midwife, or midwife? Please provide name and phone number. _____

4. Have you had any complications or problems with this pregnancy? Circle those that apply: bleeding, cramping, amniotic fluid leakage; swelling; high blood pressure, rapid weight gain, protein in urine; vision disturbances; severe nausea, vomiting, or headaches; abnormal fetal growth, heartbeat, or movements; high blood sugar; other:
   _____

5. Do you have any medical conditions? Circle those applicable: diabetes; heart, liver, kidney, or lung disorders; convulsive disorders; uterine abnormality; connective tissue or collagen diseases; other:
   _____

6. Are you currently experiencing any infection or disorder? Circle those applicable: cold, bladder, breast, scar or other infection, skin irritation, varicose veins, other:
   _____

7. Is your pregnancy considered to be high risk (due to diabetes, hypertension, multiple pregnancy, previous complicated pregnancy, asthma, Rh or genetic problems, age under 20 or over 35 years of age, fetal genetic disorders, or exposure to hazardous materials)?
   _____

8. Is there other relevant information about this pregnancy or about you that I should know?
   _____
   _____
   _____

FIGURE 8.3 Sample prenatal or postpartum client intake form. In addition to general health history and contact information, a maternity intake form needs a section with pregnancy-specific questions.

your session plan and ideas for any possible future work. Remember that a shortened version of this process must take place each time you work together.

> **REMINDER:** *Design and use an intake form and methodology that keeps you current and complete in your knowledge about your maternity clients.*

What Would You Do?

You are accustomed to taking a thorough health and prenatal history on your private practice prenatal clients. At your part-time spa job, scheduling and company policies don't easily allow for this type of client intake before your massage session begins. How can you secure the information that you need to design safe and effective sessions for your spa clients? What strategies might you try to make changes at your spa toward more relevant information gathering?

• COMMUNICATING WITH OTHER PROVIDERS AND MAINTAINING CLIENT RECORDS

Observe client/patient confidentiality standards as you consult with and build cooperation with your clients' perinatal specialists. Particularly when complications develop or when there are high-risk conditions, seek the knowledgeable, individualized insight the doctor or midwife has of your mutual "mom." (See Box 8.2 and online resources for examples of maternity healthcare releases.) You might provide your client with a release for her to return completed and signed, or you might want to ask her to request that her healthcare provider contact you directly. The more proactive method is to get your client's written permission to communicate with her doctor. Send that release along with any requests for information that you make. Periodically update clients' providers on the progress of your therapy sessions with their patient. Build a collegial relationship by your respectful demeanor, maintaining your scope of practice and professional code of ethics in all you do.

Maternity session recordkeeping addresses the same documentation, communication, and reflection needs as your general clientele records. Use whatever form of session recording you are accustomed to or required to use by your employer. Many therapists use either the Subjective, Objective, Assessment, Plan (SOAP) or Condition, Action taken, Response of client, Evaluation (CARE; Rose 2003) charting formats, depending on the nature of session goals and procedures. See examples of each in Box 8.3. Others prefer an unstructured narrative style for recording how each session progressed. Whatever your format, be sure to write the week of pregnancy or postpartum. Include her summary of any tests or prenatal assessments her doctor or midwife has made.

Box 8.3

Sample Session Records

Client No. 1 5/7/09
- S—client's second visit in 7 days. Pregnancy going well. C/o low back pain and tail bone pain when she sits. Also c/o leg pains, joint pains and a lot of anxiety. Hx of hypoglycemia, cysts on vocal chords, gastric bypass in 2003; doc is here at the hospital. Due date next week, this is first baby. Client will also try acupuncture for anxiety.
- O—Due to gastric bypass, a lot of extra skin. No tight or knotted muscles. Overall client seems overwhelmed by the physical aches, pains of pregnancy.
- A—30/30 minutes R and L sidelying. Full body massage with focus on pelvic/SI and leg work. Client had great relief from SI joint stretches and subtle rocking.
- P—Showed her how her husband can sit against her knees to relieve pressure on SI. She'll return on her due date if she hasn't delivered.

Same Client 5/27/09
- S—Client had baby on 5/15. Reports vaginal birth but long labor after water broke, resulting in baby having a fever/infection. Baby remains hospitalized. Client suffering headaches and leg swelling and nerve pain down R leg, possibly from epidural. Brought me doctor's authorization for gentle massage and lymphatic work.
- O—Client slept immediately.
- A—Combination lymph and gentle massage, but mostly lymph on legs. Incl. abdominal massage. Supine entire time with legs bolstered.
- P—Loaned infant massage DVD to help with bonding. Suggested breath awareness and deepening for daily stress reduction. Return as needed.

Client No. 2 CARE Notes
- C—Client 35+ years. Physician gave her the verbal OK for massage but promises to bring me the signed Authorization next time she comes. 21 weeks pregnant, no problems with pregnancy. C/o low back pain and the occasional headache and seeking relief from both. Loves deep work.
- A—40 minutes semireclined, 25/25 minutes L and R sidelying. Deep sculpting work at traps; enjoyed deeper pressure there. A lot of traction, scalp and occiput work in semireclined.
- R—Client able to relax immediately. Fell asleep fairly quickly. Upper traps knotted but responsive.
- E—Less back pain; no headache at start so no changes. Reminded her of water after our work. Recommended return as necessary.

In addition to session records, you may want to ask for a copy of her **birth plan** or labor preferences (see online resources for sample birth plan). These are helpful to know regardless of whether you will be massaging her during labor. Understanding her vision of her baby's birth will help you to tailor your work to help her get the best possible outcome from her plans. If you will be attending the birth as her massage therapist, you will also need to record other details you normally wouldn't know about a client. You need her address and how to get there or to the hospital or birthing center, depending on where you will meet her. Have her partner's and her doctor or midwife's names and numbers for "just-in-case" scenarios.

Regular session note formats won't accommodate the unique parameters of labor massage therapy. Try a pocket notebook to jot important facts, time, and progress reports as soon as possible after they are given. Every few hours make quick notes of difficulties, interventions, and techniques used. Within a few hours of leaving the new family, fill in the gaps and compose a more organized "story" of the labor and birth. These will help complete your records and prompt you to sift back over the difficulties and triumphs, noting any unresolved feelings or issues you might have. (See online resources for an example.) Also make note of the events in the labor that your client might need you to attend to in postpartum sessions. Some therapists like to deliver a copy of the baby's birth story from the therapist's perspective for inclusion in the mother's baby book.

● LIABILITY AND INSURANCE CONCERNS

Minimize your risk for legal actions, particularly those relevant to a maternity practice. Many of your clients may have trouble seeing their feet when they walk, can be more prone to imbalances that cause missteps and falls, and their weights can exceed 200 lb at term. You may reduce your chance of incurring physical, medical and loss liability for hazards, equipment failures, and other "slip and fall" issues if your environment accommodates these likelihoods. Be sure that your various liability insurances cover the perinatal aspects of your practice in your setting. Remember that a standard homeowner's policy doesn't cover liability if someone visiting your home for business purposes is injured (Sohnen-Moe 2008).

As discussed in Chapter 2, some sobering facts of American maternity care are very relevant to massage therapists. Patients sue more than 75% of obstetricians and gynecologists during their careers. More than 33% of them are sued more than three times. Nurses and other perinatal healthcare providers are more and more frequently being included in these lawsuits (Gilbert and Harmon 2003). At this point, massage therapists appear to have escaped this lawsuit explosion (Turgeon 2008), but it is wise to keep legal implications in mind as you conduct your business. By operating in an ethical, professional manner, and with sufficient education, you are less likely to have questionable incidents occur that could develop into litigation. (See ethics and ongoing career development discussion online.) Maintaining adequate malpractice liability insurance should be a priority protection against any possible client claims that you were negligent or failed to perform at a professional skill level.

Deciding whether you are qualified and want to accept insurance reimbursement for your maternity massage services is a complex matter, far more intricate to tackle in this book. Look for guidance from some of the resources listed online.

Enhancing Client Education

One of your best marketing tools has the equal benefit of improving your session outcomes. Self-care instruction that eases pregnancy's discomforts conveys your knowledge and your caring, which is part of developing a trusted reputation. When clients can learn how to deepen and prolong the effects of your session, they become even more ardent promoters of your work. You can incorporate this informative sharing before, during, and after sessions, with printed materials and in special educational events. You can make books and other media readily available, too.

● INDIVIDUALIZED SELF-CARE TO EASE DISCOMFORTS

Without any specific directions, massage therapy is a lesson in relaxation, but you can deliberately guide your clients to focus on the sensations of relaxation. As women prepare for labor, this can be particularly helpful for the thighs, pelvic floor, throat, jaw, and face. Explaining and guiding their breath to deeper, fuller inhalation and exhalation will teach them how to relax at any time. For daily rolling up and down and creating compression on tight erectors or gluteals, demonstrate how to use two tennis balls tied into a sock. Work with a nursing mother's posture and pillow supports to help ease neck, shoulder, and arm strain. Teach her several key zones on her feet to work with daily as preventative and maintenance daily care.

You may want to create or purchase educational handouts for your clients to take home with them. You could easily render all of the topics mentioned above into one-page instructional sheets, even if only illustrated with stick figures. Other helpful topics include the following:

- Contraction stimulation points for labor support
- Stretching to relax
- Alignment and supports for maximum sleep comfort
- Self-massage to ease nausea, heartburn, and constipation

- Connecting with baby through breath and gentle touch
- Self-massage and stretching to promote breastfeeding

Notice that all of these topics fall within the usual scope of practice guidelines for massage therapists. (MTBOK 2010)

● EDUCATIONAL EVENTS

Organizing an educational event for groups of clients can accomplish several purposes. This is a time- and cost-efficient way to teach self-care practices that you lack time for within a normal session period. Mini-workshops and classes are opportunities to invite partners and family to learn how to help each other deal with the tensions of expecting a baby. Bringing your clients together helps build connections between couples and individuals who care about maximizing their prenatal experience, another "tend and befriend experience." You can structure these events to be marketing and community relations opportunities, too. Invite a writer or a blogger in to tell the story of your class. Offer scholarships to qualified community members, and you can often get complimentary coverage in events calendars as well as help a needy woman learn how to better care for herself.

Some mini-workshop or longer class topic suggestions are as follows:

- Coping with swollen feet and legs
- Learning to relax with partner massage
- Massage for comfort during labor
- Massaging baby, older children, and your partner
- Self-massage to ease prenatal discomforts
- Daily habits to ease prenatal muscle tension

● IN-OFFICE EDUCATIONAL RESOURCES

Every wall and bookcase of your office is potentially an educational experience for your clients. Even the bathroom is a perfect place for a chart of the pelvic floor muscles! Post notices of local events of interest to childbearing women, such as lectures, screenings, and support groups. Prominently display referral numbers for services women may feel reluctant to ask about such as domestic abuse hotlines and WIC program and businesses (Women, Infants, and Children, also called the Special Supplemental Nutrition Program). Place this same information on a printed list of preferred providers that you create from your contacts and networking in the perinatal community. Give that list to every maternity client as part of her information packet.

In addition to your lending library of books, periodicals, DVDs, and music, you can get informative pamphlets to give away from the breastfeeding support group, La Leche League, SIDS (Sudden Infant Death Syndrome) Foundation, the US Department of Health and Human Services, and other agencies and businesses. You may want to offer for purchase some of these and other products that can soothe and relax her such as massage oils, belly pillows, lumbar support belts, and/or sling carriers. (See the resources listing online for lists and suggestions of places to acquire many of these items.)

> **REMINDER:** *Develop several client education activities and materials for better outcomes and as a marketing activity to attract and keep more clients.*

Expanding and Sustaining Your Business

Some of the most successful prenatal and perinatal massage therapists are double- and triple-certified providers of other forms of maternity care. Additional professional skills and the education and credentials involved can be reassuring to tentative clients and professionals. It capitalizes on the trusting relationship you build with your massage therapy client; when she needs a lactation consultant, you are the obvious choice, for example. You can market your childbirth education classes or prenatal exercise classes side by side with your massage therapy. Any given woman might be more inclined toward one than the other. Often, an exercise student also becomes a massage therapy client.

Of survey respondents, 40% are infant massage instructors and 21% are doulas, in addition to their prenatal and perinatal massage therapist certification (Osborne 2009). Other areas to consider studying and becoming certified in include the following:

- Preconception massage therapy
- Pediatric massage therapist
- Lactation consultant
- Prenatal yoga teacher
- Childbirth educator
- Ultrasound technician
- Belly caster
- Prenatal photographer
- Midwife or midwife's assistant
- Nurse

Another way to get this marketing edge is to cooperatively promote your business with one or more of these others.

For perinatal career longevity and long-term success, look to preventing burnout and managing your own self-care. Charge and organize your time appropriately. Have proper equipment, practice the body mechanics in Chapter 3, and get help at the first signs of wear and tear niggling at your joints and soft tissues. Look back to Chapter 5 to review some of the critical issues of working with the long hours and intensity of labor. Find sources for professional supervision, mentoring, and continued education and development.

My Story

I think a lot about my "image" that I portray to new clients, trying to find the balance between caring, involved focused and "professional" behavior, including what and when to share, and how I respond to client needs. I do sometimes go the extra bit for someone who may be needing special attention, especially postpartum - fitting her in somewhere, having a grandma volunteer come in to hold a baby for her, work an extra appointment in on Saturday because that feels right for me.

I have been feeling frustrated with some new therapists who are asking for advice about building practice, yet have very strict limitations—especially no evenings, no weekends. Reality here in my city is that pregnant women with money (read benefits) are usually working. We need to be available when they are if we want to attract this market. As they get closer to their due dates and begin their maternity leave they will be available for the weekday daytime appointment times, but initially you need to meet them half way.

For me, I do believe "it takes a village....," and I am proud and happy to step up and join the village. It is part of my life too and who I choose to be. That helps me when I am tired or overbooked or need a holiday. Remembering that this is important work, and I continue to work with how to do it well and long, while making it sustainable as I age. This is the stuff I spend hours talking about when I am together with my colleagues and contemporaries.

—Linda Hickey, Calgary, AB

CHAPTER SUMMARY

Developing a healthy maternity massage therapy business requires thorough theoretical and practical education and a solid foundation of practical considerations of where, when, how, and how much. Active marketing brings the right people together to support your practice growth in clients and a solid referral network. Sound practice management, coupled with activities that educate and promote business, sustains normal, healthy development of you and your business.

Test Yourself

For answers, visit the website at http://thePoint.LWW.com/Osborne-Pregnancy2e!

1. What is a target market? How would you generally describe the prenatal target market?
2. To whom do you need to address your marketing efforts when seeking to develop a prenatal and perinatal massage therapy specialization practice?
3. List types of marketing activities in the order in which they appear to be most successful in promoting maternity massage therapy.
4. What are the two most important criteria for determining what techniques to teach women and their partners in short courses?
5. List four types of obstacles to successfully marketing to pregnant and postpartum women.
6. What are the basic five pieces of perinatal information you need to know and track with prenatal clients?
7. What is the usefulness of including client education in your practice procedures and marketing plan?
8. What are three ethical issues that deserve ongoing attention as you work with childbearing women?
9. How might obtaining doctors' and midwives' releases contribute to your practice success and effectiveness?

REFERENCES

Benjamin B, Sohnen-Moe C. The Ethics of Touch. Tucson: Sohnen-Moe Associates, 2003.

Code of Ethics. Available at: http://www.ncbtmb.org/about_code_of_ethics.php. Accessed November 4, 2010.

Gilbert E, Harmon J. Manual of High Risk Pregnancy and Delivery. 3rd Ed. St. Louis: Mosby, 2003.

Massage Therapy Body of Knowledge (MTBOK). Available at http://www.mtbok.org/. Accessed November 4, 2010.

National Certification Board for Therapeutic Massage and Bodywork (NCBTMB).

Osborne C. Pre-and Perinatal Massage Therapy: Survey of Massage Therapists, 2009. www.bodytherapyassociates.com. Accessed June, 2010

Rose MK. The Art of the Chart: Documenting Massage Therapy with CARE Notes. Available at http://www.massageandbodywork.com/Articles/AprilMay2003/CAREnotes.html. Accessed November 2010.

Sohnen-Moe C. Business Mastery. 4th Ed. Tucson: Sohnen-Moe Associates, 2008.

Turgeon R. "Massage Therapy on Trial: Dealing with the Legal System." Presentation to the AMTA National Convention, Phoenix, AZ, September 18, 2008.

For additional resources, please visit http://thePoint.LWW.com/Osborne-Pregnancy2e!

Profiles of Maternity Massage Therapists

Learning Objectives

After study of this chapter, you should be able to:

1. Summarize how prenatal and perinatal massage therapists generally practice in the United States.
2. Describe several difficulties and satisfactions that therapists have experienced in their practices and places of work.
3. Create an impression of how work in various settings might feel and look.
4. Formulate a vision of yourself working with expectant women and new mothers.

In this chapter, you have the opportunity to hear the voices of wise therapists who currently practice maternity massage therapy. Some have done this work for several years, others for decades. To give you a broad picture, first you will see data summarized from a recent survey of therapists trained in prenatal and perinatal massage therapy. Through generalizations and individual practitioner profiles, you then will begin to see what is possible for your career in prenatal massage. (Note that additional practitioner profiles, along with other helpful resources, are available at the Professional Resource and Business Center on the Student site at http://thePoint.lww.com/Osborne-Pregnancy2e.) You will get a sense of the variety of practitioners doing this work and of the many venues where you could possibly work. As you read therapists' vignettes of their sessions, you will get a sense of the progression of work with a few clients. From all of this rich input, you can develop some role models for how to advance your career. So, pull up a chair with a cup of tea or your favorite beverage, and listen to these tales.

Survey Results: An Overview of How Therapists Practice Maternity Massage Therapy

As you complete your study of this book, and any additional hands-on training, you are probably beginning to wonder what the typical massage therapist actually does in her practice. After almost three decades of teaching maternity bodywork and massage, I was curious, as well. I wanted to know: who is practicing this work and where? What percentage of their practice is prenatal work? What are therapists' fees and practice settings like? Who are they engaging with collaboratively? What effects are their clients reporting to them? What are the challenges and rewards of their perinatal work? With these questions in mind, I undertook the task of surveying graduates of my childbearing-related courses.

An experienced public health researcher, Jane Serling MSPH, and I pilot tested and then finalized a questionnaire. We then mailed or emailed them to more than 3,000 therapists who had been my students, from as far back as the mid-1980s on through to the most recent certified graduates. We received 247 surveys over a 2-month period, which was a response rate of only about 8%. This low response rate was the one predominant methodological limitation. It is due in part to surveys not reaching the intended recipients, as we were unable to verify addresses or mail follow-up surveys. In full recognition that those practitioners who returned surveys are not representative of all practitioners, we continued with our task of drawing meaningful conclusions from the information that we had. These results are shown in Table 9.1.

Despite the shortcomings of this survey, the information provided by massage therapists from across the country gives us an unprecedented glimpse into the practices of those who

Table 9.1 Survey Results

Description	Percentage of Responders (%)
Demographics	
Living in the United States	95
Took the author's course since 2000	66
Preparation and education	
Have had some additional maternity-related massage therapy courses	26
Have had no other maternity-related professional training	35
Have had infant massage training	40
Have multiple areas of "specialized training, focused interest, and competency"	99
Specialization in myofascial/deep tissue work	61
Specialization in neuromuscular therapy	40
Practice setting and clientele	
Private practice	72
Spa setting	13
Medical practice or hospital	6
Chiropractic or other healthcare office	6
Maternity or women's wellness center	2
<25% of clients are maternity-related	78
26%–50% of clients are maternity-related	14
>50% of clients are maternity-related	8
Fees for 1-h prenatal session	
$61–$85	53
$60 or less	31
$86 or more	12
Use a sliding scale	2
Fees for labor massage	
Practice labor massage	19
Offer a package price for services	42
Charge hourly fee	29
Use sliding scale	29
Most common reasons clients seek massage	
Low back pain	67
Relaxation, stress reduction, help with sleeping	60
Upper back/neck and shoulder pain	48
Sacrum and pelvic pain	32
Sciatica and "similar sensations"	28
Preparation for labor (including breathing techniques)	6
Edema	4
Symphysis pubis pain	1
Effects of massage on pregnant clients	
Clients reporting a reduction in pregnancy-related pain and discomfort	95
Unsure of how clients feel after massage	3
Does massage help to begin effective labor for women past their due date?	
Unsure	~50
Yes	33
No	11
Clients returning for postpartum massage sessions in first 3 mo after birth	
<25% of clients return	66
>25% of clients return	31
Biggest reward for working with prenatal and perinatal clients	
Providing nurturing and helping women to feel more comfortable, more relaxed, and less pain	66
Empowering women by helping them to become more aware of, connected to, and trusting of their bodies	25
Contributing to the development of the mother's relationship with her baby, family, and the family of humanity	6

(table continues on page 189)

Table 9.1 Survey Results (continued)

Description	Percentage of Responders (%)
Biggest challenge in working with prenatal and perinatal clients	
Getting clients to come in for bodywork early in pregnancy	30
The medicalization of childbirth	19
Not having given birth myself	12
My own body mechanics while doing maternity massage	12
Getting clients to connect with their bodies	6
Getting women positioned comfortably on the table	6
Lack of confidence in my skills and education	6
Getting women to relax during pregnancy	4

pursued 32 hours or more of hands-on training in pregnancy massage. It paints some broad strokes for your consideration. The information from this survey may inform and inspire you as you begin or nurture your maternity massage practice.

General Massage Therapy Practices That Include Perinatal Clients

In typical massage therapy practices, therapists see clients with a variety of needs, concerns, and conditions. Pregnant and postpartum clients can be among the athletes, injured motorists, and stressed-out executives who find improved well-being and stress reduction in your care. Whether by intention, lack of opportunity, or other factors, many massage therapists only

What Would You Do?

You would like to include more pregnant women in your private practice. What additional knowledge, credentials, and/or experience do you need to prepare you for these women? What changes would make your environment, procedures, and organization of your practice more accommodating of expectant women?

My Story

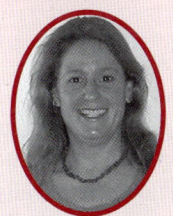

I am highly trained in prenatal and perinatal massage, and yet I only occasionally have several clients from that target market. More frequently, a client becomes pregnant, and then I have the honor of shifting into prenatal care until the birth. Sometimes that translates to more session regularity, and sometimes that means I alter the work we are doing while I am at their workplace offering on-site chair massage.

As a bodywork instructor, I often have former students who are bodyworkers themselves come to get specialized care from me when they are pregnant, which is most gratifying. I have been hoping to join one of my long-term clients in the labor room, but as yet have not been present for any births, other than my own two children. I had one client/student with whom I worked every 2 weeks for most of her pregnancy. We prepared for labor, and the plan was that she would call me for labor support. She went into labor during her anatomy final and barely finished the exam before getting to the labor room; needless to say, I never got a call. It was such joy to see her baby and to see how well she was doing a week afterward at a postpartum session. I felt that much of her calm and centeredness had been a result of her getting regular massage throughout her pregnancy.

My biggest frustration is when regular clients disappear after the birth of their baby. I know that postpartum massage is so very helpful. When they do return, I am so gratified when I not only get to see the baby but also get to help ease some of that newborn-care stress through touch. I started offering a free postpartum session for anyone who had gotten six or more prenatal sessions from me, requiring that they use it within the first month after birth. Since adding this incentive, I have been gratified to have many clients take me up on that offer.

By far, I think the two most popular techniques I practice are the SI joint releases and the quadratus lumborum rebalancing. Both are incredibly effective, and they seem to relieve clients' discomfort immediately. These techniques, along with my ability to safely administer deep tissue sculpting techniques both during pregnancy and after, have brought lots of relief to my clients. (See Chapter 4 technique manual for these techniques.)

—Shari Grayson, San Diego, CA

My Story

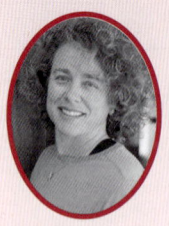

It is a joy and an honor to work with pregnant women as a massage therapist. I knew early on that I wanted to work with this demographic, so I sought certification to ensure sound practice in this work. Currently, approximately 30% of my clientele are prenatal/postpartum. These are certainly some of my most memorable therapist/client relationships.

There are many reasons why this work inspires me. When I think of each prenatal client I've had, there is a special story to tell. My first full-term client/volunteer was a fellow massage student. Her husband was on military deployment for most of her pregnancy. She had a seamless pregnancy, her water broke on my table 2 days past her due date, husband at home, and 4 hours later she had a healthy baby girl. My second prenatal client was a high-risk twins pregnancy. We did a weekly combo of yoga and massage. She was able to carry the babies for 34 weeks. A year later, the girls, mom, and dad are beaming brightly. Most recently, a dear friend and I worked together for her entire pregnancy. She successfully had a natural birth, and I was there to support her through the birthing process. Indeed, it was a joy and an honor.

Besides the obvious value of doing prenatal work, I have also noticed that my approach to bodywork, in general, has been positively affected. A heightened awareness of the process of gestation and birth has transformed the way I look upon, hear, and touch all of my clients. I believe this continues to be a catalyst for the development of my sensitivity as a bodyworker. And, it's fun to witness the parents with their bundles of joy. To date, all of my prenatal clients have come through personal referrals, and they keep coming. I imagine when I put myself out there more formally, as a prenatal massage therapist, the sky's the limit.

—Kim Kolibri, San Diego, CA

---

occasionally work with pregnant women; nevertheless, they are often enthusiastic and gratified when they can accompany a woman through all or part of her childbearing year.

Highlighting and Specializing in Prenatal and Perinatal Massage Therapy

What massage therapist hasn't had a current or former client become pregnant and want massage therapy? How many of these clients, raving about the relief they received, have spread the word to other expectant women? When their doctor or childbirth educator hears of the therapist's expertise, they often begin referring appropriate women. Before long, a skilled, knowledgeable, and caring therapist can generate a practice that specializes in prenatal and perinatal massage therapy. With continued success and desire, some of these maternity massage specialists' practices evolve. They open maternity massage therapy centers, form practice coalitions, and affiliate with other general healthcare providers. Let's take a look into some of these therapists' professional lives.

● PRIVATE PRACTICE

Great freedom, personal responsibility for all successes and failures, and convenience often lead therapists into private practice. Some conceive and nurture a maternity private practice from their career start; others fall into it organically as their perinatal clientele increases. Either way, eventually their office décor features healthy, round bellies and gurgling babies. Their libraries bulge with current and classic books and DVDs to loan, and they are often the go-to therapist in their community when complex medical conditions warrant the most knowledgeable and experienced massage therapist around.

My Story

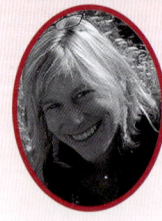

My interest in maternity massage therapy came to me, as it does many women, during my childbearing years. A practicing therapist with two babies, I became certified in prenatal and perinatal massage therapy in 1998. By ten lunar months later, I had my third child and a deeper, more personal understanding of the direct needs of this population.

While my practice was part-time and developing for the next 10 years, it included a steady flow of pregnant clients. At the same

(continued)

My Story (continued)

time, I was studying the art of labor support. I have attended over 40 births as a massage therapist/doula. I recommend doula training for therapists with a maternity massage practice. Your clients will ask you to attend their births, and do go! My ability to attend births lessened with a full-time practice, not to mention full-time motherhood. My interests in deep tissue and structural integration also grew.

I did not market myself exclusively as a prenatal therapist. Pregnant clients seemed to come in groups of two or three. Still, I've had hundreds of sessions with pregnant women with which to build experience and an understanding of the current "state" of maternity massage in my area. With focused marketing, it would not be difficult to build an exclusive practice. No one in my area has attempted this, but it would be good for those with proper training to attempt.

Although I see massage therapy gaining in general popularity, many pregnant clients came to me only once. For many, this was a "treat" or a gift from another. I did my best to focus on the moment's needs, which sometimes were far from their bodies. I did my best to "bring it back" to their bodies. For others, it was a gift for the self. Several women understood the importance of this work, and I was able to support their changing needs over the course of their pregnancies, sometimes right through labor into motherhood! I came to understand this time as just another step of the body toward maturation.

I have cared for those leaning "natural" and those preferring "technology," and I have tried to support all without judgment. I have tried to transform fear and bodily suffering with love. I love this work of maternity massage and see how it could be practiced all one's life. My interest may have started as a result of my own childbearing years, but I can see myself as an old woman still supporting women, perhaps my granddaughters! Perhaps yours.

—Sally Roach, Peoria, IL

My Story

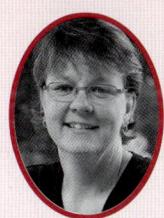

Although I began my massage career with a passion for working with clients with cancer, I sensed that I would burn out if I didn't have more of a balance: I felt I needed more joy in my practice. Happily, the life-giving work of prenatal massage presented itself to me within a year of my graduation when one of my clients became pregnant. I wanted to learn how I could help her, so I began by enrolling in a weekend-long pregnancy massage class. Subsequently, I took a 4-day intensive class that facilitated my certification in prenatal and perinatal massage—a specialty featured in my practice to this day. I became a teaching assistant in that class, and I've continued in that role for the past 10 years.

Initially, it was essential for me to overcome my fear of somehow harming a pregnant woman and her baby. Thankfully, it didn't take long for me to witness the benefits that massage brought to my pregnant clients, and they weren't shy about telling me how my work (which is a combination of massage and teaching about proper posture and positioning) made them feel much more comfortable and at ease. To integrate prenatal massage into my practice, I offered free labor support to another one of my regular clients, just to get myself some experience in the labor room. Once I attended a few births, I met midwives and doctors who became aware of my work and its value. In addition, I spread the word—at Chamber of Commerce events and community volunteer opportunities—that I specialized in prenatal massage therapy.

I also volunteered to give an in-service training for physical and occupational therapists at a local hospital on safe positioning for pregnant clients. Many of the therapists related how helpful this was for them. Now that they know me and understand my work, they refer their patients to my office.

My work serves as its own marketing strategy. Word spreads quickly from one pregnant woman to another. I've found that if I have a pregnant client who attends a prenatal yoga class, it's not long before I have many of the other women from her class in my office! Today, I have a wide range of clients and my practice feels balanced. I see mothers-to-be, athletes, the elderly, as well as many clients living with cancer—and I enjoy them all. I have other massage therapists working with me in my office, and we cover for each other when we are called into a labor unexpectedly. My prenatal massage specialization has brought about an additional benefit in terms of office décor: we have a beautiful "baby wall" in our office with photos of the little ones born to our clients!

—Nanci Newton, Hadley, MA

My Story

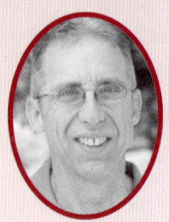

After practicing as an RN for 30 years, I became a certified massage therapist, finding deep professional satisfaction by improving health and satisfaction of one person at a time. I have always been fascinated with the miracle of life, so I sought certification in prenatal and perinatal massage therapy in 2007. Currently, about one third of my practice is with prenatal and postpartum clients.

I faced many challenges to developing a solo practitioner practice, especially without connections to a bodywork or medical referral network. Even though I still work as a registered nurse for a very large organization, there are compliance restrictions for promoting my personal business information. Being a man in a women's health specialty has additional challenges.

Building a client base required developing a professional website that appeals to women, networking with other professionals, offering packages for client returns, and promoting gift certificates for baby showers, Mother's Day, and other special occasions. My biggest referral source of pregnant clients is from the owner of a gently used maternity clothing shop. Focusing the client on her "special delivery" and promoting health during the childbearing year has fostered client loyalty and referrals.

Beginning the pregnancy massage practice was scary, but I followed the routines that we learned in my certification course. I still use these as guidelines for every session. I offered a few women discount sessions if they came for routine therapy sessions through the pregnancy and postpartum period. The addition of myofascial release and deep sculpting techniques to my practice has broadened the effectiveness of my work with these women and my general clientele.

After 2 years as a prenatal and perinatal massage therapist, these expectant clients bring the greatest professional satisfaction. One case comes to mind as remarkable. This woman was on the verge of being confined to bed rest for prenatal hypertension, so we measured her blood pressure before and after our sessions. The massage (see Chapter 4 technique manual) lowered the systolic blood pressure over 20 points and the diastolic by 10 points, allowing her to continue her daily activities.

—Steve Metzger, Sacramento, CA

● COALITIONS AND AFFILIATIONS

When qualified therapists join marketing efforts, often their practices grow exponentially. They also enjoy the stimulation and support of their colleagues. Some therapists who prefer not to or are unable to attend labors collaborate with a massage therapist colleague who does. These coalitions can be loose, more formalized, or evolve into partnerships or corporations.

As therapeutic massage and bodywork becomes more integrated into complementary healthcare, some therapists find gratifying affiliations and/or employment with group practices or centers that specialize in women's health. Their collaborations with doctors, chiropractors, naturopaths, nutritionists, acupuncturists, and others present clients with a holistic, comprehensive approach to their prenatal and postpartum care. Although they can be stimulating and successful, sometimes these larger group structures fall into common difficulties. When many people have a stake in the processes, outcomes, and bottom-line of these businesses, struggles can ensue. Here are a few therapists' stories; glean wisdom from their wide-ranging experiences.

My Story

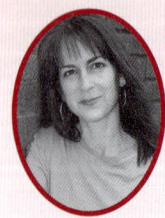

When I was 38 years old and pregnant with my third child, I took a prenatal and perinatal massage certification course. In that circle, I connected with women who were not only massage therapists, but childbirth doulas, mothers who had experienced pregnancy loss, and one woman who could not hope to have her own children. It was a moving experience and brought to life the importance of nurturing touch in this area of our lives.

It also taught me the power of bringing people together with a common cause. I realized that to do the work I wanted to do, which was support women in childbirth, I would need backup. I found

(continued)

My Story (continued)

three like-minded therapists (Monica Faux-Kota, Angela Rhinehart, and Shannon Clay-Gillette) with the level of training the work required. We connected easily and jumped right in to form our network we called Utah Prenatal Massage.

Three years later, we are an association of seven therapists, with a goal of extending throughout Utah so that, in every county, childbearing women will be able to find quality massage care. In 2010, we opened a headquarters in Salt Lake City with classroom space to help us achieve our goals. For therapists, we invite and sponsor professional birth-related courses to our area, and we offer occasional free lectures and massage practice sessions. For our associates, we sponsor a roundtable discussion group of birth and family professionals, including midwives, naturopaths, childbirth educators, and pediatricians, exploring topics such as reproductive mental health and creating bridges between conventional and alternative therapies. Education is a slow, steady process, but fundamental to our work.

We have found that as a group, we can accomplish much more to build interest in our specialty than we could possibly do alone. There is a tremendous amount of work that goes into creating a successful practice. By joining our efforts and our financial resources, we have been able to create a professional website and marketing materials for our members, as well as specialized in-take forms. Being essentially a nonprofit organization, our members work collaboratively, sharing our talents in different areas, in order to support each other's individual success. I feel fortunate to work with my cofounders and other massage therapists who share an uncommon commitment to improving birth experiences.

—Karen Salas, Utah Prenatal Massage, Salt Lake City, UT

My Story

During my time in a women's health/multidisciplinary clinic setting, I experienced both problems and successes, which I discuss below. First, though, here's what attracted me to working in the women's health center setting:

- Collaboration of disciplines: chiropractic, midwifery, massage therapy, and naturopathy
- Having maternity clients who were already clients of the center and had a previous professional relationship with the midwives.
- Desire for community, after working solo for 5 years
- Desire to boost my credibility by associating myself with esteemed colleagues
- Opportunity to expand income by hiring other therapists
- Opportunity to learn skills in clinic operations from the chiropractor that would perhaps move me out of a primary treatment role into more business management
- Shared administrative support (phone answerers, product managers, schedulers, and fee collectors) so that practitioners could just do their work

Some of the challenges we encountered while working in this setting are listed below:

- Inequitable distribution of costs among practitioners: some practitioners required much more administrative support than others, but everyone paid the same share
- Inadequate administrative support for the team of practitioners as it grew from 4 to 12
- Tripling of administrative and operating costs for all practitioners, due to the hiring of new staff to handle the increased work load
- Domination by practitioners who had invested the most financially in starting the practice in making decisions about the business; other practitioners felt more like employees

As a result of all of these issues, all but two of the original community members have left, almost all back to private practice in their own offices.

There were great successes and satisfactions:

- The team of massage therapists worked well together, with 85% of our time booked consistently by the end of the first year in operation.
- Great teamwork among the massage team, who provided effective, nurturing work to clients and mutual support that fostered their practice and skills

(continued)

My Story (continued)

- Client care improved from communication and coordination of providers to maximize effectiveness, financial resources, educational opportunities, and everyone's support.

The inclusion of massage therapy as a necessary, meaningful service for pregnant women, not just a feel-good thing to do, was a tremendous success for the profession in my area in early 2000 to 2003.

Here are my major lessons and reflections:

- I was dazzled by these esteemed professionals' interest in me and my practice, and I trusted when I perhaps shouldn't have. However, trusting feels better than realizing that I didn't trust when I should have.
- As women, we are still too new at being "out of the kitchen and into the world" to react to financial threat logically and rationally versus emotionally. Financial instability for us means our babies will starve, and we will be on the streets, energetically if not literally! So we can pull in and protect in response. How we behave in that climate is unique to individuals and their experience.
- Collaborative practices are very beneficial to the client, especially the "higher-risk" situations.

I continue to learn from this experience. I am pleased to know of similar models that are working where the right team, personalities, and clear expectations came together. I don't want to discourage anyone from pursuing this engaging practice setting; just be aware of potential pitfalls.

—Anonymous Practitioner

My Story

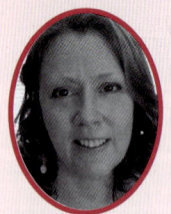

At one point in my career, my practice was associated with a multidisciplinary clinic in which I was an owner-partner for 9 years. The clinic providers I worked with included nurse-practitioners, physical therapists, chiropractors, nurse-midwives, nutritionists, naturopaths, acupuncturists, and, of course, massage therapists. One provider was an osteopath who practiced physiatry or physical medicine. On hospital rounds one morning, he was called in to consult with a high-risk obstetrical specialist. The OB had a new patient with lupus and placental abruption while expecting her first baby. She complained of significant back pain and found it difficult to get comfortable. Her pain was greatly hindering her getting the rest and restorative sleep she needed.

He asked if I could assess the patient to determine whether I could help provide comfort or pain relief. I greeted the nursing staff, introducing myself, and then talked with the patient and her husband before giving my report to the physician. I demonstrated for her the various positions that would provide comfort as well as facilitate fetal oxygen flow. I let the nursing station know that their patient would need additional pillows from now on and why.

I was also able to provide the husband with something to do in the way of relieving stiffness and soreness resulting from bed rest. I demonstrated simple techniques such as the reflexive foot work, hip/femur decompression, hip work, and kneading at the shoulders and neck (see Chapter 4 technique manual). I made sure to observe him applying them correctly. The couple was very grateful to have things to do that offered comfort as well as helped the baby.

By the time the OB had made his way to her room, we had a plan for him to approve. He was delighted that his patient could get some relief of her complaints and asked that I check back with them over the course of the next few weeks that he anticipated would be necessary before she gave birth. This afforded me the opportunity to provide other body use information to the couple, too.

I was excited to begin building a relationship with this provider. He was so open and curious about what I could offer for his patients. This type of work is not what one might expect when thinking about a prenatal massage practice, but it was one of the most rewarding episodes of my career. It took so little time and so many people were happily affected.

—Jennifer Hicks, Great Falls, MT

MATERNITY MASSAGE THERAPY CENTERS

Some therapists have created business with an exclusive or predominant prenatal, perinatal, and family focus. Often, they incorporate other wellness care services such as acupuncture or prenatal exercise. Some seek to become women's one-stop source for ways to further their enjoyment and comfort during the childbearing year. Often, these are joint ventures, loose associations, or businesses that hire a staff of qualified therapists who can serve a larger clientele.

My Story

Our client base is approximately 65% prenatal, 10% postpartum, and the remaining 25% being non–pregnancy-based massage. Our center is a two-office operation with three pregnancy massage specialists currently seeing clients. My goal is to have satellite offices around the metro Atlanta area and eventually to have a holistic wellness center that revolves around pregnant women and families.

Because we bought a thriving practice, we had a base clientele already in place; however, the constant turnover of pregnancy leads to one of our biggest challenges: the immediate and consistent need for development of new clients is never ending. We are well established within the community and with the majority of OB/GYN offices; nevertheless, we need constant contact to maintain productive relationships. This includes lobbying OB offices, brochure upkeep, and basic staff awareness. To date, we have navigated this challenge effectively, all the while remembering it is a persistent struggle. When we do all of this well, our business can weather even the worst of economies.

Another challenge, and our most difficult, is retaining our clients after their pregnancy. Because we are known as prenatal specialists, it sometimes gets lost that we are also massage therapists for everyone. One major part of this is understanding the complex transition women go through after having a baby. Time constraints, exhaustion, adjusting to motherhood, and remembering to take care of self take a big toll on most women. Although the majority of us would agree that this is the time when we truly need massage, new mothers tend to forget they need to make time for themselves. As their massage therapists, we encourage and remind them that they will need massage after the baby is born. As a business, we send a special card after the due date that includes coupons for both the new mom and the partner to encourage both postpartum and nonpregnancy massage. It has not been as successful as I would have thought, but I do believe that we have encouraged more than one new mom to take time for herself, and a dad or two also.

The best part of this job, hands down, is the look on pregnant women's faces the moment the massage is done. They are serene and relaxed and are the most grateful clients ever. You may not always relieve their problem, if there is one, in the massage, but they are always better than when they walked in. I cannot think of a better way to honor children than to help relax and soothe their parents.

—Renee Kimes, Pregnancy Massage Center, Atlanta, GA

My Story

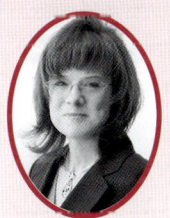

My journey into massage and the wondrous world of prenatal massage began in the 1980s, when others in my "encounter groups" acknowledged a special quality in my touch. Inspired by reading about pioneering body therapists, I sought bodywork training, and then I started working in chiropractic offices. That is where I served my first pregnant client and immediately knew that this was for me. When I became certified in maternity massage therapy in 1994, my life was about to change.

Within weeks of completing that course, a reporter wrote my story and a local TV station filmed a special report on pregnancy massage. Before long, I needed another therapist to assist with my overflow of clients. As business grew, my husband and I built a 2,000-ft² wellness spa from the ground up, in a strip mall. Intending to serve a general clientele, we wanted to also specialize in a maternity-centered practice. This business now supports five massage therapists, one esthetician, a lobby manager, a part-time receptionist, and my husband and me. We have had the blessings of press coverage and opportunities seemingly landing on our doorstep.

(continued)

My Story (continued)

Many other developments came from our clients, including them introducing us to high-risk pregnancy clinical studies, local pregnancy organizations and prenatal exercise facilities, birthing centers, and hospitals.

All of these referrals led to us becoming the referral of choice in our area, including affiliations with several local hospitals. Mixed in with those successes were many hardships, mistakes, and obstacles. Staff dishonesty and disloyalties, a theft, and our own health challenges created opportunity for deep learning for me on many levels, and we overcame them all.

—Mikki Anderson, Stressbusters Lifestyle Day Spa, Laguna Hills, CA

Collaborations with Other Maternity Professionals

Integrating prenatal and perinatal massage therapy into maternity healthcare is a growing trend. When hospitals implement complementary care within their walls or in affiliated facilities, the maternity patients (and the oncology patients) are often the first to see massage therapists. Their care adds high-touch, nurturing, individualized care to what can be high-tech, institutionalized structures. Obstetricians are beginning to recognize and employ massage therapists to help ease many of pregnancy's discomforts, particularly those that they previously could not address effectively.

Midwifery includes a broad range of professionals, from direct entry/lay midwives, certified and not, to nurse-midwives. Seeing women in private offices, small clinics, birthing centers, obstetrical offices, and hospitals, their clientele and practices varies widely. What all of these midwives share is a common history of including nurturing touch in their care of pregnant and laboring women. In addition to technical skills, in-depth knowledge, and keen intuition, many midwives massage the women in their care into birthing. The specially trained hands of a prenatal and perinatal massage therapist harmoniously work with theirs in women's care.

● HOSPITAL-BASED PROGRAMS

My Story

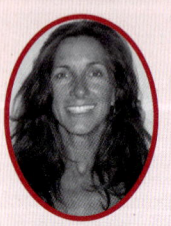

In addition to a spa and my own practice, I also currently work at a large metropolitan hospital, where I share a room with the sonogram techs. The nurses inform the high-risk moms who are in the hospital for the duration of their pregnancies that massage therapy is available. Each woman receives a brochure with various activities and options available to her during her stay, including massage therapy. With doctor clearance, patients or their family may purchase a certificate in the hospital gift shop. Between the nursing staff, doctors, and me, we have established 2 days/week with a 5-hour window available for the moms.

Most moms come to my small but relaxing therapy room. Even though it is just down the hall for them, it can seem like a vacation destination to someone confined to a hospital bed. Usually, the patient's nurse will wheel her to my room for a 55-minute session. Because most moms have multiples, many are on magnesium to stop contractions, and it makes them very warm. I cover them with sheets and nontraditional hospital blankets. I prop them with nice, fluffy pillows, providing low-light ambiance and gentle, relaxing music.

Most moms take this time as a reprieve from "all the other stuff." We exchange little conversation during the session, as most moms just need "to check out." Over the last 8 months' reviews of my work, most clients have rated their experience five on a five-point scale. Most of their physical discomfort comes from restricted activity, as well as the baby (or babies) taking up more and more room. This usually manifests in sore necks and upper ribcage pressure/discomfort, though I always address the hips and feet, as well. I document each session in a book kept at the front desk. Because of I.V.s, short time, and common sense, most all moms keep their "comfy clothing" on, and I work with no oil.

When I do go to their rooms and work with them in their beds, I bring my iPod and dock. The beds are very flexible, and this work is very easy to do while in their beds... though the change in scenery is of great value if they can make it to the "Massage Room."

—Maryfaith Schweighardt, San Diego, CA

My Story

In 1998, Longmont United Hospital's BirthPlace and the Health Center of Integrated Therapies, the hospital's complementary medicine department, had a vision of implementing more patient-centered care practices in our birthing center. In a 3-month BirthPlace massage therapy pilot program, licensed massage therapist employees provided massages to postpartum patients. The intention was offering nonpharmacological pain relief, promoting postpartum recovery, and demonstrating Longmont United Hospital's commitment to the Planetree philosophy of patient-centered care through the use of complementary therapies. (For more information about Planetree, visit their website www.planetree.org.)

Patients evaluated the pilot program with premassage and postmassage surveys that showed 100% satisfaction, with 70% of patients never before experiencing professional massage therapy. Based on the success of the 3-month pilot, Longmont United Hospital's Leadership Council supported the implementation of a 365-day program. The BirthPlace Staff creatively examined their budget with patient-centered eyes and replaced plastic lawn storks, steak dinners, and disposable baby wipes with complimentary 30-minute massage therapy sessions for every patient. The OB-GYN Medical Staff Committee provided standing written physician orders for all BirthPlace patients to receive massage therapy, which they periodically review and reapprove.

Most massages are postpartum, but there are occasional antepartum patients who also receive massage therapy. Massage therapists talk with each patient at her bedside and design and provide a treatment that addresses her unique needs. The massage therapist asks for pretreatment and posttreatment 0 to 10 patient pain ratings, documenting in each patient's medical record progress notes. Massage therapists who staff the 365-day BirthPlace Massage Therapy Program have completed advanced maternity massage therapy training. In addition, they are required to complete an annual departmental competency test.

Over the years, patients continue to report that this caring human touch is part of what brings them back to Longmont United Hospital's BirthPlace. Specifically, the massage helps them manage their pain and increases their satisfaction with their overall birth experience and care. To date, the BirthPlace Massage Therapy Program has provided over 13,000 patients with compassionate, caring and skillful maternity massage therapy. (For more information about Longmont United Hospital, visit their website www.luhcares.org.)

—Longmont United Hospital's BirthPlace Massage Therapy Program, Longmont, CO

My Story

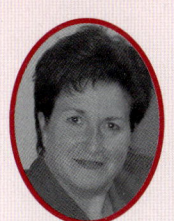

The Women's Health Resource Center provides women a location to obtain current health information, resources for health and well-being through classes and support groups, as well as supportive care for women with cancer. Massage therapy is an integral service offered, with pregnant and postpartum women receiving approximately one third of all the massages provided there. Under the direction of a nurse practitioner with over 16 years in labor and delivery, the Center enjoys a respected place in the community as a provider of medical rather than resort or spa massage services

Currently, a staff of 10 therapists works with pregnant and postpartum women, as well as other patients. They see clients on an outpatient basis, and patients who are on bed rest in the antepartum unit, all on a fee-for-service basis. This is in addition to the free sessions offered to those in the cancer and palliative care units. These therapists complete approximately 4,000 sessions annually, with only one full-time and one part-time therapy room available among them.

The founding director and ongoing coordinator, Barb Silver, NP, established the program in 1996. She attributes its initial genesis to faith, a great therapist, a cozy room, and luck. In addition, the Center's foundation is a feminist philosophy, grounded in the intention to create a compassionate, safe environment for women to heal and thrive. Ms. Silver acknowledges and values the staff massage therapists' sincere concern for women, their joy in their work, mutual respect, and highly professional and thorough training; and she pays them accordingly. Fourteen years into the program, massage therapy is a well-integrated, respected service that the doctors generally embrace.

Ms. Silver lists the biggest challenges with the massage therapy program there as doctors' shortages of time and busyness to refer more proactively, last-minute cancellations, staff and visitors coming in and out of the room during sessions, and patients' needs that take away from the scheduled massage session times. The greatest joys are seeing depressed, anxious, and tired women relax into the caring, quiet, pain-relieving effects of their sessions.

—Barb Silver, Women's Health Resource Center at California Pacific Medical Center, San Francisco, CA

WORKING IN OBSTETRICAL OFFICES

Many doctors are beginning to recognize the value of massage therapy to address the normal aches and pains of pregnancy, provide emotional support and nurturance, and contribute to healthier outcomes for mothers and babies. Joining the staff of nurses, nurse-midwives, ultrasound technicians, and other staff providers of modern maternity medicine has its satisfactions and challenges, as seen in these therapists' stories.

My Story

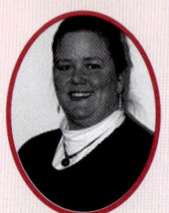

After several years of managing my private practice, I accepted a position at an obstetrical office. My new position required me to work at the obstetric office 2 days a week, providing massage for the patients of the practice. In addition, I would be on call for four births a month. Including me, there were two massage therapist/doulas on staff, and we would rotate call. I knew that a commitment to four births a month was a lot, but I didn't count on the never-ending stress of being on call 24/7, which affected my family life. With only two of us on staff, one was always a back up even after an extended birth attendance. I couldn't plan on anything firmly, except maybe that my plans were always tentative. This stress was enormous.

The sheer size of the office and stress in the space with nurses and administrative staff working to keep the practitioners on schedule was overwhelming. The size offered me definite benefits and situations in which I learned and had access to procedures that the average massage therapist/doula would miss. I had hospital clearance, which meant that, if the obstetrician wanted me to be in a surgery, I could be. In a surgical suite, I witnessed the dramatic birth of twins and a couple of cesarean sections.

I also saw the compassion that many healthcare providers (MDs, nurses, and all their associates) have for these laboring women. I really learned from working in the office with these professionals. I began to appreciate the pressure on the care team. I especially enjoyed the relationships I built with the doctors and midwives. And I saw the other side too: Sometimes, the labor and delivery floor was virtually empty, and the laboring women got loads of attention. Occasionally, they ran out of rooms due to the volume of labors in progress. You can bet that the staff was stretched thin, and the women that had us as extra attendants really appreciated us!

That said, let me say how remarkable my labor work was: it is thrilling, joyful, stressful, scary, and spiritual all at the same time. I have some amazing memories of these women and their families and the births. I am grateful to each one of them for the lessons they shared with me. Each family unit had its own challenges and triumphs, and I learned to be patient, present, and to let go of expectations and judgment.

—Liz Ellis, Chicago, IL

My Story

The seed of partnership between Mother Nurture Massage Therapy and Lowcountry Obstetrics & Gynecology (LCOB) was really planted a full 7 years ago, when I first became a patient in that practice. However, it wasn't until soon after the birth of my first child 5 years ago that I began to be called into prenatal massage therapy. The entire process of conception, pregnancy, labor and childbirth, and new motherhood was so utterly transforming for me that once pregnancy was over, I longed to remain connected to this vital process in human existence. Having always had a strong interest in massage therapy, the call to prenatal massage was loud and clear.

Before I even started classes, I knew I wanted to work in conjunction with LCOB. I loved them as a patient, and respected their balanced, caring, and open environment. I saw their busy office housing seven doctors and three nurse-midwives as an ideal place to carry on my own practice. Through the process of birthing my own child, I had become quite close with my own physician. She took great interest and helped me in so many ways to get to where I currently am.

On the OB practice manager's advice, I brought lunches in and hosted roundtables for the entire medical office and set up in their break room. It gave me valuable opportunity to drop off my printed literature, to meet with almost all the doctors, and to get my face associated with my name and logo.

Ann, the patient educator, was immediately extremely interested in what I did. Her position afforded me great access to

(continued)

My Story (continued)

every single patient in the practice, as well as every single doctor and nurse-midwife. Ann's first request of me was that I supply her with enough brochures to include with her packets, which placed my name directly into the hands of my captive audience from their doctor's office—a major marketing breakthrough. Later, I developed a 2-hour class for couples that she eventually incorporated into her childbirth education classes.

When the managing partners reorganized, they asked about incorporating my services into the office space. With a formal written business proposal, they saw that my business, Mother Nurture, was a self-contained, turnkey operation. Without any investment money or man hours needed, it was a no-risk, high-yield addition to the practice. The doctors requested that if their patients wanted a massage, they only see me to ensure their safety and the involvement of the medical team if it became necessary. A very recent consolidation there eliminated my room, but I am still receiving their many referrals for prenatal and postpartum work.

—Allison Kirk, Mt. Pleasant, NC

What Would You Do?

Who are the other massage therapists with whom you might collaborate or communicate with about your perinatal massage therapy practice? Who do you know already, what affiliations do you have, and who are potential perinatal healthcare and service providers with whom you might explore networking and making referrals?

Spa and Corporate Prenatal and Postpartum Massage

As the number of spas and their range of services expand, perinatal massage therapy has become a specialty offering on their menus. Pregnant working women escape to the therapy chairs and tables of therapists working on-site in corporate environments. Employment opportunities for qualified massage therapists are blossoming as a result. Here a few of these therapists' stories.

My Story

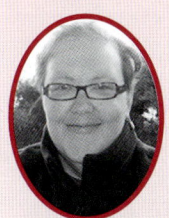

I am a massage therapist at a large tech-based company, where I have been practicing prenatal massage for about a year. Prior to working here, I had my own business and worked in spas and physical therapy clinics. I had felt competent in my skills doing prenatal massage, but, honestly I never really enjoyed it much. When this company hired me, I found that they would require certification prior to allowing me to work on their pregnant employees. With some resignation, I took a certification class, and I am so glad I did. What I learned in that class has improved and increased my skill set tremendously, but the real benefit is that I now truly enjoy working with this specific clientele.

I am very fortunate to work here because they support us so well in doing the best possible job we can for our fellow employees. They supply all our rooms with pillows and wedges, and some of our tables already come with table tilt options.

We are primarily responsible for marketing our skills and availability to our target audience, and we have a lot of latitude with which to do so. For example, we are able to place advertising posters around the office and hold what we call tech talks (lessons/discussions on any topic of interest). All of our bookings happen online, and those of us who are certified have an indicator next to our name letting employees know we are available for prenatal massage.

The population I work with is primarily engineers who sit at a computer all day long and therefore have significant upper body strain in addition to the regular discomfort that can be associated with pregnancy. Postural use affects their neck, shoulder, and upper thoracic region, often leading to carpal tunnel and thoracic outlet syndrome. Low back strain and pain in hip rotators from sitting at a desk for most hours of the day are common complaints, as well.

As with all clients anywhere, the physical relief we facilitate is valued and appreciated, but the emotional support is incalculable. I had a client who told me before our session that she had miscarried about a month prior. Though the massage I did wasn't technically prenatal, my thoughts and hers were there the entire time. If you think about it, we place the mother in fetal position for the bulk of their massage during their pregnancy. We nurture and care for them, provide emotional and physical support, allowing them to voice whatever may be on their minds without judgment. I can't think of a better job!

—Alex Bennion, Seattle, WA

My Story

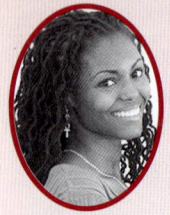

From the very start of my massage career, prenatal massage has been a passion. I attended a certification seminar where I truly obtained a deeper understanding of the expectant woman's anatomy and many techniques to relieve the discomfort of her changing form.

After working in an obstetrics office, I eventually ventured into the spa environment. I now work in a general spa that targets expectant and new moms, but prenatal massage is still only 20% of my clientele. One of the benefits there is the use of a hydraulic table, which is absolutely fantastic for the semireclining position! Another benefit is that I see my clients for a longer amount of time than at the OB office and with increased frequency. The relationship built is a long-lasting one: clients return throughout their pregnancy, postpartum, and many times bring their babies in to learn to perform infant massage themselves. I feel honored to be a part of my client's lives, and some of them I worked on through multiple pregnancies.

Word of advice: always remember the woman is your client! When she returns to you postpartum, honor her. Ask about her health and well-being first, before diving into the baby pictures! She will appreciate the fact that someone still sees her as an individual.

—Kenya Carmichael, Spa Director, Phoenix, AZ

Spotlight on Career Maternity Massage Specialists

If you are just beginning your perinatal education or have only a few years of maternity massage experience, your future in this work can be somewhat unclear. Despite your idealism, ambitiousness, and energetic enthusiasm, what lies ahead for you can be fuzzy, particularly when you peer past your first decade in the work. Every therapist's path is unique, but these highly experienced therapists' stories might provide you some glimpse of where you might be heading.

My Story

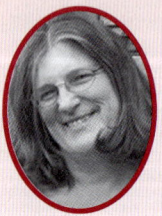

After working in many different collaborative massage settings, I feel I have "landed" where I am comfortable and independent in my own private practice clinic working with women at all stages of life. It feels like I have reached my destination for now creating a comfortable balance of work and family life that sustains me on many levels—financially, physically, and professionally.

Maternity work is joyfully intense all at the same time. It takes a balanced blend of

- Heart—our intent to walk beside women and mothers on their journeys
- Head—establishing, initiating, and managing a responsible, professional career
- Hands—learning our work and continuing to refine and integrate what we are learning into our personal application of the skill and magic of massage

Here is the list of joys in this work that I compiled over the last few days being in and thinking about my practice:

- Positively focused work rather than injury based
- The variety of presenting information: each client is different and changes dramatically
- The babies, of course!
- The satisfaction of knowing I am making a positive difference in people's lives

And here are the challenges that I regularly encounter:

- Maintaining healthy boundaries with needy clients (labor support, home visit, etc.)
- Being flexible in scheduling as clients want to increase the frequency of visits as they near 40 weeks
- Struggling to fit in home visits to bed-resting and postpartum clients
- Accommodating those beautiful babies in the room for treatment session without their distracting their mothers!

(continued)

My Story (continued)

- Remaining positive and supportive in difficult situations that arise with pregnancies
- Avoiding discussing controversial birthing issues while working on the client
- Handling the amount of laundry that this kind of practice produces

—Linda Hickey, Registered Massage Therapist, Calgary Maternity Massage Therapy, Calgary, AB

My Story

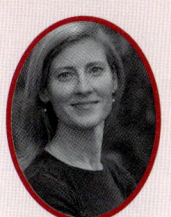

I have been extremely blessed to have many diverse opportunities to follow my passions and be of service to childbearing women and infants. My private practice started in a professional office in 1992, moved to my home, to another professional office, and then back at home as my growing family's needs changed. In addition to a private practice, I looked for a variety of opportunities to teach maternity and infant massage to new mom and family support groups, social service agencies, spas, and at massage therapy schools.

My clients teach me, and they constantly remind me of the essential healing ingredients they need: caring skillful touch, listening ears, and introspective questions to find their own answers and engage their intuition. It seems that when it comes to childbearing and babies, there is a staggering amount of information and advice (sometimes unsolicited!) to assimilate, and it can be overwhelming. I try to create a sanctuary for women and babies (and myself!).

In 2001, I was fortunate to join Longmont United Hospital's BirthPlace Massage Therapy team. In private practice and in teaching, I mostly work with healthy women and babies. In the hospital setting, I see similar healthy women and babies and also the rest of the real world: the "underbelly" of the childbearing experience, as I call it. These include the following:

- Women with little or no prenatal care
- Women with acute high-risk conditions and complications
- Young teenagers who have been raped, including incest, and are birthing their first babies
- Drug addicts who are "strung out" and withdrawing
- Women who are incarcerated but out of jail long enough to labor and birth
- Women who have been abused and whose babies are going into social service custody due to domestic violence
- Women who live in poverty
- Women whose babies have not survived

As painful as these situations are, these are the very situations that also so desperately need our caring work. Not only has it been an exquisite practice in nonjudgment and bringing the same compassion and skill to each of these women and their infants, but it also has motivated me to take better care of myself. I love being outside in nature, practicing yoga, gardening, and enjoying my family. I encourage you to find the "underbellies" in your local community and reach out to care for those women and children, and also engage regularly in the self-care practices that nurture and sustain you.

—Michele Kolakowski, Registered Massage Therapist, Certified Birth Doula (DONA), Longmont, CO

Client Vignettes

To complete your vision as to how prenatal and perinatal massage therapists actually practice, let's look at several therapists' work with individual women. Rather than formal case studies, these are loosely organized stories of these women, their pregnancies, and their therapists' responses to their needs. See online resources at http://thePoint.lww.com/Osborne-Pregnancy2e for Three Pregnancies/Three Series' Sessions (postural and technique photographs from each trimesters' work with three clients, accompanied by therapists' and clients' commentary).

My Story

Lisa first came to me when she was 12 weeks pregnant, a healthy 28-year-old having her first pregnancy. She confirmed that she currently had no physical problems and had a clean bill of health from her midwife. During her first treatment, it was apparent that a number of muscle groups were extremely tight and in spasm. Lisa had been unaware of this and the tenderness only became apparent as I was working on her. During this session, I released and stretched these muscle groups, and Lisa realized how much better she felt afterward. We agreed that she would visit once a week throughout her pregnancy during which time we would also include looking at her posture, breathing, and relaxation. I also supplied her with oil to use on her skin on a daily basis. The oil was a blend of pure vegetable oils and some extremely safe essential oils.

Throughout the pregnancy, due to the frequency of visits, I was able to resolve any potential problems before they became established. Later on in the pregnancy, I also gave Lisa instruction on perineal massage along with a safe oil to use. As well as coming for a weekly massage, she also had regular exercise every day walking her dog.

When labor started, it was 3 days early. She woke up at two in the morning with regular contractions that continued throughout the morning. During the afternoon, however, she noticed some discharge with blood at which point she decided to phone the maternity home; she was told to come in straight away. Labor was progressing normally, and at 9 PM, Lisa went into a warm bath and almost immediately the contractions increased in intensity. By 11 PM, she had a baby daughter weighing 6 lb 10 oz. During the labor, Lisa only required a very small amount of nitrous oxide and oxygen, and only sustained a very minor superficial tear to the perineum. She had massaged and stretched the perineum each day, starting approximately 4 weeks before the birth. She was absolutely delighted at how well her labor and the birth had gone, as were the midwife and those in attendance. They also commented on the beautiful condition of her skin and also the beautiful condition of the baby's skin. I next saw Lisa 6 weeks after the birth, to work with any birthing and postnatal problems.

I received the following letter from Lisa. This, along with the success of her pregnancy and labor, was such a wonderful experience and certainly was a major factor in inspiring me to specialize in prenatal and perinatal work and also to bring further education over to the UK to train other therapists, expanding the availability of the benefits of massage to as many women as possible.

"Dear Ronnie, I don't think words or the gift (water fountain for treatment room) I have chosen for you come close in showing you how much I appreciated the care I received from you during and after my pregnancy. I can't thank you enough. During my pregnancy, the massage every week was fantastic, keeping my skin soft and keeping all aches and pains away. Elidh has definitely benefited from the massage as her skin is beautiful and everyone comments on it. The gift I have chosen, I hope you will use in your massage room although the trickle of water may make your pregnant clients run to the toilet. Thanks once again, Ronnie. Your care and magic hands worked wonders."

—Ronnie Allan, Ayr, Scotland

My Story

Lea was 30 years old and in her first trimester, seeking massage therapy throughout her first pregnancy. With a history of chronic upper back stiffness and soreness, Lea found pregnancy massage much more effective than the chiropractic care she had been receiving. We implemented the sidelying position in the second trimester, and she responded quite well to relaxation and loosening of the paraspinal and pelvic muscles. By the end of the massage, the lumbar lengthening technique was very effective to bring her back into a more balanced and pain-free state (see Chapter 4 technique manual).

Monthly massages allowed her to continue her full-time accounting position. About midpregnancy, she was promoted and was given additional work responsibilities, creating more upper body pain and tension. Increased focus on the shoulders and neck was useful for her to continue her daily routines. She also was taking a pregnancy yoga class, which assisted her between massage sessions.

During the third trimester, Lea increased her frequency of massage therapy sessions to biweekly. In the eighth month, she developed aching in the right hip and leg that responded well to

(continued)

My Story (continued)

myofascial release and hip sculpting, especially in the gluteal areas and on the piriformis muscles. Lea learned an effective stretch to continue this release of these muscles by placing herself on the floor in "down-dog" position, bringing the right foot in front of the left knee and then rocking to a position in which she felt the gluteal stretch. By holding this position, the muscles were able to be released on a daily basis.

Lea was very faithful to practice Kegel exercises throughout her pregnancy and added the pelvic floor stretching from Elizabeth Noble book, Essential Exercises for the Childbearing Year. Lea also used a doula during labor, birthing a healthy boy, 9 lb 11 oz, nearly 22 inches. During her postpartum treatments, some of the pelvic and back techniques used during pregnancy were again helpful to assist her body in the transition to her prepregnancy state. In addition to the structural treatment of relaxation and pain relief, Lea enjoyed the "whole-body experience" with craniosacral techniques, scalp massage, hand/foot massage, soft music, and aromatherapy.

—Steve Metzger, RN-CMT, Sacramento, CA

My Story

Suzy sought out pregnancy massage to relieve discomforts during the third trimester for her second set of twins. She was 33 years old with 4-year-old twins and suffered from scoliosis (45 degrees). Suzy had just been released from 3 months of bed rest, and her back was in a lot of pain. With the extra weight of a twin pregnancy and the diagnosis of scoliosis from childhood, she knew that she needed to find someone certified in pregnancy massage.

Suzy was so uncomfortable that she needed assistance walking into the office and getting on the table for treatment. Deep sculpting along the back was very important to get the back muscles to relax. After the lumbar-lengthening techniques, she was able to stand and walk without pain. Because of the extra weight, Suzy's gluteal and piriformis muscles were very tight and painful. She responded well to my working with the trigger points in the hip and back (see Chapter 4 technique manual). Suzy gave birth to Joshua and Julia, healthy fraternal twins.

At her postpartum session, Suzy had a three- to four-fingerwidth gap of the recti abdominis and implemented Elizabeth Noble's "head-lift" exercises until the gap decreased. Suzy has continued to receive massage treatment after the perinatal period. The combination of myofascial release with deep tissue sculpting is very effective for pain relief and relaxation of her back, which is compromised with scoliosis (see Chapters 4 and 6 technique manual).

—Steve Metzger, RN-CMT, Sacramento, CA

CHAPTER SUMMARY

So now that the embers of this storytelling chapter are dying, and your teacup is empty, this text also is near its end. Before we close, take a few minutes to sift over the words of wisdom of these stories. Feel the professional passion and dedication of these therapists in these many venues. Soften yourself with the appreciative and relieved words of the women they have served. Then peer into your mind and your heart. Take a deep breath. Allow a vision to begin forming…

There you are in a massage therapy room in the setting where you most want to work. This room invites relaxation, exudes wisdom and competence, and is fully supplied to support your hands-on work. You are standing next to your table with a dear, round woman whose gestational energy warms you and your room. She is comfortable and receptive as she lies tenderly and professionally draped, securely positioned. You have aligned your body to feel comfortable and grounded. Your hands are powerful, yet gentle, as they effectively soothe, encourage, and guide her into relaxation and pain-free well-being. Your heart is open, compassionate, and empathetic as you listen to what has heart and meaning for her, buoying her joys and hearing her difficulties. Your mind is clear of distractions, worries, and other chatter. You observe, assess, intuit, and access all the information that you need to be safe and effective in your care.

A sense of connection and meaning begins to envelope you both. You realize that you are nurturing the birth of a mother and of her baby. You have become a prenatal and perinatal massage therapist.

Test Yourself

For answers, visit the website at http://thePoint.LWW.com/Osborne-Pregnancy2e!

1. What two types of therapeutic bodywork are most respondents to the perinatal massage therapists' survey trained and competent in?

2. In what practice setting do most respondents to the perinatal massage therapists' survey practice?

3. What are the three most common reasons respondents to the perinatal massage therapists' survey said that their clients have for coming for massage sessions?

4. What did most respondents to the perinatal massage therapists' survey say were the most rewarding and the most challenging aspects of working with maternity clients?

5. List three lessons that you learned from the stories written by the therapists in this chapter.

6. List three possible individuals, groups, businesses, or facilities that you would like to explore, possibly collaborating within your practice of prenatal and perinatal massage therapy.

7. List three ways in which you are inspired by the stories of the therapists in this chapter.

8. List three insights you have received about working in a medical setting from the stories of the therapists in this chapter.

9. Briefly describe how you would like to see yourself evolve as a prenatal and perinatal massage therapist.

For additional resources, please visit http://thePoint.LWW.com/Osborne-Pregnancy2e!

Glossary

abortion: removal of all conceptive tissues from the uterus before a viable fetus is formed.

active labor: second phase of the first stage of labor during which the cervix effaces and dilates fully to 10 cm from 3 or 4 cm.

active listening: listening in a way that makes others feel heard, feeds back what one hears to confirm accuracy of understanding and to encourage further sharing and self-exploration.

acupressure: a system of balancing the body's energy by applying pressure to specific acupoints to release tension and increase circulation. The many hands-on methods of stimulating the acupressure points can strengthen weaknesses, relieve common ailments, prevent health disorders and restore the body's vital life force. Acupressure is a form of Asian Bodywork Therapy, any form of therapeutic bodywork with its theoretical roots in Chinese Medicine Theory such as Acupressure, Amma, Chi Nei Tsang, Jin Shin Do®, Medical Qigong, Nuad Bo 'Rarn (Thai), Shiatsu, and Tuina.

amniotic fluid: liquid in which fetus floats, consisting of 98% water and 2% other organic matter excreted by the fetus.

amniotic fluid embolism: rare but extremely dangerous leakage of uterine fluids and fetal matter into maternal circulation where it can compromise lung function.

Apgar score: measurement system of the health of a newborn taken 1 and 5 minutes after birth.

aromatherapist: A healthcare provider trained in the use of volatile plant materials, also known as essential oils, with the intention of improving an individual's health, mood or cognitive functioning.

arrested labor or dystocia: when cervical dilation stops for several hours during active labor or the descent of the baby is very prolonged or stops during second stage.

Aston Patterning: system of bodywork, ergonomic analysis and movement coaching designed by Judith Aston to restore natural alignment and dynamic well-being to individuals.

augmentation: medical intervention to sustain and enhance ineffective uterine contractions after labor begins.

"baby blues": a temporary postpartum affective disorder occurring 3-4 days after childbirth that resolves itself without treatment within 1 to 2 weeks; new mothers feel anxious, irritable, emotionally oversensitive and erratic, overwhelmed and can have difficulty with normal sleep and eating.

For an extended obstetrical glossary featuring additional medical procedures, treatments, and medications, visit http://thePoint.lww.com/Osborne-Pregnancy2e!

back jack chair: a floor chair constructed of a heavy cotton duck outer cover stretched over a sturdy steel inner frame; generally laid down to a 30 degree angle when used as for a semireclining foundation for massage.

banner ad: advertisement which extends to the side (usually the top or right side) of a website.

bed rest: a partial or total restriction of activity to conserve energy and reduce strain to maternal systems when complications threaten or occur.

birth plan: a summary of a mother's priorities, concerns, and preferences for her care while laboring and giving birth, written for self-clarification and to communicate clearly with providers.

birthing pool or tub: lightweight or installed tub of sufficient depth for a laboring woman to immerse herself to enhance relaxation and reduce painful sensations.

bloody show: lightly blood-tinged vaginal secretions, usually a day or so before labor begins, that comes from small capillaries in the cervix breaking as the effacement and dilation just begins.

bodyCushion™: a positioning system of four main sections each composed of layers of shaped foam that conform to and cradle the body in a variety of positions.

body mechanics: organization and use of the body's energy and structure to perform a task.

bonding (attachment): a sense of connection and affection that unites humans in relationship and that develops with time and contact.

bow stance: standing posture with one foot forward, with a shoulder's width and two to three foot lengths between feet, and with the knees and hips flexed; modified from tai chi for massage and bodywork.

Braxton-Hicks contractions: contractions of the smooth muscle walls of the uterus occurring prior to true labor; distinguished from true labor in their irregularity in length and frequency.

breech presentation: when the fetal buttocks or feet (rather than the head) enter the maternal pelvis first; includes frank breech (buttocks at the cervix), complete breech (both buttocks and feet down), and footling breech (only one or both feet down).

bulk mailing: larger quantities of mail prepared for mailing at reduced postage.

business networking: a marketing method by which business opportunities are created through associating with like-minded or related business people either electronically or in communities. Example: LinkedIn or San Diego Birth Network.

carpal tunnel syndrome: pain, numbness, tingling, and/or weakness in the thumb, index, middle and half the ring finger; caused by irritation to the median nerve, in pregnancy usually primarily a result of edema.

ceiling-side: the side of your sidelying client's body that is available to work with.

cerebral palsy: a variety of central nervous system injuries usually incurred pre- or perinatally, or in early infancy; results in hyper- and hypotonic muscles, poor coordination and involuntary movements.

cervical insufficiency: weak, short, or structurally defective cervix that can spontaneously dilate before term in the absence of contractions, resulting in pregnancy loss.

cervical lip: the section of an otherwise fully dilated cervix that has not retracted over the fetal head, usually the anterior cervical section.

cervical mucus plug: thickened mucus that fills the cervical opening during pregnancy to prevent bacteria and any substances from entering the uterus; drops from the cervix in pre-labor or early labor phase.

cesarean section: surgical procedure through the lower abdominal wall and uterus so that the fetus can be removed from the uterus rather than passed through the vagina for birth.

childbirth education: courses that offer information, skills, and experiential activities to prepare expectant couples for childbirth.

chloasma: estrogen-induced brown or darker pigmentation forming a mask-like shape over a pregnant woman's nose, forehead, and cheeks.

circulatory massage (Swedish, European, lymph drainage, and Esalen styles): Traditional massage that employs a variety of strokes and movements to affect the skin and underlying muscular, lymphatic, and vascular systems.

colostrum: precursor of breast milk rich in protein, immunological, and intestinal tract-clearing properties.

complications: medical conditions that develop in pregnancy that may result in negative outcomes for the mother, the fetus, or both.

confidentiality: the guarantee of privacy and protection of clients' information, session progress, health, and other information.

cortisol: an adrenal hormone produced in response to stress and anxiety that influences the metabolism of proteins, increases blood pressure and blood sugar, and depresses the immune system.

countertransference: projections of a therapist onto a client of her emotional attitudes and/or past history.

cross-fiber friction: deep pressure with thumb or fingers across the axis of the muscle fiber, across specific lesions in muscle bellies, musculoteninous junctions, tendons, tenoperiosteal junctions, or ligaments; created by James Cyriax, MD, and developed by Ben Benjamin and others.

cytomegalovirus (CMV): a virus found in body fluids, spread through contact and fluid exchange that can cause many prenatal complications; the most common congenital and perinatal viral infection, affecting up to 3% of newborns.

deep tissue massage: slow specific strokes or compressions with thumbs, fingers, or elbows through fascial planes and muscles to release habitual patterns of holding in myofascial tissue; includes sculpting, structural balancing and integration, skin rolling, and other individually developed systems, many based on the principles of Ida P. Rolf.

deep vein thrombosis (DVT): formation or presence of a clot (thrombus) in a deep vein, usually the iliac, femoral, or deep saphenous veins.

deQuervain's syndrome: painful inflammation of the thumb tendons resulting in thumb, wrist, and sometimes forearm pain.

diastasis recti: softening and stretching of the midline of the rectus abdominus, the linea alba, to the point that a 3-finger or wider gap opens between the left and right halves of the muscle; caused by hormonal effects and the growing uterus pressing against the muscles.

diethylstilbestrol (DES): medication used for a variety of conditions and to prevent miscarriages that results in high percentage of grown daughters with reproductive organ anomalies and diseases; discontinued wide use in the US by 1971 when it was recognized as a teratogen, but still used occasionally into the 1990s.

dilation: the gradual opening of the uterine cervix to 10cm to allow passage of the fetus into the vagina.

disseminated intravascular coagulaopathy (DIC): complex hemorrhagic and tissue destructive condition, threatening fetal and maternal life.

doula (labor assistant): a trained and experienced attendant who provides a woman various forms of support that is non-medical and non-midwifery based; in labor a birth doula offers her continuous presence with physical and emotional caregiving to help women have the most satisfying birth possible; other doulas work primarily offering prenatal or postpartum care.

dystocia/arrested labor, dysfunctional labor/failure to progress, prodromal labor: difficult or failed progress during labor.

early labor (latent phase): beginning phase of first stage labor lasting until the cervix has dilated to 4 or 5 cm.

edema: excessive fluid retention and swelling; may be dependent, normal accumulations in the legs and feet, systemic or generalized throughout the body, and/or pitting where a depression and blanching of the skin for several seconds to several minutes after it is pressed occurs.

effacement: cervical changes of the last weeks of pregnancy or early labor that shorten, thin, and flatten the cervix.

electronic advertising: promotions done through websites, commonly in the form of banner ads, e-mail blasts and social media (such as Twitter or Facebook).

electronic fetal monitor: device that detects fetal heartbeat and another to detect maternal uterine contractions and that measures, records, and displays those readings; an external monitor is strapped around the abdomen or an internal monitor is placed on the fetal scalp and inside the uterus; can be used continuously or intermittently.

e-mail blast: an e-mail message sent to multiple recipients, intended to inform them of announcements, events, or changes.

endometriosis: growth of the inner lining of the uterus that extends outside of the uterus into the pelvic cavity with resultant pain and reproductive system dysfunction.

engagement (lightening or dropping): when the widest part of the head, or other fetal body part closest to the cervix, descends into the pelvis in preparation for labor to begin.

engorgement: painful distention of the breast caused by increased blood and lymph circulation and milk production; usually occurs 2-4 days postpartum and until production and the baby's needs balance out.

epidural: administration of anesthetic into the epidural space of the spinal column to numb the sensory and motor nerves leading to the lower body.

epinephrine and norepinephrine: adrenal hormones responsible for the flight, fright or flight response to stress, and to increasing strength and stamina for demanding situations, like pushing in labor.

episiotomy: enlargement of the vaginal opening via a surgical incision of the perineum.

essential oils: highly concentrated essences of aromatic plants.

estrogen: reproductive hormone which promotes growth of breasts and uterus, increases vascularization, relaxes pelvic ligaments and joints, swells gums and other mucous membranes, and causes skin pigmentation changes.

expansional balance: a movement concept involving the free extension of the skeletal frame in all directions in space through cycling awareness of vertical and horizontal joint expansion; originated by Michael Nebadon, and developed by Ed Maupin.

expected date of birth (estimated date of delivery) EDB or EDD: a calculation of when a baby will be born; based on last menstrual period (LMP), date of conception, and/or an obstetric ultrasound to scan, measure and date embryonic development.

femoral venous pressure: the force of the blood against the walls of leg veins.

fetal distress: problems with fetal heart rate or activity levels.

fibrinolysis: the process by which fibrin, the blood protein that coagulates to form clots, is dissolved.

fibrosis: changes in soft tissue associated with chronic congestion, contraction of muscle, thickening of fascia and increased formation of fibrous tissue; usually palpable, painful, and likely to produce areas of referred pain.

forceps: obstetrical tong-like instrument sometimes used to grasp and move the fetus during birth.

fundus: upper uterine section between the fallopian tubes.

gastric reflux (heartburn): burning and pain caused by stomach (gastric) acid injuring and inflaming the esophageal mucous linings.

Gate Theory of pain management: stimulation of the nerves that perceive pleasure, pressure, and temperature can inhibit the amount of painful stimulus perceived in the brain because these sensations travel on nerves that fire faster than those nerves perceiving pain.

genital herpes: viral infection causing painful blisters around a red base, appearing periodically on the genitals, thighs, buttocks or sacrum.

gestation: the conception and development of a baby.

gestational hypertension/hypertensive disorders/eclampsia: high blood pressure that develops during pregnancy and can proceed from mild to severe and life threatening in its severity.

gravid: pregnant; carrying a developing fetus(s).

hematological disorders: various conditions that result in reduced capacity of the blood to carry oxygen to mother and fetus.

hemorrhoids: aching, swollen mass of dilated veins in swollen anal tissue; can also occur vaginally.

horse riding stance: a standing posture with the feet parallel, a shoulder's width apart and aligned with each other directly under the flexed ankle, knee, and hip joints.

human chorionic gonadotrophin (hCG): hormone produced first by the earliest fetal cells until the placenta is developed sufficiently; this is the basis for most early pregnancy tests.

human placental lactogen (hPL): hormone responsible for glucose, carbohydrate, and other metabolic processing of nutrients; prepares mammary glands for lactation; also known as human chorionic somatomammotropin, hCS.

hyperemisis gravidarum: persistent, uncontrollable nausea and vomiting beyond the 20th week of pregnancy.

hysterectomy: surgical removal of the uterus.

induction: using medical or surgical interventions to stimulate uterine contractions before their spontaneous onset.

infertility: male or female condition resulting in an inability to conceive after one year of normal, unprotected sexual intercourse or an inability to carry a pregnancy to term.

intake: a process or form for collecting and/or recording fundamental facts about a client, taken at first visit and updated with each subsequent session.

intrauterine fetal demise (stillbirth): death of an unborn embryo or fetus at any gestational age.

intrauterine growth restriction (IUGR): fetal growth falling below the tenth percentile of expected growth norms of weight, head circumference, or length.

intrauterine pressure: the force of the uterine contents, amniotic fluid, placenta, and fetus, exerted against the interior muscular walls of the uterus.

involution: the process of the uterus shrinking to prepregnancy size and location in the pelvis, and resuming non-pregnant functioning.

keloid scar: a raised mass of scar tissue that overflows that actual original incision site.

kinesthetic awareness: the simultaneous abilities to attend to one's inner state, coordinate movement, such as massage techniques, and maintain awareness of where one is in time and space.

lability: constantly changing and unstable emotional state.

labor: process of uterine muscle contractions to thin and dilate the cervix and press the fetus and placenta through and out the vagina.

laboring mind response: rebalancing action of hemispheric brain activity to more instinctual and intuitive functions of the right brain from the logical, rational functions of the left brain.

lateral recumbent: lying on one's side; sidelying.

lift table: massage table that adjusts to variable heights by either hydraulic or electrical power.

linea nigra: a line of darker skin pigmentation that often appears on the midline of the lower abdomen in late pregnancy.

lochia: normal vaginal discharge after childbirth consisting of blood, mucus, and tissue.

low birth weight (small for gestational age, or SGA): birth weight of an infant at 2,500 grams or less.

macrosomia (large for gestational age, or LGA): a newborn weighing more than 8 lbs. 13 oz. or above the 90th percentile for birth weight and gestational age.

mastitis: inflammation of the mammary ducts and/or glands.

midwifery: a healthcare profession focused on providing prenatal care, attending births, and offering continuing care of a new mother and her baby; midwives complete a prescribed course of studies in apprenticeships, formal university programs, or a combination.

morning sickness: nausea and/or vomiting during pregnancy; primarily a response to rapidly increasing hormonal levels during the first trimester.

muscle energy techniques (MET): a method of producing relaxation of a muscle prior to stretching it by having the client use the muscle or its antagonist at 20% or so of its strength against the therapist's resistance to that action.

myofascial release: system of connective tissue manipulation involving nongliding fascial traction and stretching to lengthen and soften fascia; sometimes used in combination with other deep tissue and osteopathic techniques; developed by John Barnes and others.

myofascial trigger points: hypersensitive and hyperirritable spots most often found in taut bands and nodules in skeletal muscle; when pressed often create local and distant pain referred in characteristic patterns; the variety of systems for working with these points originate in the work of Drs. Janet Travell and David Simons.

obstetrics: branch of medicine that cares for women during pregnancy, labor and birth, and the puerperium periods.

occiput anterior: uterine position with the fetal occiput facing the mother's pubic bone.

occiput posterior: uterine position with the fetal occiput facing the mother's sacrum.

oligohydramnios: a less than normal amount of amniotic fluid; usually occurring in the third trimester.

on-site massage chair: folding, adjustable specialty chair for performing massage with a client seated while in a variety of work, medical, therapeutic or recreational settings.

oxytocin (labor stimulant): pituitary hormone that stimulates uterine contractions, release of milk into the milk ducts, and feelings of nurturing; see synthetic version under *pitocin*.

paradoxical breathing: abdomen contracts with inhalation, expands with exhalation which is the opposite of normal breathing dynamics.

parasympathetic branch of the autonomic nervous system: slows heart rate, increases intestinal and gland activity, and relaxes the sphincter muscles. The parasympathetic nervous system, together with the sympathetic nervous system (that accelerates the heart rate, constricts blood vessels, and raises blood pressure), constitutes the autonomic nervous system.

passive movements: movements of varying amplitude, intensity, and speed performed by the therapist to gently move the client's body or move specific joints; forms of passive movements include, joint mobilizations, stretching, traction, rhythmic deep tissue blends, sensory repatterning, Trager™ work, and strain/counterstrain (positional release) systems.

pelvic floor exercises (Kegels): a variety of squeezing, lifting, and releasing exercises to maintain and improve the tone and relaxation ability of both the sphincter and sling muscles of the pelvic floor; also known as Kegels after the surgeon who first designed a biofeedback device to measure and guide strengthening of these muscles.

perinatal: the time surrounding childbirth, most specifically the last five months and the month immediately after birth.

peripartum pelvic pain syndrome (PPPPS): pain in the pelvic region that started during pregnancy or within the first 3 months after delivery, and for which no clear diagnosis is available.

piriformis syndrome: pain, numbness and/or tingling in the gluteal and posterior leg regions as a result of chronic piriformis tension entrapping and compressing the sciatic nerve.

pitocin: synthetic form of oxytocin used to induce or augment labor by stimulating uterine contractions.

placenta: membranous and vascular organ that begins developing in the pre-embryonic first 7 days of pregnancy; eventually grows to 2 pounds in weight, covering a large portion of the upper uterus; provides nourishment and waste removal for the growing fetus via the umbilical cord, and also produces many of the hormones that support a normal pregnancy.

placenta previa: implantation of the placenta in the lower uterus covering or near the cervical opening (os) rather than the normal location closer to the superior end of the uterus (fundus).

placental abruption (abruption placentae): separation of the placenta from the uterine wall prior to birth of the baby.

placental accreta, increta, and percreta: defect in the vascular attachment of the placenta that allows it to attach directly or through the uterine muscles rather than to the innermost endometrium only; results in greater risk of hemorrhage and uterine rupture or inversion.

polyhydramnios (hydramnios): too much amniotic fluid, usually in the final weeks of pregnancy.

position (lie): the orientation of the fetus relative to the internal opening of the cervix; most common are occiput anterior and occiput posterior.

postpartum: the first year after birth of a baby, including the **puerperium** period of the first 4-6 weeks of extensive adjustments.

postpartum affective disorders: mental health conditions, including depression and psychosis, which can develop as a result of postpartum hormonal and brain imbalances and the stress of adapting to a newborn.

postpartum complications: medical conditions that develop in the mother, immediately after a baby's birth and up to the first year.

post-term, prolonged pregnancy, or postdatism; pregnancy that goes beyond 42 weeks.

precipitous labor: labor and birth that occurs in 3 hours or less.

premature rupture of membranes (PROM): breaking of the amniotic sack containing the baby, placenta and amniotic fluid before the onset of true labor.

prematurity: birth of a baby between weeks 20 and 37 of gestation.

prenatal: the preparatory 40-42 weeks during which a fetus is developing and growing.

presenting part: the fetal part closest to the cervix.

progesterone: hormone that prepares and maintains the uterine lining for implantation of a fertilized egg, and supports its continued development and the development of the breasts.

prolactin: pituitary hormone that triggers and sustains milk production in response to tactile breast stimulation.

prone: lying face down.

prostaglandins: hormones that affect uterine smooth muscle, vasodilatation, and constriction.

protracted labor: very slow cervical dilation during the active phase.

puerperium period: time from delivery of the placenta to about 6 weeks postpartum.

rebozo: a long scarf or shawl worn around the shoulders that Central and South American midwives also use for labor support.

reflexive techniques: massage techniques directed to cutaneous or neurological referral zones to effect either systemic change or local change at distant "referred" sites; vary from light to very deep pressure; includes many Asian bodywork techniques, connective tissue massage (*Bindegewebsmassage*), reflexology or zone therapy of the feet or hands, and trigger point (neuromuscular) therapies.

reflexology: see *Zone therapy*.

relaxin: placental hormone that works with progesterone to maintain the pregnancy and to soften connective tissue to increase pelvic flexibility.

resisted movements: see *Muscle energy techniques*.

restless leg: a movement disorder which causes an urge to move the legs and is associated with an uncomfortable or unpleasant sensation, such as pulling, drawing, crawling, wormy, tingling, pins and needles, prickly, and sometimes. Sudden muscle jerks may also occur.

Rh incompatibility (isoimmunization): blood disease resulting from conflicting maternal and fetal blood Rh factors that cause an antigen-antibody reaction.

rubella (German measles): viral infection resulting in fever, swollen glands, and rash and possible congenital defects in a fetus if mother infected during first half of pregnancy.

search engine optimization: various techniques to improve a web site's ranking in internet data analysis systems in the hopes of attracting more visitors

second stage labor: the time from the full cervical dilation until the birth.

semireclining (semirecumbent): a partially seated, partially lying position on a massage table.

sidelying (lateral recumbent): client position on the table supported on either left or right side.

Sidelying Positioning System: six part grouping of cushions engineered specifically to ergonomically support a client while lying on her side; can be adapted to semireclining position as well.

social networking: the process of building online communities through "groups" and "friends lists" that allow greater interaction on websites as well as more connectivity and interaction between web users. The most prominent examples are Facebook, Twitter, MySpace, and the business-focused LinkedIn.

somatic practices: educational and health enhancing methods of massage and therapeutic bodywork addressing the whole body through touch and/or movement, and often with attention to the emotional connections as well.

spider veins: tiny, visible capillaries with wavy, spider-like patterns, primarily on the legs (spider angioma or telangiectasias) or small blood vessels appearing superficially on the neck, thorax, face and arms that usually disappear after giving birth (vascular nevi).

spontaneous abortion/miscarriage: loss of an early pregnancy, usually before 20 weeks of gestation.

strain and counterstrain: a type of osteopathic passive movement that seeks to relieve "tender points" in soft tissues by positioning client in maximal comfort position and holding; created and developed by Lawrence Jones, DO.

striae gravidarum: reddish or darkened lines where the growing uterus and expanding underlying tissues have stretched and torn the components of the skin, particularly common on the abdomen, hips or breasts.

supervision: discussions and explorations with a more experienced practitioner or instructor or a small peer group that help improve client outcomes and practitioner self-awareness and development.

supine: lying face up

supine hypotensive syndrome: decreased blood pressure caused by the uterus compressing the inferior vena cava sufficiently to reduce venous return.

surrogacy (gestational carrier): the laboratory fertilization of embryos that are transferred to another woman's uterus for the remainder of gestation.

sympathetic branch of the autonomic nervous system: nerve network that increases heart rate, constricts blood flow to the viscera and skin while increasing it in the skeletal muscle, and prompts production of epinephrine and norepinephrine, stress hormones.

symphysis pubis dysfunction (separation): instability and/or misalignment of the articular structures at the anterior junction of the two halves of the pubic bone.

table-side: the side that a client is lying on when laterally recumbant on the table.

tai chi chuan: a martial art and exercise and meditation system based on the interplay of polarities of movement, stance and energy; originated in ancient China and developed by many modern masters of various schools of instruction and practice.

target market: a defined group of potential customers who have similar characteristics (age, location, interests, etc.) towards whom promotional efforts can be focused.

tarsal tunnel syndrome: pressure on the tarsal nerve as it passes the ankle due to extra fluid resulting in foot numbness.

tee stance: a standing posture with feet one shoulder width apart and one foot, empty of weight, about a foot length ahead of the other, weighted foot.

term: normal gestational period; 40–42 weeks.

third stage labor: the time from the birth through expulsion of the placenta.

thoracic outlet syndrome: compression of the brachial plexus, with pain, numbness, or tingling in the entire hand and along the arm.

thrombi: blood clots (singular: *thrombus*).

thromboembolisms: obstruction of a blood vessel by a blood clot carried by the circulation from the site of origin, often migrating to the lungs (pulmonary embolism).

thrombophlebitis: inflammation of a blood vessel caused by a blood clot (thrombus) within the vessel.

tidal volume: the amount of air exchanged with each breath cycle.

tilt-top table: massage table that features a top surface that is manually or electrically adjustable to various angles and heights off of the flat line of most standard tables.

toxoplasmosis: parasitic infection carried in cat feces, contaminated soil, or undercooked meat that has a high likelihood of infecting a fetus and causing congenial damage and other complications.

Trager™: a movement education approach and mind/body integration using rhythmic active and passive movements to help release deep-seated physical and mental patterns and facilitate deep relaxation, increased physical mobility, and mental clarity.

transference: a psychological reaction in which a client displaces her thoughts, feelings, or behaviors about a significant other onto her therapist.

transition phase: first stage labor's third and final phase of cervical dilation from 8 to 10 cm.

tubal ligation: surgical cutting and tying of the fallopian tubes to prevent conception.

umbilical cord prolapse: dropping of the fetal umbilical cord alongside or ahead of the presenting body part.

urinary stress incontinence: involuntary loss of urine as a result of inadequate urinary sphincter function and sufficient enough to be a social or hygiene problem.

uterine atony: lack of uterine muscle tone that can result in excessive perinatal blood loss.

uterine competence: normal structure and functioning of the uterus for maintaining a pregnancy and birthing a baby.

uterine involution: see *involution*.

uterine ligaments: thickened areas of connective tissue surrounding the uterus that support and position the reproductive system in the pelvis and connect it to the rectum and the bladder.

uterine rupture: tearing of the walls of the uterus, usually at the site of a previous scar

varicose veins: weakened areas where the valves in a vein have collapsed allowing pooling of blood.

vasodilation: increased blood flow to an area by an expansion of the blood vessels.

zone therapy (reflexology): a type of reflex massage descended from ancient natural therapies that accesses the subtle energy of the feet; uses thumbs or fingertips to compress undifferentiated nerves in the skin against bone at specific sites to create a distant specific effect and to balance and harmonize the body towards health and wellbeing; also performed on the hands.

Index

Page numbers in italics indicate figures; those followed by b indicate boxes; those followed by t indicate tables.

A

Abdominal effleurage, 127–128
Abdominal kneading, *145*
Abdominal massage
    avoidance, conditions for, 34–35, 34b
    liability considerations, 34b
    methodological precautions and contraindications, 44b
    postpartum, 144–147, *145–147*
    safety guidelines, 33–34, *33*stress reduction, 85, *85*
    trigger points, postpartum, 147–148, *147*
Abdominal vibration, *146*
Abnormal fetal growth or movement, 159–160
Active first stage labor
    back pain, 119, *119*
    epidurals in pain management, 119–121
    general technique guidelines, 118
    specific techniques for, 118
Acupressure
    for gastrointestinal functioning, 9
    for hyperemisis gravidarium, 159, *159*
    touch in labor, 18, 131t
Amniotic fluid imbalances, 159
Antepartum bleeding, 155–156
Autonomic nervous system
    parasympathetic, 4
    sympathetic, 3–4
Autonomic sedation series, 84–85, *84*

B

"Baby blues," 168
Back pain
    control, 15–16
    in labor, 119
    in pregnancy
        Braxton-Hicks contractions, 12
        peripartum pelvic pain syndrome, 12
        piriformis syndrome, 15
        symphysis pubis dysfunction, 12
        uterine ligaments, 14, *14*
    pelvic and lower
        deep tissue sculpting, 92–93, *92*
        inching on intrinsic paravertebral structures, 94–95, *94*
        lumbar lengthening, 95–96, *95*
        lumbosacral stretch or passive pelvic tilt, 91–92, *91*
        pelvic tilt reeducation, 91, *91*
        precautions, 90
        SI joint release, 93–94, *93–94*
        symphysis pubis rebalancing, 96, *96*
        technique suggestions, 90–91
    reducing residual, postpartum massage therapy, 138

Beta-endorphins, 116
Birthing pool, 118
Blood clots, 36, *37*, 44b, 142
Body mechanics, 60
Bonding, 141
Braxton-Hicks contractions, 12, 115
Breast massage, 137
Breastfeeding, 137–138, *138*
Brochures and business cards, 174–175, *175–177*
Business planning, 172, 173b

C

Carpal tunnel syndrome, 49
Cerebral palsy, 163
Cervical and pelvic floor relaxation, 130
Cervical lip, 121
Cesarean surgery
    healing from, 140–141
    operative procedures, 123–124, *123*
    scar massage, 148
Childhood sexual abuse, 164–165, *164*
Chloasma, 10, *11*
Circulatory massage therapy, 8
Circulatory system
    effects of massage therapy, 8
    normal physiological and mechanical changes in, 6–7
Client education
    educational events, 185
    in-office educational resources, 185
    individualized self-care, 184–185
Client positioning
    checklists, 51b
    prone
        safety and comfort tips, 50
        suggested supports and placement, 49
    seated, 55–56, *55*
    semireclining, 51–52, *51*, *53*
    sidelying
        requirements, 52
        safety and comfort tips, 55
        suggested supports and placement, 54–55, *54*
    supine, 50–51, *51*
Client vignettes, 201–203
Colostrum, 115
Contraction distraction, 129, *129*

D

Deep tissue massage, 8, 19, 44b
Deep tissue sculpting
    and trigger point therapy, paravertebrals, 92–93, *92*
    anterior hip, 88, *88*
    distal ribcage sculpting, 99, *99*
    lateral hip and extinguishing trigger points, 88–89, *88*
    leg and hip discomforts, 88–89, *88*
    levator scapula, 97–98, *97*
    pectoralis major, 98, *98*
    pectoralis minor, 98, *98*
    precautions, 34, 36, *37*, 44b, 98–99
    scalenes, 98, *98*
    upper trapezius, 97, *97*
Deep vein thrombosis (DVT), 36
Diastasis recti, 11, 12, 76b, 144
Disseminated intravascular coagulopathy, 36
Draping
    seated, 59
    semireclining, 56, *57*
    sidelying
        back, undraping, 56–57, *57*
        ceiling-side hip and leg, undraping, 57, *58*
        ribcage and abdomen, undraping, *57*, 59
        table-side leg, undraping, 59

E

E-mail, 178
Early labor. *See* First-stage labor
Eclampsia, 156–158, 156b
Edema, 7, *7*, 36, 157
Electronic advertising, 178
Epidurals, 119–121
Epinephrine, 116
Esalen massage, 8
Expansional balance, 61, *62*

F

Fibrinolysis, 7
Figure 8 hip mobilization, 89–90, *89*
Financial stress, 178
First trimester
    considerations and guidelines, 70–71
    early gestational period, 68
    maternal and fetal development, 68–70, *69*
    recommended bodywork, 71–72
First-stage labor
    abdominal effleurage, 127–128
    circulation support between contractions, 126–127
    contraction distraction, 129, *129*
    coping with pain, 115
    hormonal influences on uterine contractions, 116–117
    hydrotherapy, 128–129
    labor stimulation points, 129
    localized massage, 127
    precautions, 126
    relief of muscular tension and joint pain, 126
    sacral counterpressure, 128

First-stage labor (*Continued*)
  technique suggestions, 126
  techniques for early labor, 116
Foot reflexology. *See* Zone therapy

G

Gastric reflux, 9
Gastrointestinal system
  benefits, 9
  discomforts
    complaints and symptoms, 101
    precautions, 101
    technique suggestions, 101
    zone therapy, 101–103, *102–103*
Gate theory of pain control, 113
General practical considerations
  environment, 47, 47b
  equipment and supplies recommendations, 48
  equipment and supplies requirements, 47–48
Gestational diabetes, 153b, 158
Gestational hypertensive disorders
  degrees of, 156b
  eclampsia symptoms, 157–158
  pitting edema, 157, *157*
  signs and symptoms of preeclampsia, 157
  warning signs of, 157
Grounding hold, 130, *130*

H

Hip decompression, 87–88, *87–88*
Horse-riding stance, 61, *64*
Human chorionic gonadotrophin (hCG), 9
Hydrotherapy, 128–129
Hyperemesis gravidarum, 158–159, *159*

I

Inching on intrinsic paravertebral structures, 94–95, *94*
Induction and augmentation, 166, *167*
Internal rotation and rocking, hip decompression, 87–88, *87*
Internet marketing, 174
Intrauterine fetal demise, 167

L

Labor and infant care pain, 20–21, *21*
Labor complications
  induction and augmentation, 165, *166*
  labor dystocia, *38, 39,* 165
  rapid labor, 166
Labor facilitation, 17–19, *19*
Labor massage therapy
  active first stage
    back pain, 119, *119*
    epidurals in pain management, 119–121
    general technique guidelines, 118
    specific techniques for, 118
  cesarean section births, 123–124, *123*
  collaborating with midwives and medical professionals, 112
  emotional issues, 112
  first-stage labor
    abdominal effleurage, 127–128
    circulation support between contractions, 126–127
    contraction distraction, 129, *129*
    coping with pain, 115
    hormonal influences on uterine contractions, 116–117
    hydrotherapy, 128–129
    labor stimulation points, 129
    localized massage, 127
    precautions, 126
    relief of muscular tension and joint pain, 126
    sacral counterpressure, 128
    technique suggestions, 126
    techniques for early labor, 116
  improving awareness and communication, 108–109
  improving flexibility, 107
  labor and birth, 106
  labor preparation techniques, 125–126
  motivations, 109–110
  objective, 105
  partner massage instruction, 107–108
  pelvic floor preparation, 108
  practical and ethical considerations, 110–111
  prelabor, 113, 115
  preparations for labor support, 113
  relaxation and breathing, 106–107
  role of, 111–112, *112*
  second-stage labor
    resting, pushing, and birth, 121–122, *122*
    techniques, 129–130, *130*
  stages of labor, 113, *114–115,* 131t
  third stage, 122–123
  transition phase, 121, *121*
Labor preparation, 16–17, *18*
Labor stimulation points, 129. *See also* Reflex and acupressure points
Laboring mind response, 116
Leg and hip discomforts
  deep tissue sculpting, lateral hip and extinguishing trigger points, 88–89, *88*
  figure 8 hip mobilization, 89–90, *89*
  hip decompression, 87–88, *87–88*
  leg edema, 7, *7*
  precautions, 85
  structural balancing, 86, *86–87*
  Swedish and lymphatic drainage, 90, *90*
  technique suggestions, 85–86
Leg massage
  adaptations to, 38b
  blood clots, 36, *37*
  general methodological precautions and contraindications, 44b
  varicose and spider veins, 36–38, *37*
Linea alba, 11
Linea nigra, 10, *11*
Low-birth-weight, 4b, 167
Lower back pain
  deep tissue sculpting and trigger point therapy to paravertebrals, 92–93, *92*
  inching on intrinsic paravertebral structures, 94–95, *94*
  lumbar lengthening, 95–96, *95*
  lumbosacral stretch, 91–92, *91*
  pelvic tilt reeducation, 91, *91*
  precautions, 90
  SI joint releases, 93–94, *93–94*
Lumbar lengthening, 95–96, *95*
Lumbosacral stretch, 91–92, *91*
Lymphatic drainage techniques, 8, 90, *90,* 157
Lymphostatic edema. *See* Edema

M

Male massage therapists, 180
Marketing strategies
  advertising, 178
  brochures and business cards, 174–175, *175–177*
  classes, 177
  direct mail and e-mail promotions, 178
  internet marketing, 174
  printed articles, 178
  referrals and networking, 173–174
  speeches and demonstrations, 176–177
Massage table
  helping the client onto the table, 49, *50*
  padding and coverings, 49
  width, height, and model, 48–49
Mastitis, 137
Maternal and fetal development
  first trimester, 68–70, *69*
  second trimester, 73–74, *73*
  third trimester, 76–77, *77*
Maternity massage therapists
  client vignettes, 201–203
  coalitions and affiliations, 192–194
  collaborations with
    hospital-based programs, 196–197
    working in obstetrical offices, 198–199
  maternity massage therapy centers, 195
  perinatal clients, 189–190
  private practice, 190
  spa and corporate, 199–200
  spotlight on career, 200–201
  survey, 187–189, 188–189t
Maternity massage therapy
  benefits of
    improved physiological functioning, 6–11, *7, 11, 13*
    labor facilitation, 17–19, *19*
    labor preparation, 16–17, *18*
    musculoskeletal strain and pain, reduction of, 11–12, 14–16, *14*
    nurturing maternal touch, 19–20
    objective, 1
    postpartum recovery, 20–21, *21*
    stress reduction and relaxation, 2–6, *3, 5,* 6b
    touching humanity, 2
  centers for, 195
  effective methodologies, 31, 31b, 41b
  guidelines, precautions, and contraindications
    abdominal massage, 33–35, *33,* 34b
    considerations, 41–42, 41b
    eligibility, 26
    first trimester, 26
    in complicated pregnancy, 42–43, *42,* 152–170
    leg massage, 35–38, *37*
    oils and lotions, 40–41
    positioning, 30
    pressure, speed, and moderating pain level, 31–32
    prone positioning, 27–29, *28*
    reflex and acupressure points, 38–40, *38–39*
    sidelying, 30–31, *30*
    skin products and spa treatments, 41
    supine positioning, 29, *29*
    stress reduction, 6
    stress, prematurity, and low-birth-weight, 4
Miscarriage, 34–35, 42, 153b, 154, 156, 162, 167
Musculoskeletal strain and pain, reduction of
  back and pelvic pain, 12–15
  massage therapy and pain control, 15–16
  other prenatal musculoskeletal complaints, 15
  prenatal structural balance, 11–12
Myofascial pain syndromes, 16
Myofascial trigger point therapy, 8

N

Nonpitting edema. *See* Edema
Norepinephrine, 116
Nurturing maternal touch, 19–20

O

Occipital anterior (OA) position, 119
Occipital lift, 86, *86*
Occiput traction and rocking, 82, *82*
Oils and lotions, 40–41

P

Pain
    epidurals for, 119–121
    labor and infant care, 20–21, *21*
    labor back pain, 119, *119*
    leg and hip
        deep tissue sculpting, 88–89, *88*
        figure 8 hip mobilization, 89–90, *89*
        hip decompression, 87–88, *87–88*
        structural balancing, 86–87, *86–87*
        Swedish and lymph drainage, 90, *90*
    musculoskeletal, reduction of
        back and pelvic, 12–15, *13–14*
        massage therapy, 15–16
        prenatal structural balance, 11–12, *79*
    pelvic and lower back (*see* Lower back pain; Pelvic pain)
    postpartum, pelvic and back, 138
    prevention from childcare activities, 139–140
    upper body (*see* Upper body discomforts)
Paradoxical breathing, 8
Paravertebral raking, 84, *84*
Passive and active movements, 44b
Passive pelvic tilt. *See* Lumbosacral stretch
Passive relaxation of thigh adductors, 125–126, *125*
Passive wrist movements, 100, *100*
Pectoral girdle cross-fiber friction, 100–101, *100*
Pectoral girdle mobilizations, 83, *83*
Pelvic and lumbar alignment, 86, *87*
Pelvic floor (Kegel) exercises, 10
Pelvic girdle instability, 12, *14*
Pelvic girdle mobilizations, 83, *83*
Pelvic pain
    deep tissue sculpting and trigger point therapy to paravertebrals, 92–93, *92*
    in pregnancy, 12–15, *13–14*
    inching on intrinsic paravertebral structures, 94–95, *94*
    lumbar lengthening, 95–96, *95*
    lumbosacral stretch, 91–92, *91*
    pelvic tilt reeducation, 91, *91*
    precautions, 90
    SI joint releases, 93–94, *93–94*
    symphysis pubis rebalancing, 96, *96*
    technique suggestions, 90–91
Pelvic tilt reeducation, 91, *91*
Perineal massage, 108b
Peripartum pelvic pain syndrome (PPPPS), 12, *13–14*
Piriformis syndrome, 15
Pitting edema, 157, *157*
Placental abruption, 36
Placental accreta, 169
Placental increta, 169
Placental percreta, 169
Placental separation and expulsion, 122–123
Postpartum complications, 166–169, 169b
Postpartum depression, 143
Postpartum massage therapy
    extended skin-to-skin cuddling, 133, *134*
    goals and general guidelines
        breastfeeding, 137–138, *138*
        healing from cesarean surgery, 140–141, *141*
        healing from labor, 135–136, *136*
        pelvic floor and abdominal healing, 136–137
        preventing childcare strain and pain, 139–140
        providing nurturance and emotional support, 135, *135*
        structural integrity, 139
    guidelines and precautions for
        circulatory contraindications and precautions, 142–143
        infant care, 141–142
        other complications, 143
        positioning and equipment, 142
    later months and years of, 143–144
    maternal adjustments and healing, 133–134
    objective, 133
    residual pelvic and back pain, reducing, 138
    technique manual of
        abdominal massage, 144–147, *145–147*
        abdominal trigger points, 147–148, *147*
        cesarean scar massage, 148
        foot reflexology, 144
        neck, upper back and arm, 150
        seated fascia stretching, 149–150, *149*
        structural balancing for iliopsoas, 148–149, *148*
Postpartum mental illness, 167–168, *169*
Postpartum recovery
    emotional adjustments, 20
    physiological, 20
    reestablishing postural integrity, 20–21, *21*
Precipitous labor. *See* Rapid labor
Preeclampsia, 156–158, 156b
Pregnancy-related complications. *See* Prenatal complications
Prelabor, 113, 115
Premature labor, 160
Prematurity, 4
Prenatal and perinatal business
    client education
        educational events, 185
        in-office educational resources, 185
        individualized self-care, 184–185
    expanding and sustaining, 185
    management of
        communication and maintaining client records, 181b, 183–184, 183b
        intake and client interviews, 180–183, 181b, *182*
        liability and insurance concerns, 184
    private practice
        marketing strategies, 172–178, *175–177*
        overcoming obstacles, 178–180
        planning, 172, 173b
Prenatal complications
    abnormal fetal growth or movement, 159–160
    amniotic fluid imbalances, 159
    antepartum bleeding, 155–156
    biophysical factors for, 162b
    environmental factors for, 162b
    general guidelines, 153–155, *155*
    genetic concerns, 160
    gestational diabetes, 158
    gestational hypertensive disorders
        degrees of, 156b
        eclampsia symptoms, 157–158
        pitting edema, 157, *157*
        signs and symptoms of preeclampsia, 157
        warning signs of, 157
    hyperemesis gravidarum, 158–159, *159*
Postpartum support, women with unexpected outcomes
    obstetric emergencies, 166–167
    physical postpartum complications, 169, 169b
    postpartum affective disorders, 167–168, *169*
    premature labor, 160
    premature rupture of membranes, 160
    psychosocial factors for, 162b
    sociodemographic factors for, 162b
    special needs infants and fetal/infant death, 167
    special sensitivity or consideration
        being responsive to diversity, 163
        childhood sexual abuse, 164–165, *164*
        mothers with disabilities and challenges, 163–164
        surrogate mothers, 162
        women undergoing infertility treatment, 161–162
    stress reduction in, *153*
    warning signs of, 153b
    woman at higher risk of, factors affecting, 160–161, *161,* 162b
Prenatal structural balance, 11–12
Preterm premature rupture of membranes (PPROM), 160
Pricing and packaging services, 172, 173b
Print advertising, 178
Private practice
    marketing strategies, 172–178, *175–177*
    overcoming obstacles, 178–180
    planning, 172, 173b
    professional expertise, 190
Prone positioning
    checklists, 51b
    safety and guidelines, 27–29, *28*
    safety and comfort tips, 50
    suggested supports and placement, 49
    switches, 59
Puerperium, 133

R

Rapid labor, 166
Referrals and networking, 173–174
Reflex and acupressure points
    feet, legs, and hands, 38–39, *38*
    general methodological precautions and contraindications, 44b
    torso, 39–40, *39*
Reflexive techniques, 9
Release form, 181b
Respiratory system benefits, 8–9
Restless legs, 15
Rhythmic deep tissue, 93, *93*
Rhythmic passive movements, 82–84, *82–83*
Rib cage alignment, 86, *86*
Rib raking, 84, *84*
Ribcage releases, 99, *99*

S

Sacral and lumbar work, 70
Sacral counterpressure, 128
Sacral friction, 84, *84*
Sacroiliac (SI) joint releases, 93–94, *93–94*
Seated fascia stretching, 149–150, *149*
Seated positioning, 55–56, *55,* 59
Second trimester
    considerations and guidelines, 74–75, *75*
    maternal and fetal development, 73–74, *73*
    maternal developments and safe positioning, 72b
    recommended bodywork, 75–76
Second-stage labor techniques, 129–130, *130*
Semireclining, 29, *29,* 51–52, *51, 53*

Sidelying
    advantages of, 30–31, *30*
    checklists, 51b
    draping during, 56–59, *57, 58*
    positioning and stabilizing of therapists, 63–65, *64*
    requirements, 52
Sidelying
    safety and comfort tips, 55
    sleeping, 10
    suggested supports and placement, 54–55, *54*
    transitions, 59
Skin stimulation, 9–10
Somatic therapies, 31, 31b
Spas, prenatal and postpartum massage, 199–200
Speeches and demonstrations, 176–177
Spider veins, 36–38
Spinal rocking, 82, *82*
Stages of labor, 113, *114–115*
Stress reduction and relaxation
    benefits of, 4–6, *5*, 6b
    during pregnancy, 3–4
    trimester recommendations
        abdominal massage, 85, *85*
        autonomic sedation series, 84–85, *84*
        diaphragmatic breathing reduction, 81, *81*
        increasing lateral/costal breathing, 81–82
        rhythmic passive movements, 82–84, *82–83*
Striae gravidarum, 10, *11*
Structural balancing
    for iliopsoas, postpartum massage therapy, 148–149, *148*
    intention, 86
    leg and hip discomforts, trimester recommendations, 86, *86–87*
    occipital lift, 86, *86*
    pelvic and lumbar alignment, 86, *87*
    rib cage alignment, 86, *86*
Superficial abdominal effleurage, 85, *85*
Supine positioning, 29, *29*, 50–51, *51*, 59
Surrogate mothers, 162
Swedish massage, 8, 44b, 90, *90*, 100
Symphysis pubis dysfunction, 12, *14* , 75, 76b
Symphysis pubis rebalancing, 96, *96*

T

Tapotement, *147*
Tarsal tunnel syndrome, 15
Tee stance, 61, *61*
Therapist's body mechanics
    basic principles of alignment, 61, *62*
    key concepts, 60–61, *61*
    positioning and stabilizing, *61*, 63, *64*, 65
    principles for, 65b
    stances, shifting weight, and alignment, 61–63, *64*

Third trimester
    maternal and fetal development, 76–77, *77*
    maternal developments and safe positioning, 76b
    precautions, considerations, and guidelines, 77–80, *78, 79*
    recommended bodywork, 80
Thoracic outlet syndrome, 49
Thrombi. *See* Blood clots
Thrombophlebitis, 36
Traction and rocking, hip decompression, 87, *87*
Traditional European massage, 8
Transition changes
    side-to-side turn overs, 59–60, *60*
    sidelying switches, 59
    supine/prone switches, 59
Transverse cervical rocking, 82–83, *82*
Trigger points, ribcage releases, 99, *99*
Trimester recommendations
    easing leg and hip discomforts
        deep tissue sculpting, lateral hip and extinguishing trigger points, 88–89, *88*
        figure 8 hip mobilization, 89–90, *89*
        hip decompression, 87–88, *87–88*
        precautions, 85
        structural balancing, 86, *86–87*
        Swedish and lymphatic drainage, 90, *90*
        technique suggestions, 85–86
    first trimester
        considerations and guidelines, 70–71
        early gestational period, 68
        maternal and fetal development, 68–70, *69*
        recommended bodywork, 71–72
    gastrointestinal and urinary tract discomforts
        complaints and symptoms, 101
        precautions, 101
        technique suggestions, 101
        zone therapy, 101–103, *102–103*
    objective, 67
    pelvic and lower back pain
        deep tissue sculpting and trigger point therapy to paravertebrals, 92–93, *92*
        inching on intrinsic paravertebral structures, 94–95, *94*
        lumbar lengthening, 95–96, *95*
        lumbosacral stretch, 91–92, *91*
        pelvic tilt reeducation, 91, *91*
        precautions, 90
        SI joint releases, 93–94, *93–94*
        symphysis pubis rebalancing, 96, *96*
        technique suggestions, 90–91
    prenatal techniques and bodywork, 80
    reducing upper body discomforts
        arm techniques, 100, *100*
        deep tissue sculpting, 97–99, *97–98*
        pectoral girdle cross-fiber friction, 100–101, *100*
        precautions, 97
        ribcage releases, 99, *99*
        technique suggestions, 97
    second trimester
        considerations and guidelines, 74–75, *75*
        maternal and fetal development, 73–74, *73*
        maternal developments and safe positioning, 72b
        recommended bodywork, 75–76
    stress reduction
        abdominal massage, 85, *85*
        autonomic sedation series, 84–85, *84*
        diaphragmatic breathing reduction, 81, *81*
        increasing lateral/costal breathing, 81–82
        rhythmic passive movements, 82–84, *82–83*
    third trimester
        maternal and fetal development, 76–77, *77*
        maternal developments and safe positioning, 76b
        precautions, considerations, and guidelines, 77–80, *78, 79*
        recommended bodywork, 80

U

Upper body discomforts
    arm techniques, 100, *100*
    deep tissue sculpting, 97–99, *97–98*
    pectoral girdle cross-fiber friction, 100–101, *100*
    precautions, 97
    ribcage releases, 99, *99*
    technique suggestions, 97
Urinary stress incontinence, 10
Urinary system benefits, 10–11
Urinary tract discomforts
    complaints and symptoms, 101
    precautions, 101
    technique suggestions, 101
    zone therapy, 101–103, *102–103*
Uterine atony, 169
Uterine involution and fundal massage, *146*
Uterine ligaments, 14, *14*
Uterine positioning, *145*

V

Varicose veins, 7, 36–38, *37*, 44b
Vasodilation, 7

Z

Zone therapy
    for gastrointestinal system, 9
    postpartum massage therapy, 144
    precautions, 103
    procedure, 101, *102–103*